# MEMORY REHABILITATION

# MEMORY
## REHABILITATION

### INTEGRATING
### THEORY AND
### PRACTICE

## BARBARA A. WILSON

Foreword by Elizabeth L. Glisky

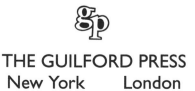

## THE GUILFORD PRESS
### New York   London

**Library of Congress Cataloging-in-Publication Data**

Wilson, Barbara A., 1941–
    Memory rehabilitation: integrating theory and practice / Barbara A. Wilson.
        p. cm.
    ISBN 978-1-60623-287-3 (hardcover: alk. paper)
    1. Memory disorders.   2. Memory.   3. Memory disorders—Patients—
Rehabilitation.   I. Title.
    RC394.M46W55 2009
    616.89—dc22

                                                                2009011603

*In memory of my beloved daughter, Sarah,*
*who died in Peru on May 12, 2000*

# About the Author

**Barbara A. Wilson, PhD, ScD,** has worked in brain injury rehabilitation since 1979, at Rivermead Rehabilitation Centre in Oxford, Charing Cross Hospital in London, and the University of Southampton Medical School. She has also been a Senior Scientist at the Medical Research Council's Cognition and Brain Sciences Unit in Cambridge since 1990. In 1996, Dr. Wilson established the Oliver Zangwill Centre for Neuropsychological Rehabilitation, a partnership between the local NHS Trust and the Medical Research Council, and serves as the Centre's Director of Research. She holds or has held several grants to study new assessment and treatment procedures for people with nonprogressive brain injury and has written over 16 books, 8 widely used neuropsychological tests, and over 260 journal articles and chapters. In addition, she is Editor-in-Chief of the journal *Neuropsychological Rehabilitation* and has served on the governing boards of organizations such as the Encephalitis Society, the Academy for Multidisciplinary Neurotraumatology, and the World Federation for NeuroRehabilitation. Dr. Wilson has received numerous awards for her work, including the May Davidson Award, an OBE in the Queen's New Year Honours List, a Distinguished Scientist Award from the British Psychological Society, Professional of the Year award from the Encephalitis Society, the British Psychological Society's Book of the Year award for *Case Studies in Neuropsychological Rehabilitation*, the Robert L. Moody Prize from the University of Texas, and lifetime achievement awards from the British Psychological Society and the International Neuropsychological Society. She is a Fellow of the British Psychological Society, the Academy of Medical Sciences, and the Academy of Social Sciences.

# Foreword

Twenty-two years after publication of her fourth book, *Rehabilitation of Memory*, Professor Barbara A. Wilson, the world's foremost expert on memory rehabilitation, has again given us an insider's view into how treatments for memory disorders are and should be designed, implemented, and evaluated. Based largely on Dr. Wilson's experiences at the Oliver Zangwill Centre for Neuropsychological Rehabilitation, which she founded in 1996 and for which she has served as Director of Research for many years, this new volume not only provides an in-depth discussion of the most successful treatment methodologies developed since the publication of the earlier book, but also serves as a comprehensive guide to setting up a holistic rehabilitation program. Although the book is focused on remediation of memory problems, Dr. Wilson has long been a proponent of a holistic approach to neuropsychological rehabilitation, stressing the importance of dealing not only with the cognitive problems associated with brain injury but also with noncognitive issues, such as the emotional and social consequences of brain damage. She also emphasizes the importance of conducting rehabilitation in a personally meaningful way, focusing on setting real-world goals and achieving relevant functional adaptations in everyday life.

This book is first and foremost a practical guide for clinicians charged with managing memory problems. It is chock full of informative case studies, illustrating how to bypass or compensate for memory difficulties and increase the probability that people will be able to function independently in everyday life. There is a strong emphasis on compensatory strategies, external aids, environmental support, and retraining of skills, and excellent chapters on assessment, goal setting, and evaluation of outcomes. It is not a one-treatment-serves-all approach, but rather an individualized approach that considers the strengths and weaknesses of each individual and how to maximize each person's potential for independent living. Although there are some guiding principles concerning the design of memory rehabilitation programs, most interventions have to be tailored to the individual and made flexible enough to meet the variable and often changing needs of patients with brain injuries.

What distinguishes this book from the earlier one, however, is the emphasis on theory. In the past two decades, the knowledge base concerning memory disorders has exploded, allowing for the development of new memory rehabilitation techniques solidly grounded in empirical and theoretical work. This has resulted in new treatment methods, based on a greater understanding of the nature of the memory impairment and of the potential cognitive strengths of each individual. Dr. Wilson has been a leader in the development of such methods, most notably the errorless learning technique, and she documents in this volume not only the benefits of that technique but also the potential for even greater benefits when errorless learning is combined with other evidence-based methods similarly grounded in contemporary theory. Throughout the book, she integrates theory with practice, providing models on which to base rehabilitation practices and theoretical justifications for treatments.

This book provides the very latest in theoretically based memory rehabilitation techniques, supported by solid empirical evidence. The specific methods will be modified and improved in years to come and new ones designed, but the approach outlined in this volume, based on theory developed from empirical studies of people with memory and other cognitive impairments, will surely stand the test of time and continue to be a model for the practice of neuropsychological rehabilitation for many years to come.

ELIZABETH L. GLISKY, PHD<br>
Department of Psychology<br>
University of Arizona

# Preface

In 1987, I published *Rehabilitation of Memory*, a book based on my PhD thesis, *Cognitive Rehabilitation after Brain Damage* (Wilson, 1984). The bulk of the work evaluated a variety of mnemonic systems to improve recall of verbal material. Although the book did surprisingly well, mnemonic strategies are not the main focus of memory rehabilitation. Mnemonics have a part to play in enhancing new learning in people with impaired memory function, but their contribution to this process is not substantial. Teaching compensatory strategies and helping people to learn more efficiently are, without doubt, the two main rehabilitation strategies utilized in memory rehabilitation. Additionally, we may need to adapt or modify the environment to help people function without dependence on memory, and this is particularly true for those with widespread and severe cognitive deficits. As well as having cognitive problems, memory-impaired people are likely to experience emotional difficulties such as anxiety and depression, which must also be addressed in rehabilitation. As time has passed and our knowledge and understanding of the processes involved in memory rehabilitation have increased, I have felt more and more uncomfortable with the 1987 book because of its failure to address many of the processes and theoretical underpinnings I now recognize as being essential for good rehabilitation practice. I therefore agreed to write this book, which attempts to reflect the true state of affairs in the field of memory rehabilitation in the 21st century.

   *Memory Rehabilitation* is about the condition and treatment of people with nonprogressive brain damage and does not, for the most part, consider work that is being conducted with patients suffering from dementia. For those requiring information about the latter group, it is recommended that they look at the work of Clare and Woods (2001), who edited a special issue of the journal *Neuropsychological Rehabilitation* entitled "Cognitive Rehabilitation in Dementia" and have since published a review of work in this area (Clare & Woods, 2004). A recent book by Clare (2008) is devoted to neuropsychological rehabilitation for people with dementia.

Memory deficits are common after many kinds of neurological damage. Some 10% of people older than 65 have dementia, with memory impairment as an almost inevitable consequence. About 34% of people with multiple sclerosis have moderate to severe memory problems, as do some 70% of people with AIDS. Of those people with nonprogressive brain injury, we can expect about 36% of survivors of severe traumatic brain injury to live with significant memory impairment for the rest of their lives. Because this means some 2,500 new cases every year in the United Kingdom and about four times this number in the United States, the prevalence is by no means insubstantial. Approximately 70% of survivors of encephalitis—a relatively rare illness—will experience memory impairment, as will some 10% of people with temporal lobe epilepsy. Survivors of stroke, cerebral tumor, myocardial infarction, Korsakoff syndrome, carbon monoxide poisoning, meningitis, and other lesser-known conditions may also experience severe memory problems.

Given such large numbers and the severity of the difficulties faced by these people in everyday life, there is surprisingly little help or guidance offered to them and their families. Many are of working age and are unlikely to return to work; many will lose independence because they cannot remember items that are essential to navigate everyday life, such as whether or not they have eaten, where they are going, or what they have just been doing. Many face anxiety, distress, and loss of self-esteem. These problems are multiplied when their families experience severe stress resulting from anxiety about the future or because of the surveillance they must provide to their memory-impaired relative, which can be hampered by almost unbearable irritations that might include hearing the same question repeated many times each day or hour.

The prevailing view of many neurologists and neurosurgeons, some psychiatrists, and a few neuropsychologists is that little can be done to alleviate problems faced by memory-impaired people. This observation likely originates from established knowledge that little can be done to restore lost memory functioning, and indeed at present no drug, surgical procedure, or exercise regimen can restore memory (although some recovery can take place, as we see later). However, acceptance of the fact that at present we can do little to restore memory functioning does not mean that nothing can be done to reduce or moderate the actual problems faced by memory-impaired people. On the contrary, they can be helped to cope with, bypass, or compensate for their memory problems; they can learn how to come to terms with their condition and its effects through an understanding of their predicament; and their anxiety and distress can be reduced. How we achieve these results is the main focus of this book.

# Acknowledgments

I am particularly grateful to all the memory-impaired people and their families with whom I have worked during my career as a clinical neuropsychologist. They have taught me so much about life, compassion, humor, and survival over adversity. I thank you all.

My thanks, too, to my husband, Mick, who has supported me throughout my career and has read my drafts and tidied up my writing. I owe a big debt of gratitude to Jessica Fish, who has always been willing to help when I panic about computers, graphs, and references, and whose specific assistance with the referencing of this book was a monumental task that I could not have managed on my own. Other people who have helped me during the process of writing this book are Ava Easton from the Encephalitis Society, who allowed me to use the photograph in Figure 7.1; Susan Kime from Phoenix, Arizona, who gave me permission to use Figure 10.1, and whose book, *Compensating for Memory Deficits Using a Systematic Approach*, has been so useful to me; Narinder Kapur, my colleague from Addenbrooke's Hospital, Cambridge, and coauthor of Chapter 4, who has always given his time, advice, and permission to use his material so freely; my colleagues from the Oliver Zangwill Centre, particularly Fergus Gracey and Andrew Bateman, for their advice, suggestions, and permission to use some of the Centre's material; Jo Cope, who helped track down some references; Jon Evans, who is always a source of kindness, diplomacy, and wisdom; Kevin Symonds, librarian at the MRC Cognition and Brain Sciences Unit, for his help with references; and Gail Robinson and Rene Stolwyk at the National Hospital, Queen Square, London, for permission to use some of their work. Table 4.1 is reproduced with the permission of Gail Robinson, who developed these strategies following discussions with Corwin Boake. Paul Ekman granted permission to use Figure 8.1 (the FEEST example). Abigail

Squire from Pearson Assessment gave permission to use Figure 3.2 (a photograph of the novel task). Thanks also to Bernice Marcopulos for helping me to obtain so many of the addresses in the Resources. Finally, I thank Psychology Press, Taylor and Francis, and Informa World (*www.informaworld.com*) for permission to reproduce the case of Jay in Chapter 10, pages 176 to 179, from an article in *Neuropsychological Rehabilitation*, and Figure 11.1, also from *Neuropsychological Rehabilitation*. If I have inadvertently left out anyone I should have thanked, please forgive me.

# Contents

CHAPTER 1. **Understanding Memory and Memory Impairments**    1

What Do We Mean by Memory?    1
Time-Dependent Memory    2
The Type of Information to Be Remembered    5
Modality-Specific Memory    8
Stages in the Process of Remembering: Encoding, Storage, and Retrieval    8
Explicit and Implicit Memory    11
Retrospective and Prospective Memory    12
Retrograde and Anterograde Memory    14
A Brief Account of the Neuroanatomy of Memory    16

CHAPTER 2. **Recovery of Memory Functions after Brain Injuries**    18

What Do We Mean by Recovery?    18
Mechanisms of Recovery    20
To What Extent Does Memory Recover?    25
Can We Improve on Natural Recovery?    29
Changes in Memory Functioning Following Intervention or Rehabilitation    30

CHAPTER 3. **Assessment for Rehabilitation**    34

What Do We Mean by Assessment?    34
What Questions Should Be Asked in Assessments for Rehabilitation?    35
Which Aspects of Memory Should Be Assessed?    38
Behavioral Assessment Procedures for Identifying Memory Problems    49

CHAPTER 4.  Compensating for Memory Deficits with Memory Aids     52
            WITH NARINDER KAPUR

            Typology of Memory Aids   54
            Which Are the Most Frequently Used Memory Aids?   55
            How Effective Are External Memory Aids?   57
            Can We Predict Who Will Use External Memory
                Aids Efficiently?   58
            Which Assessment Procedures Are Most Appropriate When
                Considering Patients for External Memory Aids?   59
            Setting Up a Memory Aids Clinic   60
            Which Types of Memory Aids Are Currently Available?   64
            How Can We Best Teach People to Use External Memory
                Aids?   67
            How Can We Best Measure the Effectiveness of External
                Memory Aids?   70
            How Can We Bring About Compliance and Generalization
                in the Use of External Memory Aids?   71
            How Will Advances in Technology Impact Memory Aids of
                the Future?   71

CHAPTER 5.  Mnemonics and Rehearsal Strategies in Rehabilitation     74

            What Are Mnemonics?   74
            Verbal Mnemonics   74
            Visual Mnemonics   77
            Motor Movements as a Memory Aid   79
            How Successful Are Mnemonics
                in Memory Rehabilitation?   80
            Advice When Using Mnemonics   81
            What Do We Mean by Rehearsal Strategies?   82
            Studies Evaluating PQRST   83
            Why Does PQRST Work?   86
            Using PQRST in Clinical Practice   87

CHAPTER 6.  New Learning in Rehabilitation: Errorless Learning,     89
            Spaced Retrieval (Expanded Rehearsal),
            and Vanishing Cues

            What Is Errorless Learning?   89
            Theoretical Underpinnings of EL Learning   89
            EL Learning Studies with Memory-Impaired People   92
            Does EL Learning Depend on Implicit
                or Explicit Memory?   94
            What Is Spaced Retrieval (Expanded Rehearsal)?   96
            Why Does Spaced Retrieval Work?   97
            Spaced Retrieval Combined with EL Learning   98
            Spaced Retrieval Alone   99
            Using Spaced Retrieval in Clinical Practice   100
            What Do We Mean by Vanishing Cues?   101

Studies Evaluating VC    101
How Does VC Work?    102
VC in Clinical Practice    104
Teaching Procedures or New Information through EL
    Learning, Spaced Retrieval, or VC    105

CHAPTER 7.  Memory Groups                                        107

Why Run Memory Groups?    107
How Should a Memory Group Be Structured?    108
Studies Evaluating Memory Groups    110
Self-Help and Support Groups    112
Memory Groups in Clinical Practice    115

CHAPTER 8.  Treating the Emotional and Mood Disorders            125
            Associated with Memory Impairment

Why Is It Important to Treat the Emotional and Mood
    Disorders Associated with Memory Impairment?    125
How Prevalent Are Emotional and Mood Disorders
    after Brain Injury?    126
Assessment of Emotional and Mood Disorders in People
    with Brain Injury    130
Group Treatments for Emotional and Mood Disorders
    in People with Memory Impairments    135
Individual Psychological Therapy for Emotional and Mood
    Disorders    138
Treatment of Emotional and Mood Disorders
    in Clinical Practice    144

CHAPTER 9.  Goal Setting to Plan and Evaluate                    147
            Memory Rehabilitation

What Are Goals?    147
Why Use Goal Setting in Memory Rehabilitation?    148
Theories of Goal Setting    151
Identifying and Setting Goals: The Art of Negotiation    152
Goal Attainment as an Outcome Measure    154
Goal Setting in Clinical Practice    155

CHAPTER 10. Putting It All Together                              163

Before Starting a Memory Rehabilitation Program    163
First Steps in Planning a Memory
    Rehabilitation Program    163
Complementing the Neuropsychological Assessment with a
    Behavioral Assessment    165
Goal Setting    170
Selecting the Best Strategies to Achieve the Goals    172
The Example of Jay    176

Generalization or Transfer of Learning   179
A Framework for Planning a Rehabilitation Program   180

CHAPTER 11. **Final Thoughts and a General Summary**                    184

Principles of Good Rehabilitation   184
Does Rehabilitation Improve QOL?   186
Combining Theory and Practice   190
Summaries of Individual Chapters   192

APPENDIX.   **Resources**                                              207

**References**                                                         231

**Index**                                                              275

CHAPTER 1

# Understanding Memory and Memory Impairments

Without the "glue" of memory, past and future lose
their meaning and awareness is reduced or even lost.
—MARKOWITSCH (2005, p. 105)

## What Do We Mean by Memory?

One simple definition of *memory* that makes sense to patients, families, and caregivers is "the ability to take in, store, and retrieve information." Although people tend to talk about memory as though it were one skill, function, or ability, saying, for example, "I have a terrible memory" or "She has a photographic memory," there are many kinds of memory and many ways it can break down. Baddeley (2004) discusses the fractionation of memory and reminds us that people with the classic amnesic syndrome have great difficulty remembering after a delay or distraction but have a normal immediate memory span, so after hearing a string of digits they can typically repeat back five, six, or seven of these in the correct order. Other people have great difficulty repeating two or more digits but have much less of a problem after a delay or distraction. Thus, a double dissociation can be found between people with a classic amnesic syndrome and those with an impaired short-term (immediate) memory store.

Memory, then, is not one skill or function but rather a "complex combination of memory subsystems" (Baddeley, 1992, p. 5). We can consider memory in terms of the length of time for which memories are stored, the type of information to be remembered, the modality the information is in, the stages in the process of remembering, explicit or implicit memory, whether recall or recognition is required, whether the memory is retrospective (for things that have already occurred) or prospective (remembering what has to be done), and whether the memory dates from before or after the injury or illness (Clare & Wilson, 1997). This chapter addresses each of these topics and provides a brief consideration of the neuroanatomy of memory.

## Time-Dependent Memory

Baddeley and Hitch (1974), influenced by Atkinson and Shriffin (1971), suggested that memory can be divided into three categories broadly based on the length of time information can be stored: *sensory memory,* which stores information for less than a quarter of a second (250 mss); *short-term store,* which holds information for a few seconds; and *long-term store,* which holds information for anything from minutes to years (Figure 1.1).

The first, sensory memory, is the system we use when we go to the cinema and perceive what appears to be a moving film. In fact, we are seeing a series of still shots but the shots are held in the brief sensory

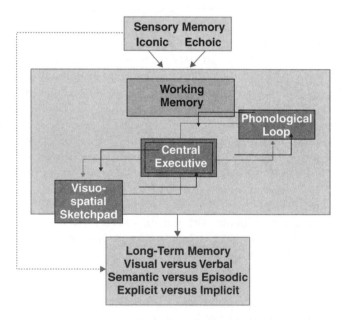

**FIGURE 1.1.** The working memory model. After Baddeley and Hitch (1974).

store and so are interpreted as moving pictures. This involves *visual sensory* or *iconic memory*. The auditory equivalent is known as *echoic sensory memory* and enables us to interpret speech sounds. In clinical practice, however, people with disorders in the sensory memory systems would present clinically as having visual or auditory perceptual disorders and would not be thought of as having a memory impairment. They are not considered in this book.

The second system, holding a few seconds memory, is what we use when we are dialing a new telephone number with perhaps seven digits. We can hold on to these seven digits long enough to dial but if the number is engaged (busy) or someone talks to us while we are dialing, the number flies away; we have lost it and have to look it up again. Psychologists refer to this as *short-term memory* (STM), but the general public thinks of STM as meaning anything from a few minutes to a few days to a few weeks, so it is best to avoid the term STM unless talking to other psychologists. *Immediate memory, primary memory*, or *working memory* are other terms in use. Primary memory and immediate memory refer to the memory span as measured by the number of digits that can be repeated in the correct order after one presentation (seven plus or minus two for the vast majority of people; Miller, 1956) or by the recency effect in free recall (the ability to recall the last few items in a list of words, letters, or digits). Baddeley (1997) prefers the terms *primary memory* when referring to the simple unitary few seconds memory system and *working memory* when referring to the interacting range of temporary memory systems people typically use in real life.

Working memory is assumed to have a controller or resource allocator, the *central executive*, which is assisted by two subsidiary systems, namely the *phonological loop* and the *visuospatial sketchpad*. The phonological loop is a store that holds memory for a few seconds but is capable of increasing this period through the use of subvocal speech. Furthermore, it can convert visual material that is capable of being named into a phonological code (Baddeley, 2004). The visuospatial sketchpad allows for the temporary storage and manipulation of visual and spatial information. In clinical practice, one can see people with damage to each of these systems. Those with a central executive disorder are said to have the dysexecutive syndrome, after Baddeley (1986) and Baddeley and Wilson (1988a). Their main difficulties are with planning, organization, divided attention, perseveration, and dealing with new or novel situations (Evans, 2005). Those with phonological loop disorders have difficulties with speech processing and new language acquisition. The few patients we see with immediate memory disorders (i.e., they can only repeat back one or two digits, words, or letters accurately) have a phonological loop disorder. Vallar and Papagno (2002) discussed the phonological loop in detail, whereas Baddeley and Wilson (1988b) and Wilson and Baddeley (1993) described a patient with a phonological loop deficit and his subsequent recovery. People with visuospatial sketchpad disorders may have deficits in just one of these functions; in other words, visual and spatial difficulties are separable (Della Sala & Logie, 2002). Although one such patient was described by Wilson, Baddeley, and Young (1999), they are rare in clinical practice and are not the typical referrals for rehabilitation.

More recently, Baddeley (2000) and Baddeley and Wilson (2002) have added a fourth component to working memory, namely the *episodic buffer*, a multimodal temporary store capable of integrating information from the phonological loop and the visuospatial sketchpad into the long-term memory store. This buffer is assumed to be particularly important in immediate memory for prose, allowing amnesic patients with good intellectual functioning and no executive impairments to show apparently normal immediate memory for prose passages that would far exceed the capacity of either of the subsidiary systems. Delayed memory is, of course, still severely impaired. When assessing an amnesic patient's immediate recall of a prose passage, it is not uncommon to find that the score is in the normal range even though, given the capacity of the short-term store, the recall should be no more than seven words plus or minus two (Miller, 1956). The episodic buffer provides an explanation for the enhanced score.

As mentioned earlier, the *long-term store* or *long-term memory* (LTM) is the system that stores information for longer periods of time ranging from minutes to decades. It is also referred to as secondary memory. The LTM store is durable with a large and possibly unlimited capacity. Unlike the phonological loop, which codes information principally by speech characteristics, the long-term system codes primarily by meaning. It is this system that is typically affected in people with memory impairments. Most have a relatively normal immediate memory, but after a delay or distraction the information is lost. The means by which information is retained for a few minutes seems to be essentially the same as that by which it is remembered for years. The divisions occurring among sensory memory (measured in milliseconds), immediate memory (measured in seconds), and longer term memory (measured in minutes, days, weeks and years) are clear-cut. This is not to say that we remember events that happened years ago as well as we remember events that happened yesterday; it is simply that there is not such an obvious distinction here as there is among sensory, primary, and secondary memory. Clinically, we tend to talk about *delayed memory, recent memory,* and *remote memory,* with delayed memory referring to events or information that occurred a few minutes earlier, recent memory referring to things that happened in the previous few days or weeks, and remote memory referring to events or information that occurred years before (Clare & Wilson, 1997). LTM can be understood or distinguished in various ways, including *semantic, episodic,* and *procedural memory; visual* and *verbal memory;* and *implicit* and *explicit memory.* These, along with other aspects of memory, are addressed in the following sections of this chapter.

## The Type of Information to Be Remembered

Memory for general knowledge, for personal experiences, and for skills or routines is dependent on different systems, each of which can be independently affected. Memory for general knowledge, such as facts, meanings of words, visual appearance of objects, and color of things, is known as *semantic memory,* after Tulving (1972). We use semantic memory when we answer questions such as the color of a banana, the capital of Egypt, whether a hippopotamus is larger or smaller than a dog, and the meaning of the word *justice.* We have a huge store of information as to what things mean, look like, sound like, smell like, and feel like. It is not necessary to remember *when* this information was acquired or *who* was present at the time. Learning typically takes place over many occasions in a variety of circumstances. Most memory-impaired people have a normal semantic memory at least for information acquired before the onset of the memory impairment. Someone with the classic amnesic syndrome, for example, will have no trouble defining words or recalling facts from his or her fund of general knowledge (Table 1.1). It may be difficult to lay down new facts, however, probably because initially one has to depend on episodic memory in order for information to enter the semantic store (Cermak & O'Connor, 1983). One densely amnesic patient has laid down almost no new facts since the onset of his amnesia from herpes simplex encephalitis in 1985. He has no knowledge of words that have entered the language since he became ill. He does not know what an e-mail is, he does not understand the terms *mad cow disease, World Wide Web,* or *Viagra* (Wilson, Kopelman, & Kapur, 2008). In contrast, another patient has learned many of these words despite a severe amnesia (Wilson, 1999). His learning, however, is slow and far from normal.

Some survivors of brain injury do exhibit semantic memory deficits, particularly after encephalitis or anoxia, although people with traumatic brain injury (TBI) can also exhibit these problems because of either damage to the semantic store or access to that store (Wilson,

**TABLE 1.1. Characteristics of People with the Classic Amnesic Syndrome and with More Widespread Cognitive Problems**

Amnesic syndrome

1. A profound difficulty in learning and remembering most kinds of new information (anterograde amnesia).
2. Difficulty remembering some information acquired before the onset of the syndrome (retrograde amnesia).
3. Normal immediate memory.
4. Normal/nearly normal learning on implicit tasks.
5. Normal/nearly normal functioning on other cognitive tasks.

More widespread cognitive difficulties

1. Immediate memory reasonable.
2. Difficulty remembering after a delay or distraction.
3. Difficulty learning most new information.
4. Events that happened some time before the insult are typically remembered better than events that happened a short time ago.

1997). Warrington (1975) argues that visual object agnosia is a visual semantic memory deficit. Some patients lose the ability to recognize living things but can still recognize manufactured objects and are said to have a category-specific disorder (Warrington & Shallice, 1984). Hillis and Caramazza (1991) and Sacchett and Humphreys (1992) describe the opposite, where people can recognize nonliving things to a much greater degree than they can living things. Impaired semantic memory is also seen in people with Alzheimer's disease (AD) alongside deficits in episodic memory (Becker & Overman, 2004). There is one group of people, however, who have particular problems with semantic memory deficits: those with progressive semantic dementia (Warrington, 1975; Snowden et al., 1992; Snowden, 2002). This condition is characterized by a "selective degradation of core semantic knowledge, affecting all types of concept, irrespective of the modality of testing" (Lambon-Ralph & Patterson, 2008, p. 61). Episodic memory deficits may be less affected. Both Snowden, Griffiths, and Neary (1996) and Graham and Hodges (1997) found that people with semantic dementia showed preserved recent memories and impaired distant memories, which is the reverse of that seen in people with AD.

Memory for personal experiences (e.g., where you spent last Christmas, when the credit card bill was paid, or what your friend asked you to do this evening) is more autobiographical and is known as *episodic memory*, again after Tulving (1972). It is more important to remember the specific occasion when the event occurred or, as Baddeley (2002) says, citing Tulving, to be able "to travel back in time" (p. 5). Episodic memory problems, like semantic memory problems, result from deficits in LTM. Although Tulving (1972) believed that semantic and episodic memory are two independent systems, Baddeley (1997, 2004) disagrees with this view. He indicates that in most situations there is a blend of the two: If one recalls what one had for breakfast (an episodic task), then this will be influenced by the semantic knowledge of what one typically eats at breakfast time. Most people with memory problems have episodic memory deficits, this being their major handicap in everyday life. Because of their magnitude, both in terms of numbers and severity of problems they face, episodic memory deficits form the main focus of attention in this book. Episodic deficits can be further subdivided into *visual and verbal recall* and *recognition,* and each of these subdivisions is discussed in detail later in this chapter.

Memory for skills or routines is known as *procedural memory.* Learning to ride a bicycle, reading words written back to front, and learning to type are examples of procedural learning. The primary characteristic of this kind of learning is that it does not depend on conscious recollection; instead, the learning can be demonstrated without the need to be aware of where and how the original learning took place. For this reason, most people with memory problems show normal or relatively normal procedural learning. H. M., the most famous amnesic patient of all time (Scoville, 1968; Scoville & Milner, 1957), was able to learn motor tasks despite a very severe episodic memory impairment. Cohen and Corkin (1981) showed that H. M. was also able to learn the complex Tower of Hanoi puzzle even though he had no recollection of ever having done the task before. Numerous other studies have demonstrated that amnesic patients can learn certain tasks. These include jigsaw puzzle assembly (Brooks & Baddeley, 1976), eyeblink conditioning (Weiskrantz & Warrington, 1979), and mirror-reversed words (Cohen & Corkin, 1981). This normal or nearly normal learning is important in rehabilitation because we can capitalize on this relatively intact skill to teach typing and computer use as well as the use of certain external memory aids. Not all studies, however, find intact procedural learning in memory-impaired patients. For example, Swinnen, Puttemans, and Lamote (2005) found that patients with Korsakoff's syndrome show some deficits on procedural learning tasks. In contrast, Cavaco, Anderson, Allen, Castro-Caldas, and Damasio (2004) reported that "preserved learning of complex perceptual–motor skills in patients with amnesia is a robust phenomenon, and that it can be demonstrated across a variety of conditions and perceptual–motor demands" (p. 1853).

Some patient groups are known to show impaired procedural learning, particularly those with Huntington's disease and Parkinson's disease (Vakil & Herishanu-Naaman, 1998; Osman, Wilkinson, Beigi, Castaneda, & Jahanshani, 2008). People with AD may (Mitchell & Schmitt,

2006) or may not (Hirono et al., 1997) show a deficit. Vicari et al. (2005) and Nicholson and Fawcett (2007) suggested that children with developmental dyslexia have impaired procedural learning, whereas Siegert, Weatherall, and Bell (2008) found a moderate impairment in people with schizophrenia.

## Modality-Specific Memory

We may be required to remember information and events in several forms, including things we have seen, heard, smelled, touched, and tasted. In memory rehabilitation, however, the main area of concern is memory for verbal and visual information. It is clear that we can remember things we can label or read, but we can also remember things that we cannot easily verbalize, such as a person's face. Because different parts of the brain are responsible for visual and verbal processing, these can be independently affected, with some people having a primary difficulty with visual memory and others with verbal memory. Many years ago, Milner (1965, 1968, 1971) demonstrated material-specific deficits following unilateral temporal lobectomy. Removal of the left temporal lobe results in verbal memory deficits, and removal of the right temporal lobe results in more impaired recall of nonverbal material, such as faces, patterns, and mazes.

If memory for one kind of material is less affected, it might be possible to capitalize on the less damaged system in order to compensate for the damaged one. For example, someone with poor verbal skills but good visual memory may be able to turn verbal material into visual information and benefit from the visual imagery techniques described in Chapter 5, while those with the reverse pattern may be able to verbalize visuospatial information such as routes. Wilson (1987) described successful treatment for patients with both verbal and visual memory deficits. Some people will, of course, have both visual and verbal memory deficits. This does not mean that they cannot benefit from mnemonics and from other memory strategies (Wilson, 1987), as we demonstrate later in this book.

## Stages in the Process of Remembering: Encoding, Storage, and Retrieval

At the beginning of this chapter, memory was defined as the ability to take in, store, and retrieve information. These are the three stages required for a memory system to function. The taking in of information is the *encoding stage*, retaining the information is the *storage stage*, and accessing the information when required is the *retrieval stage*. Although one can distinguish between these stages and patients can be found with deficits in only one system, in real life these stages interact with one another. For example, people with encoding problems show attention difficulties. Despite the fact that in some circumstances remembering is unintentional and we can recall things that happen when we are not paying particular attention to them, typically we need to pay attention when we are learning something new or when it is important to remember. People with the classic amnesic syndrome do not have encoding difficulties, whereas those with executive deficits (e.g., following a TBI or as a result of dementia) may well have them. There are guidelines we can follow to improve encoding.

First, simplify the information to be remembered, because it is easier to remember short words than long words and short sentences than long sentences even if the words and sentences are well understood by the person trying to remember (Wilson, 1989). Second, the person should be asked to remember only one thing at a time rather than three or four items, words, names, or instructions at the same time, leading inevitably to confusion. Third, make sure the person has understood the information being presented. This is usually achieved by having the person repeat it back in his or her own words. Fourth, ask the person to link the information to something already known. For example, when remembering a name, ask the person to think of someone else with the same name or a song that contains the name. Fifth, follow the "little and often rule," otherwise known as distributed practice. When people are trying to learn something, they learn better when the learning occasions or trials are spread over a period of time rather than crowded all together. Baddeley (1992) described an experiment where people were taught to type. Three groups each had 12 hrs of instruction: One group spent 1 hr a day learning for 12 days, another group was instructed for 2 hr a day for 6 days, and the third group were taught for 6 hr a day for 2 days. Those learning for 1 hr a day did better and forgot less. Distributed practice is the principle behind the spaced retrieval/expanded rehearsal technique of Landauer and Bjork (1978), described in Chapter 6. Sixth, avoid trial-and-error learning. To benefit from our mistakes, we need to be able to remember them. For people who cannot remember their errors then, the very fact of making an incorrect response may strengthen that erroneous response, so we want to avoid mistakes occurring in the first place (Baddeley & Wilson, 1994). This is the fundamental principle of errorless (EL) learning described in more detail in Chapter 6. Seventh, ensure that the people who are trying to remember or learn are not passive recipients of the information. They need to think about the material or information and manipulate it in some way. This is also known as "levels of processing," after Craik and Lockhart (1972). People who process things at a shallow level (e.g., count the number of letters in a word) remember less than those who process at a deeper level (e.g., think about the meaning of a word; Jacoby & Dallas, 1981). Baddeley (1992) suggested that deeper encoding involves elaboration, compatibility, and self reference. Elaboration involves relating the material to something already known; compatibility means that if the information is consistent with existing knowledge, then it is easier to learn (thus, football enthusiasts can remember football scores and league tables better than nonenthusiasts); and self reference means that people who relate the information to themselves remember better than if they relate it to other people.

Once information is registered in memory, it has to be stored there until needed. Most people forget new information rather rapidly over the first few days and then the rate of forgetting slows down. This is also true for people with memory problems, bearing in mind, of course, that in their case relatively little information may be stored in the first place. However, once the information is encoded adequately and enters the long-term store, testing, rehearsal, or practice can help keep it there. The best way to do this is to test the person immediately after seeing or hearing new information, test again after a short delay, and test again after a slightly longer delay. This process is continued, with the intervals being gradually lengthened. Such practice or rehearsal usually leads to better retention of information. Again, this is the principle of spaced retrieval (Landauer & Bjork, 1978), which we return to in Chapter 6. This principle can, therefore, help both encoding and storage. Other rehearsal strategies such as PQRST (**P**review, **Q**uestion, **R**ead, **S**tate and **T**est [see Chapter 5]) may also help improve storage.

Retrieving information when we need it is the third stage in the memory process. We all experience occasions when we know we know something, such as the name of a town or a particular word, and yet we cannot retrieve it at the right moment. This is known as the "tip-of-the-tongue" phenomenon. If someone provides us with a word, we can usually determine immediately whether or not it is correct. Retrieval problems are even more likely for people with memory problems. If we can provide a "hook" in the form of a cue or prompt, we may be able to help them access the correct memory. Providing the first letter of a name may well lead to the person remembering the whole name. Perhaps all of us have experienced a situation where we recognize a face but cannot place the person. This is particularly likely to happen if the person is seen in a different place than where earlier meetings occurred. Retrieval is easier for most of us if the surroundings in which we are trying to remember something are the same as those in which we first learned it. This is known as the *context specificity* principle. Godden and Baddeley (1975) showed this in an ingenious experiment. They taught deep-sea divers a list of words either on land or under water and asked them to recall the words in the same or in a different environment. Those who learned under the sea recalled better when tested under the sea. The same was true for those who learned on land (i.e., they recalled more when tested in the same environment). Forty per cent more words were recalled if the learning and testing environments were the same than if there was a mismatch between the environments. So memory-impaired people may remember better if they are in the same room with the same people as they were when the learning first occurred.

Obviously, in most situations, we want to avoid context specificity, so when trying to teach a person with memory impairments new information, we should teach that person to remember in a number of different settings and social situations. Our aim should be to encourage learning in many different, everyday situations that are likely to be encountered in daily life. Learning should not be limited to one particular context such as a hospital ward, classroom, or therapist's office.

The mood or state of mind that we are in may also influence our ability to remember. We know that people who learn things when they are sober remember them better when they are sober. This may not seem surprising. However, it is also true that things learned when a person is drunk may be remembered better when that person is drunk again. Similarly, things learned when one is happy or sad are better recalled when the original emotion is experienced again. This is known as *state-dependent learning.* Consequently, when helping a person with memory impairments to remember, we should aim to teach him or her in a number of different moods so as to avoid context specificity. This issue is further addressed in the Generalization or Transfer of Learning section in Chapter 10.

## Explicit and Implicit Memory

*Explicit memory* is similar to episodic memory; it simply means one can consciously recollect specific incidents and episodes from the past. As reported in the discussion of episodic memory, most memory-impaired people will have problems with explicit memory tasks. Such memory is vulnerable to many kinds of neurological insult and is likely to be the focus of memory rehabilitation.

*Implicit memory,* on the other hand, like procedural memory, means that no conscious recollection is required in order to show that learning has taken place. Procedural memory is a form of implicit memory enabling us to learn such skills as riding a bicycle or motor tracking tasks. Implicit memory also covers nonmotor learning such as priming. Priming is a process whereby learning is improved through preexposure to stimuli. Thus, if an amnesic patient is shown and reads a list of words before being shown the word stems (in the form of the first two or three letters of the word), he or she is likely to respond with the correct words even though there is no conscious or explicit memory of seeing the words before (Warrington & Weiskrantz, 1968). Although it has been known for decades that memory-impaired people can learn some skills and information normally through their intact (or relatively intact) implicit learning abilities, it has been difficult to apply this knowledge to reduce the real-life problems encountered by people with organic memory deficits. Glisky et al. (Glisky & Schacter, 1988; Glisky, Schacter, & Tulving, 1986) tried to capitalize on intact implicit abilities to teach people with amnesia computer terminology using a technique they called the "method of vanishing cues (VC)" (discussed more fully in Chapter 6). Despite some successes, the method of VC involved considerable time and effort both from the experimenters and the people with amnesia. Implicit memory or learning, on the other hand, does not involve effort because it occurs without conscious recollection. This, together with certain other anomalies seen during implicit learning (such as the observation that in a fragmented picture/perceptual priming procedure, if an amnesic patient mislabels a fragment during an early presentation, the error may "stick" and be repeated on successive presentations), led Baddeley and Wilson (1994) to pose the question, "Do amnesic patients learn better if prevented from making mistakes during the learning process?" This was the beginning of the EL learning studies in memory rehabilitation and is addressed in greater detail in Chapter 6.

## Retrospective and Prospective Memory

*Retrospective memory* is memory for the past, whether for events, incidents, word lists, jokes, or other experiences. This is in contrast to *prospective memory*, which is the ability to remember to do things in the future; this might be at a particular time (e.g., "At 3:00 P.M. leave for the railway station") or within a given interval of time (e.g., "In the next 15 minutes, please feed the cat") or when a certain event happens (e.g., "When you next see Jessica, give her a message from Tom"). In other words, prospective memory is remembering to do things rather than remembering things that have already happened. Ellis (1996) defined it as "the realization of delayed intentions." Retrospective memory has been covered previously in the discussion of episodic memory, verbal and visual memory, and explicit memory. Prospective memory is one of the most common complaints when people are asked what everyday memory problems they face (Baddeley, 2004). In addition, according to Baddeley, it is not clear *how* prospective memory works. It must require memory because amnesic people have great difficulty remembering what to do but young, intelligent people are often rather poor at doing things at the right time. "There is clearly an element of motivation and almost certainly one of strategy in prospective memory" (p. 9). On memory tests young people make fewer prospective memory errors than older people, but in real life older people make fewer errors because they know their limitations and compensate by writing things down or by concentrating more. Groot, Wilson, Evans, and Watson (2002) showed that prospective memory can fail because of memory failures or of executive difficulties. Indeed, there is evidence that measures of executive functioning are better at accounting for prospective memory failures than measures of memory (Burgess, Veitch, de Lacy Costello, & Shallice, 2000; Fish, Manly, & Wilson, 2008a).

There are also retrospective components to prospective memory. Fish et al. (2008) gave the example of mailing a letter. First, you must have the conscious intention of mailing the letter and unless a mailbox is immediately at hand, you must rehearse this intention until it can be executed (possible several hours later) or *intend* to remember this intention when its execution is possible. Given the many tasks you may engage in before you see the mailbox, you must store the intention in such a way that it does not impair any current activity. Then, at the appropriate time and circumstance, you must access that intention and initiate the actions associated with it. So, before leaving the house, you must remember to take the letter with you and also remember the intention to mail the letter when you reach the mailbox. In addition, you must remember afterward whether or not you mailed the letter. Ellis (1996) described these stages as encoding, retention, realization, and evaluation. Levin and Hanten (2004) also claimed that prospective memory has a declarative (explicit) component in the sense that we need to remember *what* action is to be performed and a temporal–contextual (prospective) component in the sense that we have to remember *when* and *where* the action has to be performed.

Memory-impaired people will experience difficulties with both kinds of memory. They will have problems remembering things that happened in the past as well as remembering things they are expected to do in the future. This book addresses both aspects. Chapter 4 is particularly concerned with prospective memory and Chapters 5 and 6 with retrospective memory.

## Retrograde and Anterograde Memory

*Retrograde amnesia* (RA) refers to the loss of memory before the onset of the memory deficit: that is, there is impaired recall of events that took place before any insult to the brain. (Anterograde amnesia [AA] refers to the memory difficulties that follow the neurological insult. Because AA includes the kinds of memory problems referred to previously, this is not addressed further.) As long ago as 1881, RA was of interest to clinicians. According to Ribot's (1881) law, the oldest memories are most resistant to disruption. Thus, in RA recent memories are the most likely to be lost. Although this is true for some groups of people, for example, those with Korsakoff's syndrome (Kopelman, Stanhope, & Kingsley, 1999) and those with medial temporal lobe damage (Westmacott, Leach, Freedman, & Moscovitch, 2001), it is not necessarily true for other diagnostic groups such as those with encephalitis (Kopelman et al., 1999; McCarthy, Kopelman, & Warrington, 2005) and not even invariably true for those with medial temporal lobe damage. Noulhiane et al. (2007) found all time periods were affected in a group of patients who had undergone medial temporal lobe surgery for the relief of epileptic seizures. For those with semantic dementia, the *opposite* is true in that they are likely to remember recent events better than past events (Snowden, Griffiths, & Neary, 1994; Graham, Kropelnicki, Goldman, & Hodges, 2003).

Most memory-impaired people will have both retrograde and anterograde memory deficits, with the period of RA being very variable. For some survivors of TBI it may be as little as a few minutes, whereas for some people with encephalitis it may extend back decades (Wilson et al., 2008). A few reports exist of people with an isolated RA and no anterograde deficits (Kapur, 1993, 1999; Kopelman, 2000), although some of these at least are likely to be of psychogenic origin (Kopelman, 2004). Conversely there are a few people with severe AA with no loss of memories before the insult. "Jay," described in Wilson (1999), became amnesic after a left posterior cerebral artery aneurysm at the age of 20. He could recall the tutorial he was attending and the topic being covered when he had an epileptic seizure, which led to hospital admission and discovery of the hemorrhage. Of course, it is possible that even here there were a few minutes or seconds of RA, even though "Jay" himself believed he could remember everything until the seizure. It is not easy to assess RA partly because the assessment depends on retrospective methods and imperfect tests (Reed & Squire, 1998) and because people vary considerably in their interest and capacity to recall information in tests of past knowledge (e.g., public events and famous personalities), and this is independent of the influence of amnesia. Even when testing knowledge of their own autobiography it is not always possible to assess the accuracy of their memories (Reed & Squire, 1998). Figure 1.2 illustrates RA and AA.

Why do some people show a temporal gradient and others do not? Ribot (1881) believed that older memories were more integrated with existing memories than recent memories, which is reflected in the view of Squire and Alvarez (1995), who suggested that the hippocampus is crucial in laying down new memories but is less involved in old memories. This is known as the consolidation theory and is consistent with the temporal gradient seen in some patients. In support, Reed and Squire (1998), suggested that "damage to the hippocampal formation produces limited RA and that additional temporal cortical damage is needed to produce severe and extensive RA" (p. 3944). Nadel and Moscovitch (1997), on the other hand, believed that the hippocampus is crucial to memories from all periods of the lifespan. This is known as the multiple trace theory and is consistent with the lack of temporal gradient seen in some patient groups. Evidence can be found for both these points of view, although Westmacott and Moscovitch (2002) suggested that the two views are, in fact, compatible because the multiple trace theory is correct for explicit memories while the consolidation theory explains both semantic memory and implicit memory, as these do show a tem-

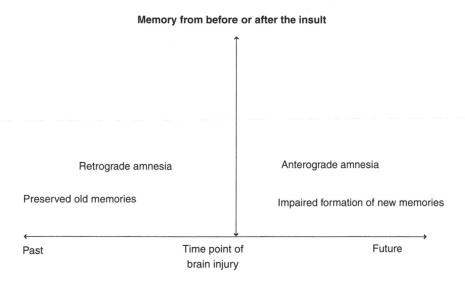

**FIGURE 1.2.** An illustration of retrograde and anterograde amnesia. From Markowitsch (2003). Copyright 2003 by Oxford University Press. Reprinted by permission.

poral gradient. This idea was further supported by Steinvorth, Levine, and Corkin (2005), who found that medial temporal lobe structures are required for recalling events from the distant past as well as the recent past, whereas semantic memory is independent of these structures.

In clinical practice, AA is the greatest handicap for memory-impaired patients and the main focus of rehabilitation, although occasionally people do need help with recall of their earlier autobiographical knowledge. If there is no (or mild) AA, then it is possible to reteach factual knowledge from the past. When this occurs, patients may say they "know" the event happened but they have no sense of familiarity with the events in questions (Hunkin et al., 1995). For recovery from psychogenic amnesia, see Kopelman (2004).

## A Brief Account of the Neuroanatomy of Memory

A landmark in the neuroanatomy of memory dates to 1953, when Scoville performed surgery on a man with intractable epileptic seizures (Scoville & Milner, 1957). At the age of 27, H. M. received bilateral temporal lobe ablations in an attempt to stop the seizures that had been occurring for many years. Once H. M. had recovered from surgery, it became apparent that he was unable to learn new information, had RA, and showed all the characteristics of the classic amnesic syndrome. Eight psychotic patients who had received similar operations were also reported. Severe amnesia developed after removal of the hippocampus, but if this was spared amnesia did not develop. The authors concluded that an intact hippocampus was necessary for normal memory functioning. Although this was not the first description of the neuroanatomy of memory, it certainly stimulated considerable research into memory functioning. H. M. is probably the most famous amnesic patient of all time and is still the subject of research. Many papers about H. M. have appeared between 1957 and 2007.[*]

Of course, the hippocampus and the surrounding areas are not the only brain structures involved in memory. Sensory memory is probably processed by the respective cortical sensory memory systems (Lu & Sperling, 2003). Several cortical areas appear to be involved in working memory, including a network of prefrontal cortex-based domain-specific buffers that act as work spaces for the storage and manipulation of information (Feredoes & Postle, 2007); the auditory cortex (Rader, Holmes, & Golob, 2008) and parietal areas (Arnott, Grady, Hevenor, Graham, & Alain, 2005; Hong, Lee, Kim, & Nam, 2000). According

[*]Henry Molaison died at the age of 82 on December 2, 2008.

to Markowitsch (2003), "Information for the declarative and episodic memory systems enters the brain via the sensory channels, and is then stored online or short term in cortical association areas, particularly those of the lateral parietal cortex" (p. 730). The hippocampus, part of the limbic system, is crucial for memory to enter the long-term store, but other structures are also important. The parahippocampal gyrus, the uncus, the fornix, the mammillary bodies, and the thalamus are all implicated in episodic/explicit memory (Markowitsch, 2003). Left-hemisphere damage will particularly affect verbal memory and right visual memory (Milner, 1965, 1968, 1971).

Semantic memory is typically associated with atrophy in the temporal lobes, with the left hemisphere more affected than the right, the inferior lobe more affected than the superior, and the anterior part of the lobe more affected than the posterior (Chan et al., 2001). As stated, sensory memory enters through the sensory organs and once there it may be encoded implicitly as primed information involving the sensory cortex (Naccache & Dehaene, 2001) or as procedural memory, which is dependent on the basal ganglia and possibly the cerebellum (Eichenbaum & Cohen, 2001). Markowitsch (2003) believed that most of the limbic structures are involved in consolidation and storage, with the frontotemporal cortex being crucial for retrieval. Prospective memory depends on both memory and executive functioning and can, therefore, be disrupted by damage to the hippocampal and parahippocampal areas, affecting memory, and also the prefrontal cortex, affecting executive abilities. RA has been addressed in the discussion of the consolidation and the multiple trace theories. It is associated with medial temporal lobe, particularly hippocampal, deficits, and very severe RA may require additional temporal cortical damage (Reed & Squire, 1998). One of the most severe cases of amnesia ever reported is that of C. W. (Wearing, 2005; Wilson, Kopelman, & Kapur, 2008). C. W. has very little recall of the 45 years before the onset of his amnesia from herpes simplex encephalitis, and he certainly has significant cortical damage in addition to almost complete loss of both hippocampi.

Given the number of structures and networks involved, perhaps it is hardly surprising that memory problems are frequently seen after so many kinds of brain damage. To what extent can we expect recovery of memory functioning after an insult to the brain? This is the topic of the next chapter.

CHAPTER 2

# Recovery of Memory Functions
# after Brain Injuries

## What Do We Mean by Recovery?

The term, *recovery* can be interpreted in several different ways (see Table
2.1). Almli and Finger (1988) discussed some of the definitions of recovery. They suggested it is a complete regaining of the identical functions
that were lost or impaired after brain injury. Few memory-impaired
people achieve recovery in this sense. Jennett and Bond (1975) defined
"good recovery" on the Glasgow Outcome Scale (GOS) as "resumption
of normal life even though there may be minor neurological and psy-

---

**TABLE 2.1. Some Definitions of Recovery**

1. Postlesion reinstatement of specific behaviors disrupted by the brain injury
   (LeVere, 1980)—*impossible for most survivors of brain injury.*
2. Complete recovery of the identical functions lost or impaired by the brain
   injury (Almli & Finger, 1988)—*impossible for most people with severe brain injury.*
3. Resumption of a normal life with minor neurological and psychological
   deficits (Jennett & Bond, 1975)—*sometimes achievable for those with organic memory
   problems.*
4. Return to normal or near-normal levels of performance (Laurence & Stein,
   1978)—*unlikely for most memory-impaired people once past the acute stage.*
5. Reduction of persistent behavioral deficits through special training or
   pharmacological or other interventions (Braun, 1978)—*this encompasses
   rehabilitation.*
6. Diminution of impairments in behavioral or physiological functions over time
   (Marshall, 1985)—*we can and do see this.*
7. Partial recovery of function with considerable substitution of function (Kolb,
   1995)—*what most of us in rehabilitation expect to see.*

---

chological deficits" (p. 483). This is sometimes achievable for those with organic memory problems. Laurence and Stein (1978) suggested that recovery is a "return to normal or near-normal levels of performance following the initially disruptive effects of an injury to the nervous system" (p. 370). Again, this is unlikely for most people with memory impairment once the acute stage has passed.

More likely to apply to those with organic memory deficits is the definition from Marshall (1985), who interpreted recovery as "impairments in behavioral or physiological functions that abate as time since injury increases" (p. 201). Braun (1978) stated that recovery has occurred "when persistent behavioral deficits are reduced by special training or by pharmacological, surgical, or other independent manipulations" (p. 178). This definition, with its emphasis on *reduction of deficits* would, to some extent, encompass rehabilitation. Perhaps the most precise and certainly the strictest definition is that by LeVere (1980), who defined recover as "the post lesion reinstatement of the specific behaviors that were disrupted by the brain injury" (p. 298). However, it is very unlikely that the majority of improvements made by memory-impaired people through a combination of natural recovery and rehabilitation would fulfill this criterion. According to Kolb (1995), on the other hand, recovery typically involves two processes—partial recovery of lost functioning together with considerable substitution of function (i.e., compensating for the lost function through other means)—and this feels more comfortable to those of us working in rehabilitation because it includes (1) natural recovery and (2) the compensations for lost functioning that are targeted in rehabilitation programs.

The most common cause of brain damage and subsequent memory impairment in people younger than 25 is TBI. People incurring such injury usually undergo some, and often considerable, recovery. Accepting Teasdale and Jennett's (1974) definition of coma—"not opening the eyes spontaneously or to stimulation, not obeying commands and no verbal response"—then once people have opened their eyes, they are no longer in coma. Because people with severe TBI have usually opened their eyes within a period of 4 weeks or so, they are no longer in coma. Therefore, by about 4 weeks post injury, people with TBI may be in the vegetative or minimally conscious state (Giacino et al., 2002), or they may be fully conscious, the most likely outcome for the majority of these patients. Further recovery will almost certainly still take place, and this is likely to be fairly rapid in the early weeks and months post injury, followed by a slower recovery that can continue for many years. A similar pattern may be seen after other kinds of nonprogressive injury such as hypoxia, encephalitis, and cerebrovascular accident. In these latter cases, however, the recovery process may last months rather than years.

It must be stressed that, although some partial resolution of deficits may occur, this will be minimal for many patients. The adoption of a *compensatory* approach provides the best chance of reducing everyday problems and enhancing independent living and quality of life (QOL) for the majority of those with organic memory.

## Mechanisms of Recovery

Several authors have considered the mechanisms by which recovery can occur (Almli & Finger, 1992; Kolb, 1995, 2003; Robertson, 1999). The most frequently postulated mechanisms have been resolution from edema or swelling of the brain, diaschisis (whereby lesions cause damage to other areas of the brain through shock), plasticity or changes to the structure of the nervous system, and regeneration or regrowth of neural tissue. Changes seen in the first few minutes (e.g., after a mild head injury) probably reflect the resolution of temporary damage that has not caused structural damage. Changes seen within several days are more likely to be due to resolution of temporary structural abnormalities such as edema or vascular disruption or of depressed enzyme metabolic activity. Recovery after several months or years is less well understood. There are several ways in which this might be achieved, including diaschisis, plasticity, and regeneration.

The term *diaschisis* was introduced by Von Monakov in 1914 and means "shocked throughout." Von Monakov described remote functional changes, gradual regression, and a "wave of diaschisis" following neuroanatomical pathways (Feeney & Baron, 1986). Modern usage of the term refers to depression of regional neuronal metabolism and cerebral blood flow caused by dysfunction in an anatomically separate but functionally related neuronal region (Brunberg, Frey, Horton, & Kuhl, 1992). These authors suggest that diaschisis occurs in 50% of patients with well-defined hemispheric lesions. In short, diaschisis assumes that damage to a particular area of the brain can result in neural shock or disruption elsewhere in the brain. The secondary neural shock can be adjacent to the primary insult or farther away. In a study of a 67-year-old stroke patient with an amnesic syndrome following a left thalamic infarction, Stenset et al. (2007) showed that cortical diaschisis corresponded to the areas of corticothalamic fiber loss. Whether the shock occurs close to the initial damage or farther away, it follows a specific neural route. Similar, but not identical, to this procedure is the idea of inhibition. In inhibition the shock is more diffuse and affects the brain as a whole. Robertson and Murre (1999) interpreted diaschisis as "a weakening of synaptic connections between the damaged and undamaged sites, contingent on the reduced level of activity in the lesioned area" (p. 547). Because cells in the two areas are no longer firing together, synaptic connectivity between them is weakened, and this results in the depression of functioning in the undamaged but partly disconnected remote site.

Brodtmann, Puce, Darby, and Donnan (2007) studied three stroke patients who had sustained damage to the visual system. Using functional magnetic resonance imaging (fMRI), they showed that initially the patients displayed absent or significantly reduced activation in ventral extrastriate sites but 6 months later activation had been restored. The authors suggested this revealed evidence of ipsilesional cortical diaschisis within these sites and that diaschisis may play an underrecognized role in visual recovery after stroke.

Plasticity implies anatomical reorganization based on the idea that undamaged areas of the brain can take over the functions of the damaged areas. Postulated in the 19th century by Casal (1888; Azmitia, 2007), it fell out of favor, and until recently this idea was discredited as an explanation for recovery in adults. Views are now changing, however. Jang, You, and Ahn (2007) evaluated the effects of a comprehensive neurorehabilitation program provided for a 25-year-old man with significant motor problems associated with right hippocampal sclerosis, temporal lobectomy, and amygdalotomy. The patient received 8 months of treatment. Motor difficulties were the focus of treatment, and both motor tests and fMRI were used to determine the restoration of motor function and neuroplasitic changes. The motor tests showed that the man had improved on functional reaching, grasping, and hand manipulation skills. He maintained this improvement at 6-month follow-up. Furthermore, the fMRI investigations showed that before treatment there was asymmetry of the contralesional sensorimotor cortex activation, which was restored to normal symmetry after rehabilitation. The authors suggest that "comprehensive neurorehabilitation may facilitate restitution of normal symmetry of cortical activation, thereby enhancing motor function." This case provides the first neuroimaging evidence about a long-term comprehensive neurorehabilitation: induced neuroplasticity (p. 117). We do not know what happened to this patient's memory functioning.

In a thought-provoking article, Robertson and Murre (1999) suggested that plastic reorganization may occur initially because of rapid alterations in synaptic activity taking place over seconds or minutes followed by structural changes over days and weeks. The authors focused in particular on those individuals who will only show recovery after rehabilitation. They believed that there are three types of brain-injured patients: those who will recover without help, others who show no significant change even with help, and those who do reasonably well provided they receive assistance. They referred to this as a triage of spontaneous recovery, no recovery, and assisted recovery. Robertson and Murre suggested that those in the no-recovery group should be taught compensatory strategies and those in the spontaneous recovery group do not need help because they will get better anyway, so those in the assisted-recovery group are those who can help us answer questions about plasticity. Robertson and Murre also believed that the severity of the lesion relates to the triage, so patients with mild lesions experience spontaneous recovery, those with moderate lesions require assistance, and those with severe lesions will see no recovery. My own view is that this is only partly true, because one can have relatively mild lesions in particular locations that may cause more problems in everyday life than more severe lesions in other locations. Thus, individuals with severe lesions in the hippocampus but with no other cortical damage may lead independent lives (see, e.g., "Jay," in Chapter 4 of Wilson, 1999, and Chapter 10 in the current text), whereas those with mild frontal lobe lesions may be unable to cope without help (Shallice & Burgess, 1991).

Regeneration in the central nervous system can occur and is more likely early in life although it can occur in adults (Eriksson et al., 1998; Kolb, 2003). The view held for many years that cerebral plasticity is severely restricted in the human adult brain is no longer true. Eriksson et al. (1998) found postmortem evidence for neurogenesis in the hippocampus of the brains of five adults who died of cancer. The authors were cautious about the implications of their findings, and the extent to which we can harness the brain's regeneration ability to achieve functional gains is by no means clear. We still have no evidence that memory exercises can improve memory functioning in general, even though exercise may increase the likelihood of recovery in spinal cord patients (Rojas, Vega, et al., 2008).

Robertson (2002) suggested that recovery is rapid for deficits that are subserved by multiple circuits, such as unilateral neglect, and slowest for deficits that are subserved by a more limited number of circuits, such as hemianopia, because fewer alternative pathways are available to take over the functioning of the damaged pathways. This could be why language functions appear to show better recovery over time than memory functions (Kolb, 1995). Vargha-Khadem, Carr, et al. (1997) reported on a boy with Sturge–Weber syndrome who was mute until the age of 9 years, when he underwent a hemispherectomy. He then developed clearly articulated, well-structured, and appropriate language. At the age of 15, he had the language skills of an 8- to 10-year-old. In contrast, in another report, three individuals with childhood amnesia retained considerable memory deficits into adulthood (Vargha-Khadem, Gadian, et al., 1997).

Age at insult, diagnosis, number of insults sustained, and premorbid status of the brain are just a few of the likely factors influencing recovery. Age, often thought to be an important variable, is perhaps less clear-cut than many believe. There is a fairly widespread view that younger people recover from injury to the brain better than older people. This is known as the Kennard principle after Kennard (1940), who showed that young primates who sustained lesions to the motor and premotor cortex had better recovery than adults sustaining the same lesions. It is not always true, however, that brain damage occurring earlier in life leads to better recovery. Even Kennard herself recognized this. Hebb (1949) also suggested that injuries occurring early in life will sometimes result in a worse outcome than those occurring later. Once severity, etiology, and other demographic variables are taken into account, age is not always a good predictor of outcome, and young people sustaining a severe TBI early in life tend to do worse than older people in terms of social deficits and behavior problems (Thomsen, 1984).

Kolb (2004) presented some interesting views on age, indicating that a better outcome in younger compared with older people is to be expected if the cerebral cortex is damaged when neurogenesis is still ongoing and the reverse is true if there is damage during the time of neural migration. He suggested that for humans injury during the last stages of pregnancy and around birth lead to poor outcome because this is the time for maximum migration. Injury during the next 18 months or so will lead to a better outcome because this is the time of maximum synaptogenesis. Kolb pointed out, too, that other factors affecting early injury are location of the damage and the behavior of interest. Thus, early damage to language areas usually results in complete recovery of language but at the expense of executive deficits. So age is just one factor to consider when trying to predict recovery.

With regard to memory functions, it seems that neither children nor adults are likely to recover from the amnesic syndrome. We have already seen that three people who developed amnesia in childhood remained amnesic in adulthood (Vargha-Khadem, Gadian, et al., 1997). Broman, Rose, Hotson, and Casey (1997) describe a boy who became amnesic at the age of 8 after suffering cardiac arrest. He was monitored for 19 years, during which his memory functions showed no sign of recovery. Vargha-Khadem, Gadian, and Mishkin (2001) studied 11 children with childhood amnesia and found that regardless of age of onset there was a marked dissociation between episodic memory, which was severely impaired, and semantic memory, which was relatively well preserved. They also found a discrepancy between recall, again severely impaired, and recognition, which was relatively intact.

Some studies have shown that very premature infants are more likely to have memory difficulties later in childhood. Isaacs et al. (2000) studied 11 adolescents with very low birth weights (born at or before 30 weeks gestation) and compared them with eight adolescents born full term. Investigations involved both neuropsychological assessments and magnetic functional imaging procedures. All participants were regarded as neurologically normal. The prematurely born group not only had significantly smaller hippocampi (despite equivalent head size), but they also scored poorly on a test of everyday memory functioning: the children's version of the Rivermead Behavioural Memory Test (RBMT; Wilson, Ivani-Chalian, & Aldrich, 1991). The parents of these adolescents were also asked to complete a memory questionnaire about their children's difficulties, and once again the preterm children were found to have more problems than those born full term. The authors concluded that "the reduced hippocampal volumes and deficits in everyday memory have previously been unrecognized, but their prevalence in a group of neurologically normal children is striking" (p. 713). Ment and Constable (2007), using fMRI, found changes in the neural networks involved in language and memory for preterm children.

Another factor influencing outcome is the cause of the injury or the diagnostic condition. People who sustain a moderate or severe TBI (the most common cause of brain damage in people younger than 25) usually undergo some, and often considerable, recovery. As indicated previously, this is likely to be fairly swift in the early weeks and months after the injury followed by a slower period that can last for years. A typical pattern is an initial period of coma when the patient is not opening the eyes, not obeying commands, and not responding verbally (Teasdale & Jennett, 1976). This is followed by a period of posttraumatic amnesia (PTA), when the patient is confused and disoriented, suffers from retrograde amnesia, and seems to lack the capacity to store and retrieve new information (Schacter & Crovitz, 1977). The next stage is emergence from PTA, when the patient may well be left with a number of motor, cognitive, emotional, and behavioral problems that may resolve or partially resolve over time. Variations on this pattern may be seen in other diagnostic conditions such as encephalitis, hypoxic brain damage, and cerebrovascular accident.

## To What Extent Does Memory Recover?

So much for general mechanisms of recovery. What about recovery of memory functioning? There is no doubt that some recovery of lost memory functioning does occur in the early weeks and months after nonprogressive brain damage. People who survive a severe TBI may have considerable memory loss in the early days but may make a complete or almost complete recovery insofar as their memory functions are concerned. The same pattern is true of some people who survive herpes simplex encephalitis, stroke, and hypoxic brain damage. Although people with progressive conditions such as AD or Huntington's disease will not recover, deterioration occurs at different rates, and such people should not be excluded from memory rehabilitation (see, e.g., Clare, 2008; Clare & Woods, 2001, 2004). Many people will not recover, however, although they may show some improvement over time. So what should we tell relatives of memory-impaired people who ask about the level of recovery or how much improvement to expect? Most health care professionals will probably say something along the lines of "Things are likely to improve, but we don't know by how much and the patient may not get back to the same level as before the accident/illness." We try to tread a thin line: We do not want to give false hope, but we do not want to sound too pessimistic and destroy all hope.

What evidence is there for recovery of memory after brain injury? As we saw earlier, "recovery" means different things to different people: Some are solely concerned with recovery of cognitive functions, others focus on survival rates, whereas others consider only biological recovery such as repair of brain structures.

What can studies investigating the recovery of memory functioning tell us? The picture is a little confusing. Lezak (1979) reported significant recovery of memory functioning during the first year; Victor, Adams, and Collins (1989) found that about 74% of a sample of 104 patients with Korsakoff's syndrome showed some degree of recovery over a 3-year period and 21% showed a substantial degree of recovery; and Wilson (1991) found marked improvement in 33% of people referred for memory rehabilitation 5 to 10 years earlier. Wilson and Baddeley (1993) described a man with a severe STM deficit who made a substantial recovery even though the memory deficit had been stable for at least 2 years. This man, a mathematician, was initially considered to have possible AD because he scored badly on the mental arithmetic portion of the Wechsler Adult Intelligence Scale. His poor score was due, of course, to the fact that he could only recall two digits or words and thus could not hold on to the questions long enough to compute the answers (Baddeley & Wilson, 1988a). This patient's forward digit span of two when first seen (and for a 2-year follow-up period) improved to a normal seven when seen several years later (Wilson & Baddeley, 1993). In contrast, we know that families of people with brain injury report significant memory problems several years after the initial insult (Brooks, 1984; Brooks, Campsie, Symington, Beattie, & McKinlay, 1987; Oddy, 1984; Stilwell, Stilwell, Hawley, & Davies, 1999), and some studies of individual patients show almost no recovery over many years. The most famous amnesic patient in the world, H. M. (Scoville & Milner, 1957), appears to have shown no recovery since his operation in 1957 (Freed et al., 1998; Ogden, 1996). H. M. had bilateral surgical hippocampal lesions. Another amnesic patient, C. W. (Wilson, Baddeley, & Kapur, 1995), who had survived herpes simplex encephalitis, showed no recovery over a 10-year period. This is still true 23 years post illness (Wilson, Kopelman, & Kapur, 2008).

Sim, Terryberry-Spohr, and Wilson (2008) examined the recovery of memory functioning after mild TBI in 419 high school athletes (mean age = 15.69 years). Interestingly, this group had undergone neuropsychological assessment before the sports season began. Fourteen had sustained a concussion during the season and were consequently reassessed at 2, 5, 6, and 10 days postinjury. Another 14 uninjured matched control students were reassessed at the end of the school year. Impairments in reaction time, processing speed, and delayed memory were seen in the concussed group. Reaction time and processing speed deficits returned to baseline levels by day 6 postinjury, but the memory impairments did not resolve until day 10.

Szakács, Kálmán, Barzós, Sas, and Janka reported on the recovery of a densely amnesic woman who had sustained a ruptured aneurysm on the anterior communicating artery with massive bleeding. A computed tomography (CT) scan showed a lesion in the left hippocampus and fornix. After some early recovery, she was left with severe AA and disorientation. Another CT scan weeks later showed hydrocephalus, requiring insertion of a ventriculoperitoneal shunt. Gradual but continuous improvement of memory occurred, with total recovery after 1 year.

Kapur and Graham (2002) reviewed recovery of long-term episodic memory functioning and considered both single-case and group studies. They assessed the shrinkage of RA in individual patients with traumatic injury (which can be seen as one of the characteristics of PTA) and also regarded patients with transient global amnesia. These conditions are temporary, so we expect some, or perhaps substantial, recovery to take place depending on the length of the PTA (Wilson, Evans, Emslie, Balleny, Watson, & Balleny, 1999). Indeed, this is confirmed in the group studies reported by Kapur and Graham (2002). They concluded, however, that recovery of memory function "remains a relatively uncharted map in the geography of cognitive neuroscience" (p. 245). Thus, we only have very tentative answers when we ask questions about recovery.

Kertesz and Gold (2003) provided another review of recovery. Although this review is concerned particularly with recovery from aphasia, the authors briefly considered recovery of memory and also reflected on recovery from different diagnoses (e.g., TBI and encephalitis) likely to give rise to memory problems. Like Kapur and Graham (2002), they looked at shrinkage of RA and at recovery from PTA, pointing out that prognosis of LTM impairment is correlated with the length of PTA. They had little to say on recovery of memory functioning in people no longer in PTA but with more stable memory deficits.

One fascinating account of recovery and readjustment over time is provided by Luria (1975) in *The Man with a Shattered World*. This is essentially the story of Zasetsky, a man injured by a gunshot wound to the left temporoparietal area of the brain, who spent 25 years trying to write his story, make sense of his world, and learn to regain some of his lost skills. He described how his memory functions improved to some extent but from "the wrong end," as he put it.

> During the weeks immediately after I was wounded I couldn't remember my first or last name or patronymic, or even the names of my close relatives. Only later was I gradually able to remember a few things, mostly about my childhood and elementary-school years. My memories came back from the wrong end—that is, it's become easier for me to remember things that go far back—the buildings where I went to kindergarten and elementary school, the games I played, the faces of children and teachers I used to know. But I've either forgotten or have a great deal of trouble remembering anything about the recent past—even what life was like on the front. (in Luria, 1975, p. 85).

This is a compelling and insightful account of RA. Zasetsky's recovery was very limited, but his determination and spirit fill one with awe.

There is some evidence suggesting that females recover better from insults to the brain than males. As long ago as 1987, it was suggested that female animals may be protected against the effects of brain injury at certain stages of their cycle as a result of estrogen and progesterone (Attella, Nattinville, & Stein, 1987). This was confirmed by Roof and Hall (2000). Potentially important for rehabilitation, progesterone has been given to survivors of TBI, with some suggestion that this leads to a better outcome (Wright et al., 2007). In addition, studies have looked at the long-term outcome for females and males after TBI. There are conflicting reports: Ratcliff et al. (2007) suggested that females fare better, whereas others, such as Farace and Alves (2000) and Ponsford et al.

(2008), found that the outcome for women was worse. The latter study controlled for Glasgow Coma Scale score, age, and cause of injury. The authors found that females had a lower rate of survival and a lower rate of good outcome at 6 months postinjury, suggesting that this reflected the lower rate of initial survival. They found no evidence that females did better and some evidence that they did worse.

At this point, it is worth mentioning the concept of *cognitive reserve*. This stems from Katzman et al's. (1988) study of 137 postmortem examinations of elderly people (mean age = 85.5 years). Seventy-eight percent had dementia and 55% had AD. Ten of the best functioning people with signs of AD were as good as the top percentage of the control subjects without AD. These high-functioning people with AD brain pathology had heavier brains and more neurons than the controls. Two possible explanations were postulated: They either had incipient AD but escaped the large loss of neurons or they started with larger brains and a greater number of large neurons and thus a greater *reserve*. This is the first time the term was used in the literature in this context.

Cognitive reserve, then, refers to the fact that people with more education and higher intelligence may show less impairment than those with poor education and low intelligence (Stern, 2007). Richards and Deary (2005) suggested that this reserve can buffer the effects of neuropathology such that the greater the reserve the more severe the pathology must be to cause functional impairment. Whalley, Deary, Appleton, and Starr (2004) proposed that it can explain the great variation in people with similar degrees of damage. In talking about people with AD, Starr and Lonie (2008) operationally defined cognitive reserve as "the hypothesized capacity of the mature adult brain to sustain the effects of disease or injury without manifesting clinical symptoms of AD, but sufficient to cause clinical dementia in an individual possessing less cognitive reserve" (p. 27). The concept can also apply to people with TBI (Kesler, Adams, Blaser, & Bigler, 2003), mild TBI (Dawson, Batchelor, Meares, Chapman, & Marosszeky, 2007), temporal lobe epilepsy (Helmstaedter & Kockelmann, 2006), and cerebrovascular infarcts (Elkins et al., 2006).

The person who has probably written most about cognitive reserve is Stern. In 2006 he suggested that there are two mechanisms by which cognitive reserve might work: neural reserve and neural compensation. In neural reserve the more efficient preexisting brain networks of those with high intelligence or more education are less susceptible to disruption; in neural compensation other networks may compensate for the disrupted ones. So individuals with high intelligence may process tasks in a more efficient way. Consequently, in cases of AD, task impairment manifests itself later in the disease in people with such cognitive reserve. Stern (2007) also suggested that most clinicians are aware of the fact that any insult of the same severity can produce profound damage in one patient and minimal damage in another. This may explain differences in recovery after nonprogressive brain injury. As Symonds (1937, p. 1092) said in an often-quoted remark, "It is not only the kind of head injury that matters but the kind of head." Stern (2007) argued that there is no direct relationship between the degree of damage and the clinical manifestation of that damage.

## Can We Improve on Natural Recovery?

The following comments in this section are taken from Wilson (in press). Earlier we saw that some regeneration can take place in the adult brain; one area of research trying to increase the likelihood of this happening is the implantation of stem cells. Stem cells of the adult human brain support regeneration in the hippocampus through neuronal replacement (Conover & Notti, 2008) Although there is some controversy as to how much, if any, functional recovery may take place through the replacement of stem cells, it is certainly one area of research that could enhance recovery of memory (Zeitlow, Lane, Dunnett, & Rosser, 2008). Animal studies have shown that it is possible to regenerate cells in the dentate gyrus through the provision of specific learning tasks (Griesbach, Hovda, Molteni, Wu, & Gomez-Pinilla, 2004) or enriched environments (Dhanushkodi & Shetty, 2008; Döbrössy & Dunnett, 2001). Given these findings, it might be possible to enhance natural recovery through enriched environments and focused rehabilitation strategies. Furthermore, such programs might indeed lead to neurogenesis in the human brain (see McMillan, Robertson, & Wilson, 1999, and Ogden, 2000, for further discussion).

Imaging procedures could allow us to see whether it is possible to improve memory functioning per se rather than relying primarily on compensatory approaches and to see whether any observed behavioral changes result in structural changes to the brain (Levin, 2006). Grady and Kapur (1999) suggested that imaging studies may enable us to measure specific changes occurring in the brain during recovery and, therefore, allow us to determine whether recovery is the result of (1) reorganization within an existing framework, (2) recruitment of new areas into the network, or (3) plasticity in regions surrounding the damaged area.

A few studies have used imagery techniques to study recovery from brain injury. One of the first articles in this area reported changes in regional cerebral blood flow (rCBF) after cognitive rehabilitation for people who had sustained toxic encephalopathy after exposure to toxins (Lindgren, Österberg, Ørbæk, & Rosén, 1997). Later the same year positron emission tomography was used to identify the neural correlates of stimulation procedures implemented in the rehabilitation of people with dysphasia (Carlomagno et al., 1997). Laatsch, Jobe, Sychra, Lin, and Blend (1997) and Laatsch, Pavel, Jobe, Lin, and Quintana (1999) used single photon emission CT to evaluate rCBF during recovery from brain injury. The authors suggested that specific changes in rCBF appeared to be related to both the location of the injury and the strategies used in cognitive rehabilitation.

Continued improvements in the three patients in the Laatsch et al. (1997) study were documented in rCBF, functional abilities, and cognitive skills up to 45 months postinsult. A further study by Laatsch, Thulborn, Krisky, Shobat, and Sweeney (2004) showed that improvements following cognitive rehabilitation could be detected by fMRI.

In 1998, Pizzamiglio et al. used functional imaging to monitor the effects of rehabilitation for unilateral neglect. The brain regions most active after recovery were almost identical to the areas active in control participants engaged in the same tasks. This appears to support the view that some rehabilitation methods repair the lesioned network and do not simply work through compensation or behavioral change.

Baxter, Spencer, and Kerrigan (2007) described a patient with nonparaneoplastic limbic encephalitis who had severe AA with subsequent recovery. They used fMRI to show increased hippocampal activation before and after recovery. Does this happen after memory rehabilitation? We do not yet know the answer to this question, but there is a growing interest in determining (1) whether attempts to restore memory functioning and attempts to help people compensate result in structural changes to the brain and (2) whether any changes seen are different depending on the approach used. In reality, of course, the two approaches are not mutually exclusive, and a combination of the two may prove to be the most practically useful.

## Changes in Memory Functioning Following Intervention or Rehabilitation

Rehabilitation is a process whereby people who are disabled by injury or disease work together with professional staff, relatives, and members of the wider community to achieve their optimum physical, psychological, social, and vocational well-being (McLellan, 1991). Insofar as memory rehabilitation is concerned, rehabilitation may encompass (1) trying to restore lost functioning, (2) modifying or organizing the environment and thus avoiding the need for memory, (3) helping people to learn more efficiently, or (4) teaching patients to compensate for their problems. Although the terms *recovery* and *compensation* are sometimes used interchangeably, they are different (Kolb, 2004), as discussed in the first section of this chapter. Nevertheless, given that restoration of episodic, explicit memory is unlikely in the majority of cases once the acute period has passed, the other approaches are more likely to lead to change in everyday memory functioning. Because these approaches are the main themes of this book, they are considered in more detail later. Some of the ways we can help memory-impaired people are shown in Figure 2.1.

Because this book does not cover the treatment of semantic memory disorders, this is covered only briefly here. Few studies have tried to teach lost semantic knowledge to people with a damaged semantic memory system. Of those, Graham, Patterson, Pratt, and Hodges (2001) have perhaps carried out the most systematic work. They suggested that

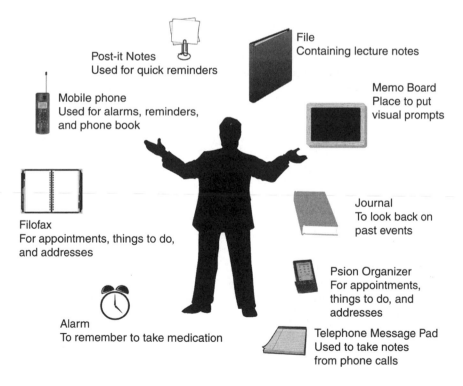

**FIGURE 2.1.** Some compensatory memory aids. Reprinted with permission from the Oliver Zangwill Centre.

the predominant, and most socially isolating, symptom typically seen in semantic dementia is anomia, or word-finding difficulties, in conjunction with a deteriorating central semantic system. In one study, they demonstrated that repeated rehearsal of the names of concepts paired with pictures of them or real items resulted in a dramatic improvement in the ability of D. M., a patient with semantic dementia, to produce previously difficult-to-retrieve words on tests of word production. Although the substantial improvement shown by D. M. suggests that rehearsal with pictorial and verbal stimuli could be a useful rehabilitative strategy for word-finding difficulties in semantic dementia, the experiment also revealed that constant exposure to items was necessary in order to prevent the observed decline in performance once D. M.'s daily drill was stopped.

Snowden and Neary (2002) also looked at the relearning of object names in two patients with severe anomia associated with semantic dementia. They found that some relearning of lost vocabulary is possible in semantic dementia. In both these studies, however, patients' learning was confounded by deterioration in their condition. Given the difficulty of measuring new learning in people who are deteriorating, Dewar, Patterson, Wilson, and Graham (in press) assessed the learning and generalization of new semantic information in people with semantic memory problems after nonprogressive brain damage. They taught the names of 10 famous people to two patients who had survived herpes simplex encephalitis. Stimuli comprised 10 photographs and 10 semantic facts. Mnemonics were used following an EL learning procedure incorporating VC and expanded rehearsal in much the same way as the procedure used by Clare, Wilson, Breen, and Hodges (1999) in their work with a man with AD. The patients also practiced each day at home. Recall of all items was tested at the beginning of each session. Maintenance and generalization were assessed at the end of training. Both patients improved relative to baseline in naming the photographs, but recall of the semantic fact was less robust. There was some evidence of subsequent maintenance of learning after cessation of practice, and one patient demonstrated some generalization to new photographs of the famous people used in training. Another patient with prosopagnosia (an inability to recognize familiar faces) was also taught to recognize the faces of family and friends using a similar procedure (Dewar & Wilson, 2006). Following multiple baseline tests to ensure that practice alone was not causing improvement, eight faces were selected for training. Two faces were trained at each weekly session in addition to home practice. Recall of all faces was tested at the beginning of each session. Maintenance and generalization of learning were also assessed. The patient was able to correctly name the faces following training. There was evidence of generalization of learning to different (profile) photographs and learning was maintained in the absence of practice. Although many questions remain to be answered in this area, there is evidence that people with semantic memory deficits can relearn new information.

Another area not addressed elsewhere in this book is the field of animal studies. There is evidence that recovery can take place in rats after specific treatment procedures. Loukavenko, Ottley, Moran, Wolff, and Dalrymple-Alford (2007), for example, provided enriched environments to rats that had sustained lesions to the anterior thalamic nuclei. The rats subjected to the enriched environments showed substantial recovery of severe, and otherwise long-lasting, spatial working memory deficits. Dhanushkodi and Shetty (2008) also found memory improvement in rats subjected to enriched environments.

The next chapter addresses assessment of memory, before we come to the heart of the book: rehabilitation of episodic memory deficits. For now, suffice it to say that there is increasing evidence that rehabilitation can improve the independence and QOL of memory-impaired people, and supporting evidence is presented elsewhere in this book.

CHAPTER 3

# Assessment for Rehabilitation

## What Do We Mean by Assessment?

*Assessment* is concerned with judgment, estimation, appraisal, analysis, and evaluation. An assessor is someone who helps with the processes involved in judging, estimating, and so forth. A good definition for psychologists, provided as long ago as 1962 by Sundberg and Tyler, is that assessment is the systematic collection, organization, and interpretation of information about a person and his or her situation. It is also concerned with the prediction of behavior in new situations (Sundberg & Tyler, 1962). The way this information is collected, organized, and interpreted will depend on the reason the assessment is required in the first place: If one is interested in theoretical aspects of memory, one would assess in a different way than if the concerns were more to do with whether a person being assessed could live independently or return to work. For example, if we wanted to answer a theoretical question such as "Is there a distinction between short-term and long-term memory?", we would look for people with one kind of deficit but not the other. Thus, we might give a large group of brain-injured people forward digit span tasks together with delayed recall of prose passages. We would then look for double dissociations among the sample. We would hope to find some people with very poor scores on digit span but normal performance on delayed recall of prose passages (these would be very rare) and others with normal performance on digit span but impaired scores on delayed recall of the passages (these would be much easier to find). Such evidence would show there are two separate systems. Of course, this has already been demonstrated (Shallice & Warrington, 1970). On

34

the other hand, if we wanted to know whether a person could live independently, the assessment is more likely to involve the administration of tests known to predict independent living such as the RBMT (Wilson, Cockburn, & Baddeley, 1985), which has been demonstrated to predict both independence (Wilson, 1991) and employability (Schwartz & McMillan, 1989) in memory-impaired people. Such a quantitative evaluation would need to be supplemented with observations of the person in certain situations. We might want to identify tasks required for independent living such as cooking, self-care, managing money, and so forth and observe whether these tasks can be achieved at certain times of the day and under varying loads of distraction. Preferably an occupational therapist and a clinical neuropsychologist would combine resources to carry out such an assessment.

One could also argue that assessments are carried out in order to answer questions. Certain questions can be answered through the use of standardized tests, others need functional or behavioral assessments, and others may require specially designed procedures. We discuss standardized and functional assessments later. To determine whether a patient might require a specially designed procedure, one could question whether he or she has specialist knowledge. For instance, if a farmer has lost the ability to recognize people's faces, we might want to know whether he can still remember his cows. The musician Clive Wearing (Wearing, 2005), was once the world's expert on Orlando Lassus, the Renaissance composer. Since the onset of his amnesia in 1985, he not only had almost no episodic memory but he had also lost some of his semantic knowledge. Tests were designed to see whether he could remember his musical knowledge (Wilson et al., 1995), and it was thereby discovered that, although he could play and conduct, much of his semantic knowledge about musicians had been destroyed or was inaccessible.

## What Questions Should Be Asked in Assessments for Rehabilitation?

In addition to questions about the nature and severity of memory difficulties, most neuropsychologists will want to know about cognitive functioning in general, the level of premorbid functioning, emotional and psychosocial problems, and the main concerns of the patient, the family, and other caregivers. For the purposes of this chapter, these questions are separated into those that can be answered by standardized tests and those that are best answered through behavioral or functional assessments.

*Standardized tests can help us answer the following questions:*

- What is this person's general level of intellectual functioning?
- What was the probable level of premorbid functioning?
- What are this person's cognitive strengths and weaknesses?
- How does this person's memory functioning compare with that of same-age people in the general population?
- Is the level of memory functioning consistent with what one would expect from this level of intellectual ability?
- Is the memory problem global or restricted to certain kinds of material (e.g., is memory for visual material better than for verbal material)?
- To what extent are the memory problems due to executive, language, perceptual, or attention difficulties?
- Does this person have a high level of anxiety?
- Is this person depressed?

These and similar questions are typically addressed by clinical neuropsychologists and can, to a large extent, be answered through the administration of standardized tests provided these have been adequately normed and shown to be reliable and valid. A cognitive map showing the strengths and weaknesses of one person with severe visuoperceptual and memory problems is illustrated in Figure 3.1.

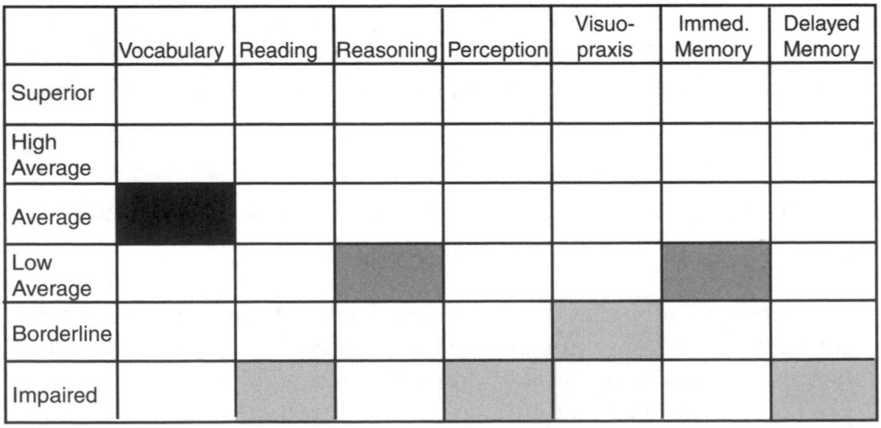

| | Vocabulary | Reading | Reasoning | Perception | Visuo-praxis | Immed. Memory | Delayed Memory |
|---|---|---|---|---|---|---|---|
| Superior | | | | | | | |
| High Average | | | | | | | |
| Average | ■ | | | | | | |
| Low Average | | | ▓ | | | ▓ | |
| Borderline | | | | | ▓ | | |
| Impaired | | ▓ | | ▓ | | | ▓ |

**FIGURE 3.1.** A map of cognitive strengths and weaknesses. Adapted from Lezak (1976). Copyright 1976 by Oxford University Press. Reprinted by permission.

There are many other important questions, however, particularly those regarding treatment, that cannot be answered by such tests. *Standardized tests are very limited when it comes to answering the following questions:*

- How are the memory difficulties manifested in everyday life?
- What problems cause most concern to the family and the memory-impaired person?
- What do we know about the cultural background and level of support available?
- What coping strategies are used?
- Are the problems exacerbated by depression or anxiety?
- Is this person likely to be able to return to work (or school)?
- Can this person live independently?
- What kind of compensatory aids did this person use premorbidly?
- What kind of memory compensation strategies are being used now?
- What is the best way for this person to learn new information?

These and similar questions require a different approach because, although standardized tests can shed some light (e.g., someone with a severe memory impairment and widespread cognitive deficits is unlikely to return to university), they cannot answer most of them directly. A more behavioral or functional approach through observations, self-report measures (probably from relatives or caregivers), and interviews will better answer these treatment-related questions. A better way of looking at this is to recognize that standardized and functional assessment procedures provide complementary information: The former allows us to build a cognitive map of a person's strengths and weaknesses while the latter enables us to target areas for treatment.

Middleton (2004) considered assessment of memory problems in children. According to Middleton, there are six lines of inquiry to be followed: (1) Find out about the underlying pathology; (2) consider the child's age, developmental level, and cultural background; (3) determine the general level of cognitive functioning and any comorbid problems; (4) assess for functional difficulties through careful interviewing; (5) observe carefully how the child copes or fails any memory or learning tasks; (6) use results from psychometric tests. Although structured in a different way, the views put forward by Middleton (2004) are similar to the approach outlined previously.

The actual tests selected will depend on the experience and preference of the assessor. In the next section, we consider which aspects of memory should be assessed and make some suggestions as to the tests available to measure these aspects followed by a discussion of the functional or behavioral approach to assessment.

## Which Aspects of Memory Should Be Assessed?

What should be included in a clinical memory assessment? This depends, of course, on the purpose of the assessment or which questions one is trying to answer. If one simply wishes to determine whether or not there is evidence of organic memory impairment, then the Wechsler Memory Scale—3 (WMS-3; Wechsler, 1997) and a measure of premorbid functioning such as the National Adult Reading Test (Nelson & Willison, 1991) or Spot-the-Word test from the Speed and Capacity of Language Processing Test (Baddeley, Emslie, & Nimmo-Smith, 1992) would probably be sufficient. If the results were consistent with the picture of organic memory impairment (i.e., a normal forward digit span with poor delayed recall below that expected for the person's predicted level of premorbid ability), then the question is answered. In many circumstances, however, a more detailed and fine-grained assessment will be required, particularly when the referral is for rehabilitation. To attempt rehabilitation, we need to know more specifically the strengths and weaknesses of an individual's memory functioning. We need to know precisely which kinds of memory are intact and which are impaired and how severe the impairment is. Most of what follows immediately derives from the classification of memory described in Chapter 1.

Table 3.1 provides a guide to the range of memory functions that should be assessed. Some of these areas can be readily assessed with existing tests, whereas others require some ingenuity on behalf of the tester. Immediate memory for verbal material is almost always assessed in any clinical examination through forward digit span. Norms can be found in the WMS-3. Backward digit span is not a good measure of immediate verbal memory, although it is often used to measure attention. Immediate visuospatial span can easily be measured by Corsi blocks (described by Milner, 1971) or by the tapping tasks in the WMS-3. If one is looking for a purer measure of visual memory, then the Visual Patterns Test (Della Sala, Gray, Baddeley, & Wilson, 1997) can be used, because some have reported a double dissociation between the visual and spatial aspects of immediate memory (Della Sala, Gray, Baddeley, Allamano, & Wilson, 1999). The patient with the visuospatial sketchpad deficit mentioned in Chapter 1 (Wilson, Baddeley, & Young, 1999) scored normally on Corsi blocks but was very impaired on the Visual

**TABLE 3.1. What Aspects of Memory Should Be Tested in a Memory Assessment for Rehabilitation?**

1. Immediate memory (including verbal, visual, and spatial short-term memory).
2. Delayed episodic memory (including verbal recall, visual recall, and recognition).
3. New episodic learning (including verbal, visual, and spatial learning).
4. Implicit memory (including, perhaps, motor, verbal, and visual aspects).
5. Remote memory (including personal autobiographical memory and memory for public information; this will help determine the length of retrograde amnesia).
6. Prospective memory (including remembering to do things at a specific time, within a certain interval, and when a certain event occurs).
7. Semantic memory (including visual and verbal aspects).
8. Orientation (for time, place, and person).

*Note.* Adapted from Wilson (2004). Copyright 2004 by John Wiley and Sons. Adapted by permission.

Patterns Test because she had a normal spatial immediate memory with an impaired visual immediate memory.

Wilson (2004) discussed other ways in which immediate memory can be assessed, including:

1. The recency effect in free recall whereby testees are requested to recall a list of words. If the last few words are consistently recalled correctly (the recency effect), then one can conclude that immediate verbal memory is normal (Baddeley, 1992).
2. Pattern recognition tasks similar to the Visual Patterns Test (Della Sala et al., 1997) which was based on work by Phillips (1983).
3. The Token Test (De Renzi & Vignolo, 1962), which is normally used to assess spoken comprehension but is also sensitive to immediate memory deficits.

There are four main classes of delayed episodic memory tests: verbal recall, verbal recognition, visual recall, and visual recognition. One test derived from Baddeley and Hitch's (1974) model of memory is the Doors and People Test assessing recall and recognition (Baddeley, Nimmo-Smith, & Emslie, 1994). The advantage of this test is that all four sections are of equal difficulty, unlike other tests in which recognition subtests are typically easier than recall subtests. The Doors and People Test includes one subtest of each of the four components together with delayed visual and verbal recall. Thus, one can calculate a number of different measures such as (1) overall memory functioning, (2) forgetting, (3) verbal memory (combining both recall and recognition), (4) visual memory (combining visual recall and recognition), (5) recall (combining verbal and visual recall), and (6) recognition (combining verbal and visual recognition). Even in the United Kingdom where it originated, this is not the most widely used test but it does have certain features to recommend it.

Prose passages are used very frequently in memory assessments and are certainly sensitive to memory impairment. Passages can be found in the Wechsler scales, the RBMT (Wilson et al., 1985; Wilson, Clare, et al., 1999), and the Adult Memory and Information Processing Battery (AMIPB; Coughlan & Hollows, 1985). The most widely used test of recognition, at least in the United Kingdom, is probably the Recognition Memory Test (RMT; Warrington, 1984). This includes recognition memory for faces (visual recognition) and words (verbal recognition). The Camden (Warrington, 1996) includes recognition subtests for words, faces (both of which are shorter versions of the RMT), topographical scenes, and pictures. The RBMT and the RBMT–Extended Version (RBMT-E) also include pictorial and face recognition subtests together with immediate and delayed recall of a new short route. A new version of this test, the RBMT-3 (Wilson, Greenfield, et al., 2008), with improved visuospatial recognition subtests, has recently been published.

The best known visual recall tests are the Visual Reproduction subtest from the WMS, the Rey–Osterrieth Complex Figure (Rey, 1941), the Benton Visual Retention Test (BVRT; Benton, 1974), and, to a lesser extent, the AMIPB, which has a complex figure analogous to the Rey–Osterrieth. One of the problems with all of the visual recall tests is that they are, to some degree, verbalizable. Apart from the BVRT, participants are asked to copy the figure first and then recall after a delay, so recall can be affected because of dyspraxia, unilateral neglect, or planning problems as well as poor memory. When interpreting the results of any assessments, we need to be aware of such problems. The Doors and People Test reduces these problems by (1) asking testees to copy the material before the test so that any difficulties with execution can be detected and (2) making it very difficult to verbalize because, although the material is verbalizable (a door for the recognition task and a cross for the recall task), *all items are doors or crosses* so the verbal label is of limited help. I was a control subject when this test was being developed and tried to use my verbal skills, which I thought were better than my visual skills. I muttered to myself such observations as, "A brown door with a round top and a brass handle," but this was no help whatsoever because all the doors in the recognition plate were brown with round tops and brass handles and each plate was similarly organized.

New episodic verbal learning is often measured by paired-associate learning. The old WMS-R included both verbal and visual paired-associate learning tasks. In the verbal subtest, eight pairs of words were presented: Four were easy to learn because of a logical connection (e.g., baby–cry) and the remaining four were difficult because there is no logical connection (e.g., obey–inch). Although everyone finds the nonconnected pairs more difficult, people with memory impairments find the difficult pairs almost impossible to learn. In the visual paired-associates subtest, those with memory deficits find the learning very difficult. In the WMS-3, however, the paired-associate learning subtests have been replaced with a new verbal test and the omission of the visual subtest. The new verbal paired-associate learning consists of eight unrelated pairs (e.g., insect–acorn). The word pairs are repeated across four trials with the order varying. After each trial, the patient is given the first word from each pair and is asked for its partner, enabling the examiner to calculate a learning slope. After a delay, one recall trial is given using the initial word from each word pair. There is a recognition trial of 24 word pairs.

Other new learning tasks are readily, available, with the best known probably being the California Verbal Learning Test (CVLT; Delis, Kramer, Kaplan, & Ober, 1987) and the Rey Auditory Verbal Learning Test (Rey, 1964). Although both are useful tests to have available, the CVLT may have certain advantages, the main one being that category cues are provided to aid recall (e.g., "Tell me all the fruits you can think of"). Apart from the visual paired associates in the WMS, few tests measure nonverbal learning. The new RBMT-3 includes one subtest to assess the ability to learn a new skill: the Novel Task subtest. Many memory-impaired people can learn new skills because this involves procedural memory, which is typically unaffected by organic memory impairment. However, the Novel Task subtest is not a procedural memory task because it involves episodic new learning. The person being tested uses different colored pieces to make a particular shape. The examiner demonstrates how the pieces can be put together to make the shape using a prescribed order. The examinee then tries. The procedure is repeated twice more, for three learning trials altogether. This is followed later by a delayed recall trial. An illustration of the Novel Task subtest can be seen in Figure 3.2.

Although the new Novel Task subtest of the RBMT-3 is not, strictly speaking, a pure visuospatial task, because the instructions are given verbally as well as demonstrated and the testees can talk themselves

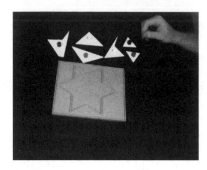

**FIGURE 3.2.** The novel task from the Rivermead Behavioural Memory Test—3. From Wilson, Greenfield, et al. (2008). Copyright 2008 by Pearson Education Ltd. Reprinted by permission.

through it, it certainly includes a large visuospatial component and can be given to people with language problems. The demonstration appears to be critical and the task sensitive to learning difficulties (Greenfield, Nannery, & Wilson, 2007). In addition, different diagnostic groups show different degrees of difficulty, with TBI patients learning more than people with encephalitis or stroke and, not surprisingly, people with AD learning least (Greenfield, 2005). The combination of verbal and visual instructions found in the Novel Task and the new Route Learning subtests, replicates the kinds of situations faced in real life, and the RBMT is, indeed, a test of everyday, real-life memory functioning.

One very easy way to assess nonverbal learning is to administer the span plus two task (Wilson, 2004). Once a person's span has been established with the WMS Visual Tapping subtest, Corsi blocks, or the Visual Patterns Test, the examiner can add two to the span and repeat the sequence until it is correctly reproduced. Thus, if a typical span of five is achieved, a sequence of seven taps is administered and the same sequence repeated until it has been reproduced correctly, preferably on three consecutive occasions to make sure it was not a fluke. Although no norms are known to exist, most people would learn span plus two in three trials and almost certainly in five trials. Someone with a severe amnesia would not learn in 50 trials (and would not remember how many times they had been tested).

Implicit memory is rarely formally measured as part of a neuropsychological assessment even though it is of great interest to memory researchers. Not only are there no standardized published tests of implicit memory, but it is also unclear how implicit memory relates to the rehabilitation needs of brain-injured patients. Having said this, as long ago as 1988, Baddeley and Wilson believed that poor implicit memory was a bad prognostic sign. Furthermore, we know that most memory-impaired people have normal or nearly normal implicit memory, so it seems sensible to measure this and to capitalize on it as far as possible. This, indeed, is what Glisky et al. (1986) and Glisky and Schacter (1988) tried to do when teaching amnesic patients to use computers. We return to this in Chapter 6. Implicit learning is believed to be why memory-impaired people learn better when prevented from making mistakes during the learning process (Baddeley & Wilson, 1994; Page et al., 2006). This is another reason why it is a good idea to try to evaluate it. It should be made clear, however, that implicit memory is not a unitary concept: Like STM and LTM, it can be fractionated into a number of subtypes, including motor, perceptual, auditory, and verbal implicit memory. Wilson et al. (1996) showed dissociations among auditory, motor, and perceptual implicit memory tasks.

In the absence of formal tests, one can still look at some aspects using patients as their own controls. For motor memory, one can set up a tracking task on a computer. Even densely amnesic people improve over time on this, even though they may not always remember they have done the task before. One can see whether there is an improvement over time even though the score cannot be compared with that for a control group. Assessing visual implicit memory is typically carried out through perceptual priming in the form of fragmented pictures (Warrington & Weiskrantz, 1968). The pictures are degraded from a greater to a lesser degree.

Nannery, Greenfield, Wilson, Sopena, and Rous (2007) described a procedure whereby seven pictures are shown in total and each picture has seven fragments followed by the complete picture. The first fragment is the most degraded, and individuals are asked to guess what it might be. Then a slightly less degraded picture is presented and participants are asked if they can now identify it. The third fragment is then presented and so on, with the final picture showing the complete object. Three trials are given. Savings are seen on the second trial. Of course, people can use both episodic and implicit memory to recall the pictures, but for very amnesic people, with very little episodic memory, savings occur and they identify the pictures earlier in the sequence (Wilson et al., 1996).

One of the easiest ways to assess verbal implicit memory is to use a stem completion task. A set of complete words is presented and read by the examinee. A stem in the form of the first two or three letters of the word is then presented and the person asked to think of the first word that comes to mind beginning with the stem. Thus, if the list of words starts with BLANK, THUMB, QUEST, etc., the stems would be BL_____, TH_____, QU_____. The response is more likely to be the word presented earlier even for amnesic people, who have no explicit recall of the original list (Graf, Squire, & Mandler, 1984). A set of materials has been produced and some unpublished norms collected on the performance of people with and without brain injury. Essentially, the people with brain injury perform worse overall than those without brain injury but the pattern of response is similar. This was also found in a previous study with regard to fragmented pictures (Wilson et al., 1996).

The 1996 study provides some norms for a group of 136 control participants and 16 people with amnesia on three implicit memory tests: mirror tracing (a motor tracking task), perceptual priming (fragmented pictures), and Korean melodies, an auditory priming task originally developed by Johnson, Kim, and Risse (1985). In this last task, melodies heard several times were preferred to melodies heard only once; most people were unaware that certain melodies were repeated. This study found that the amnesic people were indistinguishable from the control participants on the Korean melodies task but were poorer on the motor tracking and the perceptual priming tasks. Nevertheless, the *pattern* of learning was similar: It was just at a lower level overall. It was also found that "normal" performance, compared with that of controls, on one type of task did not guarantee such performance on another task. Three-way dissociations were seen, with some being good at any one of the tasks and poor at the others.

The next aspect of memory to be discussed is *remote memory*. Again, this is not often formally assessed in clinical practice despite having important implications for rehabilitation and real-life problems. Baddeley and Wilson (1986) suggested that people with a long RA and loss of autobiographical knowledge are more likely to be anxious, angry, and depressed or exhibit behavior problems. They believed this was because, in order to know *who* we are, we need to have a past. Baddeley and Wilson (1986) and Wilson (1999) described such patients. Most people with remote memory loss will have problems with both personal and public knowledge, although there are reports of one without the other (Hodges & McCarthy, 1993; Kapur, 1993, 1999). Kopelman, Wilson, and Baddeley (1990) published a semistructured interview to assess autobiographical knowledge.

For measurement of public events, tests of famous faces and famous events from different decades are typically used, but it is difficult to find a readily available test for this. Although Butters and Albert (1982) published an RA battery, the main problem is that tests have to be updated every year. In addition, some people who were famous in one decade remain famous long after they died. Princess Diana, for example, died in 1997 but her face is still seen frequently years later. In contrast, someone who died much more recently, such as Robin Cook, the British politician, in 2005, will be less well known. In addition to differences in exposure levels, such tests involve differences in the level of interest, with some people having a much greater interest in politics or sport than others, and cultural differences. Attempts have been made to develop easier tests of remote memory such as Kapur's Dead and Alive Test (Kapur, Thompson, Cook, Lang, & Brice, 1996), but the same problems apply and testers resort mostly to developing their own materials specific to individual needs.

Prospective memory is another area that is rarely formally assessed despite the fact that one of the most frequent complaints of memory-impaired people is that they forget what they need to do. Mateer, Sohlberg, and Crinean (1987) found that both people with and without brain injury rated themselves as having more difficulty with prospective memory tasks than with any other kind of memory problems. This led Sohlberg and Mateer (1989a) to publish the Prospective Memory Screening Tool to measure people's ability to carry out prospective memory tasks after 60 seconds, 2 minutes, 10 minutes, 20 minutes, and 24 hours. Looking at situations more analogous to everyday life, the RBMT, the RBMT-E, and the RBMT-3 all include prospective memory tasks whereby participants are requested to remember (depending on the version used) to ask about their next appointment(s) at a prespecified time, to remember to deliver one or two messages, or to remember to collect one or two belongings at the end of the test. These items appear to add to the sensitivity of the test when used with older people (Cockburn & Smith, 1989) and with the identification of early AD (Beardsall & Huppert, 1991). More recently, a new test of prospective memory has been used, namely the Cambridge Prospective Memory Test (Wilson, Emslie, Foley, et al., 2005), which includes both time-based and event-based tasks. Following a pilot study (Groot et al., 2002), the test was modified and now comprises three time-based and three event-based tasks. Norms have been collected from 212 controls and a group of people with brain injury. Considerable differences, as reflected in the scoring, were found between age groups and groups of different ability levels.

Patients with semantic memory deficits are likely to have problems expressing themselves and recognizing objects. This aspect of memory functioning can be assessed in a variety of ways, including word comprehension, category fluency, and general knowledge. Hodges, Patterson, Oxbury, and Funnell (1992) described a semantic memory battery designed to assess semantic knowledge in patients with progressive conditions. One set of items is used to assess input to and output from a central store of representational knowledge. There are three living categories and three man-made categories. Knowledge is measured in a number of ways, for example, fluency, naming, picture–word match-ing, picture sorting, and naming to description. Wilson (1997) adminis-tered the battery to a group of people with nonprogressive brain injury and found results broadly similar to those of Hodges et al. (1992) with dementia patients. Unfortunately, a formal published version of this very useful test is not yet available.

One published semantic memory battery that is available is the Cat-egory Specific Names Test (McKenna, 1998) in which people are asked to name objects and match objects to their spoken names in four seman-tic categories. Another test useful for determining semantic memory deficits is the Pyramids and Palm Trees Test (PPT; Howard & Patter-son, 1992). This test determines the degree to which an individual can access meaning from pictures and words. Testers can establish whether difficulty in naming or pointing to a named picture is due to difficulty retrieving semantic information from pictures, difficulty retrieving semantic information from words, or, in the case of a naming failure, difficulty retrieving the appropriate spoken form of the word. The test is suitable for measuring picture and word comprehension in people with aphasia, visual agnosia, and general semantic impairment such as might be seen in AD. Because of its simple forced-choice format, the PPT is suitable for people with severe problems such as global aphasia, where it may be the only practicable way of testing semantic knowledge.

Finally, there is orientation for time, place, and person. This should always be included in any assessment and is easy to do because both the Wechsler scales and all versions of the RBMT include orientation items.

## Rivermead Behavioural Memory Test

Before moving on to the more functional assessments, I will say a few words about the RBMT because this is a test that addresses everyday life functioning and can help plan for rehabilitation. I argue, however, that it is not sufficient on its own because, although it can highlight some of the areas that one might want to tackle in a treatment program, it does not specify with sufficient precision the nature and extent of the every-day problems in such a way that we can set appropriate goals (addressed in Chapter 9). I also suggest that the RBMT is insufficient on its own for the assessment of memory. As an ecologically valid test, it provides an indication of whether memory difficulties are causing problems in real life, whereas tests such as the WMS-3 inform us of how the problems affect the structure of memory. The two types of tests are, therefore, different but complementary.

The original RBMT was published in 1985 (Wilson et al., 1985). It was designed to (1) predict everyday memory problems in people with acquired, nonprogressive brain injury and (2) monitor change over time. It comprises tasks analogous to everyday situations that appear to be troublesome for memory-impaired people. There are four parallel versions, and the test has been translated into 14 languages, with norms established for ages ranging from 5 to 96: Norms for elderly people appeared in 1989 (Cockburn & Smith); for adolescents in 1990 (Wilson, Forester, Bryant, & Cockburn); for children aged 5 to 10 in 1991 (Wilson et al.).

In the original RBMT validation study, 80 brain-injured patients were observed by their therapists for a period of time ranging from 30 to 55 hours. The correlation between therapists' observations of everyday memory failures and scores on the RBMT was a highly significant .75 (Wilson, Cockburn, Baddeley, & Hiorns, 1989). In addition to the two studies mentioned earlier showing that the RBMT is a good predictor of independence and employability (Wilson, 1991; Schwartz & McMillan, 1989), Kotler-Cope (1990) found that the RBMT was a better measure of everyday memory than the WMS–Revised (Wechsler, 1987), and Pérez and Godoy (1998) found the RBMT to be as robust as the WMS for discriminating between patients and controls.

The RBMT has been used with people with nonprogressive brain injury and with other patient groups. Beardsall and Huppert (1991) found that certain subtests of the RBMT were better than other tests for diagnosing dementia. Wilson and Ivani-Chalian (1995) found the children's RBMT useful for assessing memory functioning in adults with Down syndrome. In addition, Isaacs et al. (2003) found that the children's version of the RBMT discriminated between adolescents who were born prematurely at very low birth weights and control participants despite being matched for IQ and immediate memory. In particular, the pre-term-born children were poor at the route finding and the prospective memory subtests.

Moradi, Neshat-Doost, Taghavi, Yule, and Dalgleish (1999) found that the RBMT discriminated between children and adolescents with and without posttraumatic stress disorder (PTSD). According to Lezak, Howieson, Loring, and Hannay (2004), others have found the RBMT to be a useful instrument in characterizing memory disorders ranging from basal forebrain disease (Goldenberg, Schuri, Gromminger, & Arnold, 1999) to cardiac failure (Grubb et al., 2000), Parkinson's disease (Benke, Hohenstein, Poewe, & Butterworth, 2000), multiple sclerosis (Cutajar et al., 2000), and limbic encephalitis (Bak, Antoun, Balan, & Hodges, 2001).

Although the RBMT has proved useful, it was designed as a screening test and, as such, is insufficiently sensitive to detect mild deficits. To enhance the test's sensitivity, we decided to increase the level of difficulty by doubling the amount of material to be remembered. Versions A and B of the original test were combined to make version 1 of the RBMT-E and versions C and D were combined to make version 2 of the RBMT-E (1999).

When developing the RBMT-E, we wanted to determine whether brain-injured people who scored in the normal or nearly normal range on the original RBMT would have deficits when assessed on the RBMT-E. To address this question, 45 neurologically impaired people were given both the original and the extended versions in counterbalanced order. Of the total sample, 35 were in the poor–normal memory range on the original RBMT standardized profile score and 36 were in the poor–normal range on the screening score. Thus, the RBMT-E separated those with reasonable RBMT scores into good, average, poor, and impaired subgroups.

Because some of the subtests were too difficult (RBMT-E) or too easy (RBMT) for certain patients, we decided to develop another version—the RBMT-3—to overcome the difficulty level by modifying some of the subtests and adding a new subtest, the Novel Task described earlier. This assesses the ability to learn a new skill, an accomplishment critical for everyday functioning. By increasing the breadth of the memory functions assessed, the test now offers a more comprehensive assessment. Finally, we wanted to update and improve the norms. The new test is now available (Wilson, Greenfield, et al., 2008).

### Additional Tests

The tests described previously are only a few of those available. For a more detailed list and description, see Lezak, Howieson, Loring, Hannay, and Fischer (2004); Strauss, Sherman, and Spreen (2006); Mitrushina, Boone, Razani, and D'Elia (2005); and others. These books describe a wide range of neuropsychological tests and not just those concerned with memory. The assessment of mood and emotion is equally important, and measures for this are covered in detail in Chapter 8.

One last point for discussion involves the issue of effort: Is the person being assessed trying hard enough? Is there a question of malingering or an attempt to distort test performance? This is more likely to be an issue for medicolegal situations, but for those who believe effort should be measured, Bush et al. (2005) published a position paper for North American neuropsychologists and, at the time of writing, the

British Psychological Society is drawing up a similar paper for British assessors.

## Behavioral Assessment Procedures for Identifying Memory Problems

As useful as standardized tests are for building a cognitive map of a person's strengths and weaknesses, they are insufficient for planning rehabilitation. We need the tests to provide information whether patients will be able to understand instructions, remember things in a certain format, have problems reading, and so forth. We must not ask patients to do things that are cognitively impossible for them, so we need information from neuropsychological tests. However, standardized tests will not tell us what problems are most distressing for the patients and their families, what coping methods are used, what is the best intervention strategy to adopt, or how to determine whether our treatment programs are effective, so we need to complement our standardized tests with other forms of assessment. We can do this from observations, self-report measures, and structured interviews.

Two seminal papers on behavioral assessment—by Baer, Wolf, and Risley in 1968 and by Kanfer and Saslow in 1969—heralded the beginning of a more formal approach to behavioral assessment. Before this, it had been less formal and more indirect, being part of behavior modification where the main concern was on new treatment strategies. In the 1970s and 1980s, emphasis shifted to (1) the identification and measurement of variables that control behavior, (2) the selection of successful treatment techniques, and (3) the evaluation of treatment (Nelson & Hayes, 1979). The distinction between behavioral assessment and behavioral treatment is often difficult because the two blur into each other. If we are measuring how often an amnesic patient repeats a particular question, for example, we are almost certainly doing this to find a way to reduce the repetitions. If we then find a way that might achieve this, we will measure the repetitions while we implement the treatment strategy, so measurement or assessment and treatment are part and parcel of the same process. Like standardized assessments, behavioral measures are also concerned with the systematic collection, organization, and interpretation of details about patients and their situation; the difference here is the way in which this is implemented. In essence, a behavioral assessment is concerned with the analysis of a person's behavior, its antecedents, and its consequences. This is often described as an ABC assessment or a functional analysis. To return to the example of the amnesic patient repeating the same question, we need to establish whether this occurs in response to a verbal trigger, such as a remark made to the patient, or whether it is more likely to happen when a particular member of staff is on duty or at certain times of the day. Then we need to know what happens afterward in response to the question. Is it answered or ignored, or is the person shown how to answer the question by being taken, for example, to a wall calendar? Does the patient calm down or get more agitated when he or she is answered? In such ways we can look at antecedents and consequences.

Mischel (1968) pointed out some differences between the two types of assessment. The standardized tests tend to tell us what a person *has.* Thus, a person may *have* a global amnesia, Broca's dysphasia, or unilateral neglect. In contrast, a behavioral assessment tends to tell us what a person *does.* Thus, a memory-impaired person may ask the same question 15 times each hour, fail to put on his or her wheelchair brakes, or be unable to find his or her bed on the ward.

Another difference is that in standardized tests the observed behavior is seen as a *sign*, so an inability to recall a prose passage after a delay is a sign of organic memory impairment, whereas in a behavioral assessment the observed behavior is seen as a *sample*, so we are sampling, for example, "question-asking behavior" or the "putting on of wheelchair brakes" behavior.

Implicit in the traditional approach is the view that the results from an assessment are a reflection of the underlying problem, cause, impairment, or personality trait. Implicit in the behavioral approach is the assumption that behavior is a result of environmental circumstances. The former kind of assessment assumes that the behavior observed is relatively stable; a person's IQ will not fluctuate a great deal if measured in the morning or the evening. Sometimes this is true for memory-impaired people too. An amnesic patient will be unable to recall a prose passage whatever the circumstances but sometimes the behavior is variable. For a person with more moderate deficits, fatigue, anxiety, and stress can increase the problems, and the amount of this variability needs to be established. Whereas a traditional assessment is performed once, the more functional assessments are typically carried out several or many times in different situations. In standardized tests, the relationship with treatment is *indirect* because one does not, or should not, treat someone in order for that person to pass a test. As mentioned, behavioral approaches have a much more *direct* relationship to treatment: For example, some memory-impaired individuals will need to stop repeating the same question, whereas others who use wheelchairs will need to learn to apply the wheelchair brakes and others may need to find the correct bed on the ward.

Finally, standardized assessments are typically performed before treatment. They may sometimes be conducted during or after treatment, but *they are not part of the treatment process itself*, whereas behavioral assessments can be seen as an essential item in this process.

Further details on behavioral observations, self-report measures, and interviews follow in Chapter 10, when we discuss the process of planning a rehabilitation program. Additional assessments to determine who is likely to benefit from external memory aids are considered in Chapter 4.

CHAPTER 4

# Compensating for Memory Deficits with Memory Aids

## with NARINDER KAPUR

The ultimate goal of rehabilitation is to enable people to function as independently as possible in their own most appropriate environment (McLellan, 1991). In the early days or weeks after brain injury, most people, including therapists and psychologists, are looking for recovery and some restoration of lost functioning. Once recovery has stopped or slowed down, we tend to adjust our expectations and help people compensate for their difficulties. Anderson (1996) suggested that attempts to restore lost functioning stem from a belief in a major degree of neural plasticity, whereas compensatory strategies are based on the assumption that we cannot restore lost functioning so we need to teach people how to cope better with their difficulties. Robertson and Murre (1999) put forward somewhat similar views, arguing that compensatory strategies should be the treatment of choice for people who are not expected to recover, whereas for those who *are* expected to recover (e.g., those with milder lesions) trying to enhance the rate of recovery may be more effective. This may be true for some cognitive functions such as language and attention, but it would not appear to be true for memory, where there is little evidence of major improvements in function once the initial period of spontaneous recovery has passed (Kapur & Graham, 2002; Wilson, 2004). Indeed, Robertson himself noted that "in the case of memory rehabilitation, there is yet no evidence for direct

**Narinder Kapur, PhD,** is a consultant clinical neuropsychologist at Addenbrooke's Hospital, Cambridge, United Kingdom.

and lasting improvement of memory through restitution-oriented therapies. Hence, compensatory approaches to memory problems appear to be, for the time being at least, the treatment of choice" (p. 704).

We have already discussed recovery of function in Chapter 2. This present chapter, as already stated, focuses on compensatory aids. Zangwill (1947) defined compensation as "reorganization of psychological function in order to minimize or circumvent a particular disability" (p. 63). He argued that compensation for the most part took place spontaneously, without explicit intention by the patient, although in some cases it could occur by the patient's own efforts or as a result of instruction and guidance from the psychologist/therapist. The examples of compensation offered by Zangwill include giving a person with expressive speech impairment a slate to write on or teaching someone with a right hemiplegia to write with his or her left hand.

Although external memory aids are arguably the most efficient strategies for memory-impaired people, it is not always easy for them to use such aids. Efficient use of many external memory aids involves a degree of motivation, patience, planning, problem solving, concentration, learning, and, indeed, memory, so the people who need them most often have the greatest difficulty in learning how to use them. This chapter describes the most commonly used external aids and their use. Examples of the successful use of aids in people with severe memory deficits are provided, and the setting up of a memory aids clinic is discussed.

The provision of memory aids needs to be seen in the context of other attempts to improve memory functioning in patients with brain dysfunction. The teaching of cognitive strategies, such as association and rehearsal techniques, is covered in Chapters 5 and 6. Changes in behavior may also benefit memory, such as reducing the workload, establishing regular routines, and always putting items back in the correct place. More general advice relating, for example, to fatigue, anxiety, and alcohol and drug use may benefit memory functioning indirectly. External memory aids represent a somewhat distinctive form of intervention in that greater reliance is placed on an external object or part of the environment rather than purely cognitive or behavioral strategies initiated by the memory-impaired individual. The primary focus of this chapter is on portable or installable memory aids. The design of buildings or equipment may function as a form of memory aid, and these "environmental memory aids" are discussed in more detail elsewhere (Wilson & Kapur, 2008) and in Chapter 11, but we include here Table 4.1 to illustrate how environmental management strategies may help confused and agitated patients in the acute stage.

This chapter focuses more closely on practical aspects of the application of external memory aids in memory rehabilitation settings. The

**TABLE 4.1. Environmental Management Strategies to Cope
with Confused and Agitated Patients in the Acute Stage**

1. Reduce the level of stimulation in the environment.
   - Avoid overstimulation and visual distraction.
   - Monitor room temperature for comfort.
   - Room should be in area of low traffic but able to be monitored easily.
   - Limit visitors and orient visitors regarding strategies.
   - During therapies, eliminate or reduce activities that cause annoyance,
     frustration, and overstimulation.
   - Avoid excessive touching and handling.

2. Reduce the patient's confusion.
   - Provide consistent staffing.
   - Avoid moving rooms.
   - Allow one person to speak at a time.
   - Communicate clearly and concisely (i.e., one idea at a time).
   - Keep a consistent schedule for therapies and activities (i.e., routine).
   - Reorient to place, time, and purpose throughout the day.
   - Keep area well lit during the day and dark and quiet at night.
   - Promote sleep.

3. Tolerate restlessness and agitation as much as possible.
   - Review with staff specific strategies to be used for each patient and "crisis
     intervention" techniques.
   - Allow patient to thrash about in floor bed.
   - Allow mobile patient to pace around the unit supervised.
   - Allow confused patient to be verbally inappropriate.

*Note.* Reprinted with permission from Gail Robinson, National Hospital, Queen Square, London, who developed these strategies following discussions with Corwen Boake.

reader is referred to recent articles for more detailed consideration of experimental studies of external memory aids (Kapur, Glisky, & Wilson, 2002, 2004; Sohlberg, 2005; Sohlberg et al., 2007) and to books by Kime (2006) and Bourgeois (2007) for practical approaches to implementing compensatory strategies using external memory aids. Although we are more concerned with people with nonprogressive conditions, we direct readers to a recent special issue of the journal *Technology and Disability*, "Technology in Dementia Care" (Hagen, 2007), which includes such topics as cost–benefit analysis of assistive technology and the use of technology to improve QOL for people with dementia.

## Typology of Memory Aids

Compared to conceptual frameworks for memory systems in general, and to specific systems such as working memory, autobiographical memory, and semantic memory in particular, there have been relatively few, if any, attempts to offer a typology of memory aids. This is regrettable because having at least a rudimentary model of the enhancing effects of memory aids may help to gain a better understanding of the ways in which memory aids are effective and how their effectiveness can be improved. It is unlikely that simply mapping external memory aids onto existing conceptual frameworks for memory systems would be helpful: For example, thinking in terms of episodic memory aids and semantic memory aids does not seem to make intuitive or practical sense.

As a first approximation, it appears that external memory aids can be divided into those that act as alerting cues, offering a cue at a particular time and in a particular place, and those that take the form of representational aids, in that they provide a stored representation of information that is not tied for its value to a particular temporal or spatial context. Alarms that help prospective memory would seem to fit neatly into the former category, while notepads and Dictaphones are ready examples of devices that store information for later use. The most widely used form of representational memory aid is the written language and electronic variants of writing. Paintings, photographs, sculptures, and gravestones can also be seen as representational memory aids. However, some devices may be multimodal, blurring this simple distinction. For example, satellite navigation devices store representations of the outside world but also provide alerting cues at certain points in space.

## Which Are the Most Frequently Used Memory Aids?

Most people without neurological memory deficits use memory aids (Harris, 1980; Long, Cameron, Harju, Lutz, & Means, 1999; West, 1995); lists, notes, and calendars are used most often. Park, Smith, and Cavanaugh (1990) found that psychologists involved in memory research typically wrote things down to help them remember. What about people with neurological memory impairment? Evans, Wilson, Needham, and Brentnall (2003) surveyed 94 memory-impaired survivors of brain injury to identify the most commonly used memory aids. As can be seen in Table 4.2, nonelectronic aids are the overwhelming choice of tool for people with memory problems: Of 44 different aids used, 35 (79.5%) were nonelectronic. The most widely used electronic aids were an alarm clock for wake-up purposes (used by 38 [40.4%] patients), followed by a watch with the date or timer (used by 17 [18.1%] patients). The top four memory tools were (1) a wall calendar or wall chart ($n$ = 68 [72.3%]); (2) a notebook ($n$ = 60 [63.8%]); (3) a list ($n$ = 59 [62.8%]); and (4) an appointment diary ($n$ = 51 [54.3%]).

**TABLE 4.2. Memory Aids and Strategies Used by People with Brain Injury**

| Strategy | Number (percentage) of sample using the strategy |
|---|---|
| 1. Wall calendar/wall chart | 68 (72.3) |
| 2. Notebook | 60 (63.8) |
| 3. List | 59 (62.8) |
| 4. Appointment diary | 51 (54.3) |
| 5. Asking others to remind | 46 (48.9) |
| 6. Mental retracing | 45 (47.9) |
| 7. Alarm clock (for wake-up) | 38 (40.4) |
| 8. Objects in unusual place | 33 (35.1) |
| 9. Notes in special places | 32 (34.0) |
| 10. Repetitive practice | 28 (29.8) |
| 11. Writing on hand | 23 (24.5) |
| 12. Making associations | 20 (21.3) |
| 13. Watch with date/timer | 17 (18.1) |
| 14. Daily routine | 17 (18.1) |
| 15. Personal organizer | 16 (17.0) |
| 16. Journal | 15 (15.9) |
| 17. Daily timetable | 14 (14.9) |
| 18. Alarm clock/timer | 9 (9.6) |
| 19. Visual imagery | 9 (9.6) |
| 20. Weekly routine | 9 (9.6) |
| 21. Alphabetical searching | 7 (7.4) |
| 22. Electronic organizer | 7 (7.4) |
| 23. TV guide (annotated) | 7 (7.4) |
| 24. Pillbox with day/time | 6 (6.4) |
| 25. First-Letter mnemonics | 5 (5.3) |
| 26. Pager | 5 (5.3) |
| 27. Recipe card or book | 5 (5.3) |
| 28. Pleasantness rating | 3 (3.2) |
| 29. Key chain | 3 (3.2) |
| 30. Pocket phone book | 3 (3.2) |
| 31. Mobile phone | 3 (3.2) |
| 32. Dictaphone/tape recorder | 2 (2.1) |
| 33. Rhymes | 2 (2.1) |
| 34. Knot in handkerchief | 2 (2.1) |
| 35. Orientation of medication | 2 (2.1) |
| 36. Dictionary | 2 (2.1) |
| 37. Chunking | 1 (1.1) |
| 38. Information on key ring | 1 (1.1) |
| 39. Home filing system | 1 (1.1) |
| 40. Home accounts | 1 (1.1) |
| 41. Instructions for work on wall | 1 (1.1) |
| 42. Organizer handbag | 1 (1.1) |
| 43. Buying small quantities | 1 (1.1) |
| 44. Clock calendar combination | 1 (1.1) |

*Note.* From Evans, Wilson, Needham, and Brentnall (2003). Copyright 2003 by the International Neuropsychological Society. Reprinted with permission.

These findings are reasonably similar to an earlier study of 43 memory-impaired people who had received rehabilitation for memory problems 5 to 10 years previously (Wilson, 1991). Of the 43 participants, 29 (67.4%) used notes or notebooks and 25 (58.1%) used wall charts or wall calendars. In both studies, some participants had devised their own rather idiosyncratic memory device. For example, in the 1991 study, one man used a special watch to remind him of a drop in body temperature, because he had hypothalamic damage that could have caused him to suffer from hypothermia. Another woman tore the tops from packets of items she needed to replace and put the tops on the kitchen table to remind her to take them with her when she went shopping. In the 2003 study, one man put instructions for work on the wall to remind him what had to be done, and another person only ever bought small quantities of food in case she forgot to use up all her stock. Thus, it can be seen that nonelectronic aids are widely used and very variable.

Most people used more aids at follow-up than they had used before the onset of the brain injury. In Wilson (1991), a mean of four aids were used before injury compared with 7.39 postinjury. Likewise, Evans et al. (2003) found a mean of 2.45 aids were used preinjury versus 6.8 postinjury. In both studies, there is a relationship between the use of aids and independence, suggesting that being independent in the context of a memory impairment requires the use of memory aids. Two provisos may be worth keeping in mind: (1) The estimates of preinjury/illness memory aids were retrospective and may have underestimated or otherwise distorted estimates because of the length of time since use of the aids; and (2) those individuals who were more independent may have had higher levels of general cognitive functioning or educational attainment, and this may also have contributed to their frequent use of memory aids.

## How Effective Are External Memory Aids?

In the case of everyday adjustment, both studies described previously (Wilson, 1991; Evans et al., 2003) directly or indirectly assessed the efficacy of memory aids. Wilson (1991) found that people living independently (defined as living alone, in paid employment, or in full-time education) were more likely to be using six or more aids and strategies than those who were not independent ($X^2 = 10.87$, $p < .001$). Evans et al. (2003) examined more closely the efficiency of the aids/strategies by asking an independent other to rate their use (1 = *rarely effective*, 2 = *sometimes effective*, 3 = *usually effective*). It appears that the most widely used aids are not necessarily the most effective at least as rated by caregivers. Although we need to be cautious, some strategies appear to be used by a small number of people but to good effect. These include both electronic and nonelectronic aids. Of the nonelectronic aids, tying a knot in a handkerchief (or the American equivalent of tying a string round a finger) was not effective, whereas following a weekly or daily routine, making lists, and asking others for reminders received high ratings. Remembering to take medication is an important everyday goal of some memory-impaired individuals: Van Hulle and Hux (2006) reported that a wristwatch alarm and a digital voice reminder were effective in improving compliance in three individuals with TBI.

In the case of laboratory- or clinic-based measures, a number of relevant studies have been described elsewhere (Kapur et al., 2004; Sohlberg, 2005). More recent studies have confirmed the value of cuing, even if it is content free, in enhancing prospective memory (Fish et al., 2007). O'Connell et al. (2008) showed that a group of individuals with attention–deficit/hyperactivity disorder could be taught a self-alerting technique, with the benefit of biofeedback, and that this improved performance in a sustained attention task involving remembering to inhibit a response to a particular cue. Fish et al. (2008b) reported that an electronic pager was more effective than a checklist in encouraging a patient with bilateral frontal lobe pathology to implement everyday intentions and suggested that this was achieved by encouraging goal-monitoring behavior. Gentry (2008) assessed the effectiveness of an off-the-shelf personal digital assistant, the Palm Zire 31, and found that a group of patients with multiple sclerosis showed improvements in cognitive independence, mobility, and social integration after being trained to use the device. It is worth noting that formal memory test scores did not show an improvement over the same period. In a similar study with head-injured patients, Gentry, Wallace, Kvarfordt, and Lynch (2008) found similar improvements in the areas of mobility, cognitive independence, and occupation. Several studies have demonstrated the effectiveness of a paging system, NeuroPage, to help survivors of brain injury compensate for everyday memory and planning problems (Wilson, Evans, Emslie, & Malinek, 1997; Wilson, Emslie, Quirk, & Evans, 2001; Emslie et al., 2007; Fish et al., 2008c).

## Can We Predict Who Will Use External Memory Aids Efficiently?

We know that some memory impaired people use external aids well and easily while others experience great difficulty. What determines whether aids are used efficiently? Wilson and Watson (1996) described a framework for understanding compensatory behavior in people with neurological memory impairment. This framework, developed by Bäckman and Dixon (1992) and further modified by Dixon and Bäckman (1999), distinguishes four stages in the evolution of compensatory behavior: origins, mechanisms, forms, and consequences. Wilson (2000) used this framework to consider compensation for a variety of cognitive deficits. Evans et al. (2003) investigated factors that predict good use of compensatory strategies. The main predictors appear to be:

1. Age—younger people compensate better.
2. Severity of impairment—very severely impaired people compensate less well.
3. Specificity of deficit—those with widespread cognitive deficits appear to compensate less well than those with more focal deficits.
4. Premorbid use of strategies—those who had used some compensatory aids premorbidly appear to compensate better after their brain injury/illness.

This area requires further evaluation. If we can predict who is likely to compensate without too much difficulty, we can target our rehabilitation to help those who are less likely to compensate spontaneously. Clinical experience tends to suggest other variables that are likely to be important, including insight and motivation, support from family members and work colleagues, and absence of major sensory, motor, or psychiatric disability. Stapleton, Adams, and Atterton (2007) noted that of five individuals with TBI who were given mobile phones as a memory aid, the two individuals who did not successfully use the mobile phone to remember to carry out target behaviors had marked memory impairment and some executive dysfunction and required 24-hour care.

## Which Assessment Procedures Are Most Appropriate When Considering Patients for External Memory Aids?

Various forms of assessment are required to help determine those patients who will benefit most from external memory aids. A formal neuropsychological assessment will provide information on key factors such as the severity of memory impairment and the presence of major executive dysfunction. A clinical assessment will be helpful to gauge previous use of aids, insight, motivation, memory demands in work, and support that will be available from caregivers/family members and work colleagues. This assessment will also point to major problems in mood, temperament, or anxiety and other factors such as tiredness, alcohol/ drug abuse, sleep disturbance, and so on. that could interfere with a rehabilitation program. It may also be useful to gather simple measures of the degree of stress caused by memory difficulties and caregivers' stress as a result of looking after and living with a memory-impaired person. Basic memory questionnaires completed by the patient and by an informed observer will help to confirm information from an interview as to the main everyday memory difficulties. Structured questionnaires will also help to gather information on existing cognitive-behavioral strategies and the external aids or other techniques that the person is using. A further assessment that we have found useful in clinical practice is a memory problem-solving inventory, in which written scenarios are presented, such as "How would you remember to mail a letter?" and "How would you remember to send a friend a birthday card?" The clinician should have an idea of the range of strategies that could be used to solve these problem situations, and the plan would be to repeat administration of such an inventory after intervention with memory aids. Having gathered information on the key memory lapses that require intervention, one would ideally proceed to gather a record of the frequency and related circumstances of these lapses. This diary itself requires a degree of memory and concentration, and it is here that a caregiver will be invaluable. It may be that providing a patient with a notebook or simple Dictaphone or perhaps a memo pad that can be attached to a fridge door with a magnet will help improve compliance in keeping a record of memory lapses. Periodic telephone calls will also help to ensure that patients and caregivers are being diligent in recording everyday memory lapses.

As Scherer (2005) has pointed out, successful use of external aids in helping to achieve goals for memory-impaired individuals will depend on a good match between a number of variables, including insight and motivation; past use of memory aids; cognitive, emotional, and motivational profile; everyday demands on memory; family/work support; and the various cognitive and behavioral strategies and types of memory aids that are available as part of the resources of the clinician.

## Setting Up a Memory Aids Clinic

Memory aids clinics would seem a logical consequence of memory rehabilitation efforts, but it was a surprise to one of the authors of this chapter (Narinder Kapur) that there were few, if any, precedents for such a clinic when he set one up. The absence of such clinics may have been for several reasons: the relative scarcity of many external memory aids before the 1990s; the difficulty in finding about and purchasing aids, which only became possible in the late 1990s with the growth of the Internet; the absence of ready sources of funding for the purchase of memory aids in many health care settings; and the relative paucity of publications on the role and effectiveness of memory aids.

In 2003, the first memory aids clinic in the United Kingdom, and possibly in the world, was set up at Addenbrooke's Hospital, Cambridge (Figure 4.1).

It is said that for something to be successful it needs a good idea, good resources to back it, and good people to take the idea forward. Fortunately, these elements were in place when this memory aids clinic was set up. In collaboration with Professor Michael Kopelman and Ms Bonnie-Kate Dewar, we also helped to set up an equivalent memory aids clinic at St. Thomas's Hospital, London, in 2006.

## Funding

Most developments in health care settings require a business plan, but we did not have such a plan when we set up our clinic in Cambridge. Through sources such as private patient income, support from Microsoft Research as a result of a research collaboration, and personal financial input from the head of the clinic (Narinder Kapur), we were able to put together the resources necessary to purchase material items and basic infrastructure. A dedicated testing–treatment room was made available by the hospital and was the site of the memory aids clinic. It was used for routine neuropsychological assessments and housing of test materi-

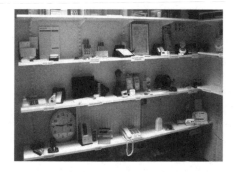

**FIGURE 4.1.** Part of the Cambridge Memory Aids Resource Centre. Reprinted with permission from Narinder Kapur.

als and a range of memory aids. The material costs of maintaining a memory aids clinic depend on patient traffic. Currently, we see about 100 patients a year in the clinic, and we give them memory aids free of charge. One would need to allow approximately $10,000 to set up and supply the clinic with a broad range of aids and $100 per patient expenditure on aids. Staffing costs are, of course, extra (see later discussion).

It is possible that a memory aids clinic could be set up initially as a research project, funded by a medical research source, and the results of the study then used to persuade local stakeholders to invest in the clinic. A further means of gathering funds is to persuade a patients' charity, such as those dealing with multiple sclerosis, epilepsy, stroke, AD, TBI, or encephalitis, to fund the clinic for their patients for a 3-year period, with a promise from the health care provider or local health care commissioners to continue that funding after the 3-year period.

## Staffing

Ideally, a memory aids clinic with 100 patients should have a full-time qualified clinical psychologist, one full-time assistant psychologist, and a part-time secretary.

## Range of Aids and Support Materials

The clinic and resource center should be in the same location and should house a wide range of memory aids. These include "concept aids," which are seldom given out to patients but are kept for demonstration purposes to indicate current trends and developments in technology. For example, advanced mobile phones are usually too expensive to give routinely to patients but may be useful to have on display. A second type of memory aid may occasionally be given out but only for select cases: location detection memory aids that help people find items such as lost keys. The third type of external memory aid can be given out frequently: White boards, Post-it Note materials, simple electronic reminders, and Dictaphones. The aids need to be displayed in meaningful groupings, with appropriate signage on the display shelves. If possible, paste a note beneath each memory aid, indicating when and from whom (website, telephone number, e-mail address) it was purchased and the cost.

Memory aids will need dedicated brochures given to patients for back-up explanations and use instructions. These should be available as part of the display materials. In addition, providing external memory aids will usually be only one part of an overall holistic rehabilitation program; other support literature (e.g., dealing with concentration difficulties; coping with stress, anxiety, and depression; anger management;

returning to work after a brain injury/illness) should be available for patients and caregivers.

The memory aids resource center will be your "showcase" for visitors, some of whom will be financially responsible for purchases, so it is important that it looks as impressive as possible. The resource center should also house a range of spare batteries and simple materials such as screwdrivers and double-sided tape for making impromptu memory aids.

## Audit

Audit should be built in to the running of the memory aids clinic to show that it is both efficient and cost-effective. Value is often defined as output divided by cost, and anyone running a memory aids clinic needs to be able to demonstrate value, especially if starting with seed funding and seeking more substantive funding at a later stage. Audit instruments will include not only standard assessment procedures such as reduction in memory lapses but also other measures such as work, domestic or leisure goals, reduction of stress for the patient and caregiver, and improved self-esteem. Gathering long-term follow-up data on the continued use of aids after 1 to 2 years is also important. The costs of care, savings in health care measured in outcomes such as better medication compliance, and income generated by the individual returning to work all need to be computed so as to provide some idea as to whether the clinic has been cost-effective (cf. Turner-Stokes, Disler, Nair, & Wades, 2005).

## Finding and Purchasing Memory Aids

The Internet is invaluable not only for tracing the wide range of memory aids that are now available but also for the ease of purchasing and shipping these aids. It may be necessary to pay with your own credit card and also try to put in place some means of reimbursement for the purchases you have made.

## Cataloging of Aids

Although ideally one would keep an inventory of memory aids, the range and cost of available aids will change every few months, so this may not be feasible logistically. It is, however, important to keep a note of past aids purchased, from whom, and so on and also a catalog of aids that are currently available. Categories of memory aids may include Post-it Note materials; notebooks, diaries, or filofaxes, or personal organizers; electronic reminders; pillboxes; White boards; location detectors; mobile phones; audio recording devices; photographic devices; and navigation devices.

### Advertising for Business

Generally, once it is known that a memory aids clinic is in operation, there should be no shortage of referrals. However, if necessary, communication with local patient organizations may be helpful. It is important to give some general idea as to exclusion criteria to restrict the number of unsuitable referrals. Promotion on local radio and TV shows or in newspapers may also help to increase publicity for the memory aids clinic.

### Research and Development

It is important to have some form of research activity as part of the running of the memory aids clinic. In Cambridge, we were fortunate that Microsoft Research had a major research laboratory based in the city and were developing a prototype camera-based memory aid that was intended to improve autobiographical memory. This research collaboration helped to fund the resources in the memory aids clinic and also provided staff who were able to spend a day a week in the clinic or related clinics.

### Compliance and Generalization

Showing a patient one or two memory aids in the clinic and supplying them for use at home or at work is fine, but how can one ensure compliance? This question needs to be kept to the fore. Ideally, if staffing resources permit, one or two home or work site visits as well as regular phone calls, should be made. The use of virtual reality procedures, perhaps with embedded images of the patient's home or workplace, may also be worth considering as part of the goal of transitioning the use of aids from the clinic to the community.

## Which Types of Memory Aids Are Currently Available?

### Information Display Items

We live in a visual world, with much of the human brain devoted to visual processing, so visual display items that provide memory-related information are useful memory aids. They need to be in the field of view of the user and not subject to the vagaries of gaze. Types of display items that are often used as memory aids include day/date clocks, White boards, and labels on cupboards. A refrigerator door with messages or reminders could also be classified as a form of information display memory aid. Calendars with space for messages or lists of things to do also fall into the category of information display materials. Some digital frames can display time/day/date together with preprogrammed items, and these may also be worth considering.

## Electronic Reminders

A wide range of electronic reminder alarms are available. They include electronic timers, multi-alarm reminders (with ±30 alarms that can be set at half-hour settings), mobile phones with alarm features, pagers, watches with a range of alarm features, and pillboxes with built-in multiple electronic alarm settings. Electronic reminders may be part of the design of a building, as in the case of "smart homes" (Boman, 2007).

## Location Detection Devices

Location detection devices have been designed to help individuals remember where they put things. In a newer variation of this, an alarm will sound if something is left behind. Usually, an item is tagged with an electronic receiver, and when the emitting device sends a radio signal the tagged item will emit a loud sound. Some devices have a visual display panel indicating the proximity of the item that is lost.

## Way-Finding Aids

Satellite navigation devices have been a major development in external aid support for those who have difficulty finding their way to a destination. Such devices now come in various forms: as built-in components of automobiles, as stand-alone devices that can be located near the dashboard of a vehicle, and as devices that can be integral features of personal digital assistants or mobile phones and can be used while the person is walking about. These devices invariably have spoken commands in addition to dynamic visual cues. Static road maps and suggested routes can also now be downloaded to mobile phones, laptop computers, and so on, and screen or print versions of these may also be useful as navigational memory aids. It is also worth noting that for those patients with marked memory impairment or confusion resulting from other cognitive deficits, navigating within a residence may be problematic. In these instances, navigational aids may take the form of supportive architectural design, strategically located landmarks, icon and text-based signs, and so on (Warner, 2000; Zeisel, 2006).

## Electronic Storage Devices

Devices such as personal digital assistants, mobile phones, landline phones, cameras, and computers may provide a means of information storage, including photographs, contact details, and "journal" records of past autobiographical events. Audio recording may be a feature of mobile phones, but dedicated, easy-to-use Dictaphones with large storage capacity and connectivity with computers have become available in recent years. A photophone (Figure 4.2) has large buttons on which a photograph of a significant person is pasted. When the memory-impaired individual wants to call this person, he or she just presses the button with the photograph and the number is speed-dialed automatically.

## Post-It Note Materials

Post-it Note materials are among the most widely used external memory aids, by both those with brain injury and the general population. A variety is now available that is useful for indexing pages. Post-it Note tape is available in three widths, the widest of which (2.6 centimeters) is invaluable for labeling, using as a temporary notepad, or using as a cue/sign in a strategic location. Post-it Notes are available in dispensers, and one of these, with a pen next to a telephone, can make it easier for patients to jot down messages that can then be readily transferred to a White board, refrigerator door, and so on.

## Diaries, Filofaxes/Personal Organizers, Stationery Items

Some individuals, especially elderly people, prefer to use stationery items such as filofaxes/personal organizers and diaries rather than electronic personal digital assistants. For these people, there are many items of varying sizes, with varying preprinted inserts, that may help them keep track of things to do or messages.

## Mechanical and Other Storage Devices

Pillboxes, one of the most common type of mechanical memory aids, will be a staple item to have stocked in a memory aids resource center.

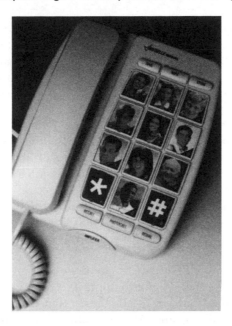

**FIGURE 4.2.** A telephone memory aid that automatically dials the number of the person displayed. Courtesy Narinder Kapur.

These vary in size, transparency of material, and number of compartments, depending on the medication regimen. Many pillboxes now come with built-in electronic reminders. Other, often overlooked forms of storage items include clothing with a number of pockets to store memory aids and related material while on the move. Handbags/purses with well-organized compartments are also helpful. The latter may be particularly important for patients with marked memory impairment and will help to avoid distressing episodes at the checkout counter while shopping when cash or credit card items cannot be readily found.

## How Can We Best Teach People to Use External Memory Aids?

Although the application of many external memory aids looks straightforward, the use of each involves a degree of memory and concentration, so those who need memory aids the most may have the greatest difficulty learning how to use them. Glisky, Schacter, and Tulving (1986) taught people with amnesia to remember computer-related terminology through the method of VC, which involves the systematic reduction of letters (described in Chapter 6). Glisky (1995) taught an amnesic patient a considerable amount of information about a word-processing task. These two studies are not teaching people to use computers per se but rather are teaching them about the *use* of computers. One of the first reports of a systematic attempt to teach the use of a nonelectronic organizer was that of Sohlberg and Mateer (1989c). They described a systematic structured training sequence to teach the use of a memory book and provide an example of this training sequence with a memory-impaired patient. The patient's book comprised five color-coded sections (although the authors pointed out that the number of sections could be decreased or increased as necessary): (1) orientation, (2) memory log, (3) calendar, (4) things to do, and (5) transportation. The training sequence involved three processes: acquisition, application, and adaptation. In the first stage, the patient was taught the use of each section of the book, then taught to apply it to situations encountered at the rehabilitation center, and finally taught to use it in real life.

Although Sohlberg and Mateer believed that patients need to have explicit knowledge of the features of the organizer before using it in real-life situations, Kapur et al. (2004) felt that explicit recall is not always necessary provided that the organizer is used accurately. This view is supported by the experience of "Jay," described in Wilson (1999), who could use a data bank watch very accurately but had no explicit knowledge of *how* to enter messages into the watch. Zencius, Wesolowski, Krankowski, and Burke (1991) found that training patients to use a memory book was more effective in improving everyday performance than other methods. For Donaghy and Williams (1998), a modified version of the training suggested by Sohlberg and Mateer improved performance.

Kime, Lamb, and Wilson (1996) provided some details regarding the successful training of a severely amnesic patient in using a date-book (an organizer) so that she was able to return to independent living and eventually to paid employment. The patient, A. B., sustained multiple injuries in an automobile accident at the age of 22. Three months later, she went into status epilepticus and suffered anoxic brain damage, resulting in a very severe amnesia. Almost 2 years after the accident, A. B. was admitted to a rehabilitation center, where she was found to have very severe deficits on neuropsychological tests of memory and in everyday memory. After several days, she could not remember the names of the therapists treating her, the purposes of each session, the location of the bathroom, or indeed the fact that she had participated in the

rehabilitation program for the past few days. One of the main strategies used to help A. B. was the provision of a datebook/organizer and
a watch alarm that chimed every hour to remind her to refer to the
organizer. The organizer contained five sections: (1) daily time log, (2)
instructions for using the watch (see Figure 10.1), (3) the location of
the different therapists, (4) names of the therapists, and (5) maps of the
rehabilitation center and of the apartment complex where A. B. lived
during her stay at the center. In addition, there was a separate section
for each therapy session, including a brief description of the purpose of
the session and the name of the therapist running that session. Later,
additional sections were incorporated as required, namely letters she
had written, people to whom she had talked, films she had seen, and a
calendar of future events.

Initially A. B. was resistant to using the watch alarm and was embar-
rassed at having to carry the organizer. Nevertheless, she was prompted
to use this during each therapy session and also at home with her mother's help. To help her learn how to use the book, different therapists
would provide A. B. with messages and assignments. For the first few
weeks of the program, A. B. was always accompanied by a therapist or
a family member. Whenever the watch sounded, the person with A. B.
would ask her to check her book and carry out the appropriate action.
Thus, if the alarm sounded at 10.00 A.M. and A. B. did not respond, her
chaperone would remind her that the alarm was a signal to check her
datebook. When A. B. found the correct entry, the chaperone would
ask, "What are you supposed to do now, A. B.? Yes, phone your mother."
Once the correct action was completed, A. B. was asked to initial the
action to show that it had been carried out. Written procedures were
produced for every multistep activity A. B. was required to perform,
such as setting the watch. Trial runs were performed to ensure that the
steps were detailed enough for A. B. to follow them independently. At
first A. B. needed help with all these actions: For example, for the first
33 days, she initialed actions only when prompted by a member of staff
or her mother. She then began taking on responsibility herself. Later in
the action record section, A. B. began to write notes to herself to do specific tasks or record specific conversations. After this, she was encouraged to enter cross-references to previous notes or entries to facilitate
recall. Finally, A. B. was encouraged to make notes on a monthly plan-
ner to promote confirmation and completion of tasks. The main goal
of this training was to ensure that A. B. generalized the intervention
techniques to home and would be able to live independently. The main
outcome measures were: (1) the percentage of occasions A. B. checked
her datebook when the alarm chimed; (2) the number of entries in the

action record in her datebook; (3) the number of cross-references in her datebook; and (4) the number of separate entries in her monthly calendar. In fact, A. B. was not allowed to fail at any of the tasks, so the training probably worked through an EL learning procedure, which is described in Chapter 6.

Measures were taken at four different times during the rehabilitation process: the first 21 days after the introduction of the datebook, the last 21 days before discharge from the program, 4 months postdischarge, and 13 months postdischarge. There was a significant improvement in the first and second 21-day measures. Her performance did not decline significantly once she left the rehabilitation center apart from the monthly calendar, which decreased and then increased again. A. B. was able to return to employment initially in a voluntary capacity but later as a paid employee.

Some aids require very little training. NeuroPage, for example, requires the user to press a button when the message appears, and a trial run is carried out during the first meeting. If the user cannot press the button and act on the message, then the system is probably not suitable for that person. The cognitive prostheses described by Cole and Dehdashti (1990) and Cole (1999) are typically learned within three half-hour training sessions. For those familiar with mobile telephones, very little learning is required to respond to messages received by telephone. In the Fish et al. (2007) study described previously, each patient received a short training session (~30 minutes) using the cues to aid prospective memory performance.

## How Can We Best Measure the Effectiveness of External Memory Aids?

The measures used to gauge the effectiveness of external memory aids are similar to those that apply to memory rehabilitation interventions in general: diaries of memory lapses, preferably kept by both the patient and the caregiver; rating scales and memory-symptom inventories; problem-solving inventories combining various scenarios that could involve the use of memory aids; and other indirect measures, such as blood levels associated with certain medications when a patient has difficulty remembering to take medication. Other measures may indirectly reflect the success of intervention: work-related goals (e.g., return to certain levels and amounts of work); greater independence in performing activities of daily living; reduced stress for the caregiver and the patient; improvements in measures of anxiety and depression; increased social and recreational participation; and so on.

## How Can We Bring about Compliance and Generalization in the Use of External Memory Aids?

Instructing a patient on the use of memory aids in the clinic is all very well, but how can one ensure that the aids will be used, and used effectively, once the patient returns to domestic and work settings, and that they are still being used after several years? Home or work site visits will help in seeing where memory aids are located and in reorganizing any practical difficulties in implementing their use. Such visits may also encourage the patient to use external memory aids in community settings. In the case of the type of teaching carried out in the clinic, role-play sessions should ideally occur in environments such as kitchens, work stations, and so on, that are similar to those target settings where the aids will be used. The use of virtual reality systems when teaching the use of memory aids, ideally with photographs from home and work settings that are embedded in virtual reality software, may help to bridge the gap between the clinic and the community, and this remains an area to be explored in the future.

## How Will Advances in Technology Impact Memory Aids of the Future?*

### Smart Homes

Wilson and Evans (2000) and Cheek, Nikpour, and Nowlin (2005) noted the emergence of "smart houses," where appliances are centrally controlled and include reminder functions that help prevent memory lapses (e.g., ensuring equipment is turned on or off). For example, refrigerators—typically one of the most commonly visited sites in a household—with built-in reminder and Internet facilities on the door are already on the market. Chan, Estève, Escriba, and Campo (2008) have reviewed a number of smart home projects and associated monitoring systems. They offered the following conclusions: "Smart homes need to integrate more fully their construction, computing infrastructure, and service delivery aspects. The proposed solution must match or exceed the patient's standard of living. User habits and intentions should be studied in more detail and respected whenever possible. Further research is needed into legal and ethical problems, user and provider acceptance, and user and provider requirements and satisfaction" (2008, p. 76).

---

*This section is adapted from Wilson and Kapur (2008). Copyright 2008 by Cambridge University Press. Reprinted by permission.

## Mobile Phones

Mobile phones have become more sophisticated in terms of the range of functions that they perform and in the degree to which they can integrate with other devices, such as computers. Most mobile phones now have personal digital assistant features, and these may include, for example, a voice recorder, a diary, various alarm features, a camera, and a satellite navigation system. Although few mobile phones appear to have been designed with memory impaired or neurologically disabled people in mind, there are some with real or virtual QWERTY keyboards that may be easier to use for text entry purposes (Wright et al., 2000). Teaching memory-impaired patients to use mobile phones requires some thought and planning (Lekeu, Wojtasik, Van der Linden, & Salmon, 2002). The use of mobile phones to receive text message reminders has been shown to improve clinic attendance rates (Leong et al., 2006). Stapleton et al. (2007) found that a mobile phone could be helpful for some brain-injured patients as a means of prompting them to carry out certain targeted behaviors.

## Cameras

Devices that automatically keep a photographic record of activities during the day, such as Microsoft's SenseCam (Berry et al., 2007), may help to act as a pictorial diary to enable events to be reviewed and rehearsed at regular intervals after downloading onto a computer. The images may also act as cues to help retrieve forgotten memories. The advantages over general photographic devices is the automaticity of image production and the ability to readily categorize and retrieve images that are subsequently stored on computer. More generally, there may be developments in software that will enable video and other photographic records to be easily archived and readily retrieved and thus allow blogging to be interfaced with sophisticated data retrieval systems.

## Location Detection Devices

Location detection devices to help find lost items at home have become more sophisticated in recent years, with radiofrequency- and radar technology-based devices now available in the market. It is possible that, in the future, radiofrequency identification devices may become miniaturized to the extent that they can be attached to items that are easily lost (e.g., eyeglasses) or to household items in general so that the owner can instantly locate the item.

## Virtual Reality

Virtual reality procedures are beginning to impact on the discipline of neurorehabilitation (e.g., Merians, Poizner, Boian, Burdea, & Adamovich, 2006), and in the field of cognitive rehabilitation virtual reality software is being increasingly used to help bridge the gap between treatments in the clinic setting and activities in the patient's home environment. Such software may also have a role in providing more ecologically valid assessments of areas such as prospective memory functioning. A few promising pilot studies have been carried out (Rose et al., 1999; Rose, Brooks, & Rizzo, 2005; Schultheis & Rizzo, 2001; Zhang et al., 2003), but more work needs to be done before the full benefits of virtual reality can be ascertained.

## Advanced Brain Imaging

In general, advances in brain imaging and in memory rehabilitation have traveled along separate paths, with little in the way of cross-fertilization of data or ideas. There is, however, every reason to promote such interactions and to expect that they may occur in the future (cf. Strangman et al., 2008). Advanced structural and functional brain-imaging procedures may help to identify those individuals who might benefit from certain forms of memory rehabilitation (Strangman et al., 2008). Structural imaging, both in the form of gray matter status and fiber tract integrity, may provide a detailed profile of brain pathology and which areas are spared; and it is possible, for example, that comprehensive measures of frontal lobe or limbic–diencephalic integrity will help to predict which patients could benefit from mnemonic strategy training as opposed to external memory aids. As in the case of language rehabilitation (Peck et al., 2004), functional brain-imaging paradigms before and after a period of memory rehabilitation may provide useful information regarding the neural mechanisms underlying any changes that have taken place as the result of treatment (cf. Behrmann, Marotta, Gauthier, Tarr, & McKeeff, 2005; DeGutis, Bentin, Robertson, & D'Esposito, 2007). More speculatively, there is the prospect of online fMRI-mediated teaching of encoding and retrieval strategies, if we can generalize from some recent developments in neuroimaging (Weiskopf et al., 2004; Yoo et al., 2006).

In Chapter 11 we provide a selection of websites from which memory aids can be purchased.

CHAPTER 5

# Mnemonics and Rehearsal
# Strategies in Rehabilitation

## What Are Mnemonics?

Mnemonics are systems that enable us to remember things more easily. Sometimes the term is used to describe anything that improves memory, including external memory aids, but more often it refers to internal strategies that are consciously learned and require considerable effort to put into practice (Harris, 1984). The most widely used artificial mnemonic is a method for remembering how many days there are in each month of the year. Most British and American people use a rhyme to do this ("Thirty days has September ..."). In other parts of the world, many people use their knuckles, with the knuckles themselves representing the long months and the dips in between representing the short months. Still other countries use suffixes and prefixes to remember the long and short months. Every country using our calendar system has a mnemonic for remembering months of different lengths. Some examples of mnemonics can be seen in Table 5.1.

## Verbal Mnemonics

Other types of verbal mnemonics include first-letter mnemonics, in which the initial letters of words in a sentence are used to recall information in a particular order. For example, many people in the United Kingdom use the mnemonic EGBDF when learning the notes on the lines of a musical staff. The letters are incorporated into a sentence such as "Every good boy deserves fruit." After leaning the sentence, one uses

**TABLE 5.1. Some Examples of Mnemonics**

A first-letter mnemonic (to remember the colors of the rainbow—red, orange, yellow, green, blue, indigo, violet)
    Richard of York gives battle in vain

A mnemonic using numbers (to remember the value of pi—the number of letters in each word is counted to remember that pi = 3.14158265358979323845) [a]
    Pie: I wish I could remember pi. Eureka, cried the great inventor.
    Christmas pudding, Christmas pie is the problem's very center.

A rhyming mnemonic (to remember how to convert from Centigrade to Fahrenheit) [b]
    From centigrade to Fahrenheit
    Will keep you puzzling day and night
    A simple rule that you can state
    Is multiply by one point eight
    The other thing that you should do
    Is add another thirty-two
    (so multiply by 1.8 and add 32).

---

[a]With thanks to Alan Baddeley.
[b]Constructed with Alan Baddeley.

the initial letters for notes, so the note on the first line is *E*, the note on the second line is *G*, etc. My granddaughter recently taught me a first-letter mnemonic for remembering the order of the planets from the sun: "My very elderly mother just sat upon a new pin" (Mercury, Venus, Earth, Mars, Jupiter, Saturn, Uranus, Neptune, Pluto). A variation on this theme is to use a whole word to remember the information so that the notes in the spaces of the musical staff spell out the word *face*. Harris (1984) suggested that first-letter mnemonics are useful only when the material to be remembered is well known but difficult to recall in the correct order. They can however, be used to learn new material (Wilson, 1987). Another variation can be used to remember a list of digits such as a credit card number: One can make up a sentence in which each word consists of a number of letters corresponding to the numbers to be remembered. For example, the number 6,734 can be "Mother (six digits) courage (seven) was (three) here (four)." Wilson and Moffat (1984) argued that first-letter mnemonics work for two reasons: (1) Because the information is being chunked and chunking has long been known to increase recall (Miller, 1956) and (2) because it reduces the number of competing responses.

    Elaboration or making words into a story is another method used to improve recall for people with and without brain injury (Crovitz, 1979; Gianutsos & Gianutsos, 1987; Wilson, 1987). Crovitz used the "airplane list," in which 10 words are embedded in a story with each word linked to the next. Wilson (1987) compared the story method with three other methods. The list of words to be remembered was *umpire, nose, iceberg, vase, elephant, refugee, skylark, imp, tree,* and *yak* (the first letters of these make the word *university*, as the first-letter mnemonic system was one of the methods studied. For the story method, the words were made into a story based on the procedure used by Crovitz (1979):

> "The first word is *umpire* and you can remember that any way you like. The second word is *nose* because the umpire was hit on the nose by a ball. The third word is *iceberg* because the umpire crashed his nose into an iceberg. The fourth word is *vase* because an ancient Egyptian vase was balanced on the iceberg. The fifth word is *elephant* because an elephant picked up the vase with his trunk. The sixth word is *refugee* because a refugee was escaping on the elephant's back. The seventh word is *skylark* because a skylark was flying round and round the refugee's head. The eighth word is *imp* because a mischievous imp trapped the skylark in a net. The next word is *tree* because the imp climbed up a tree to hide. The last word is *yak* because a big yak came up to the tree to scratch his back."

It can be seen immediately that this method combines both verbal and visual techniques, and this may be why it was the most successful of the four methods compared by Wilson (1987). The other methods were first-letter cuing (described previously), method of loci (described next), and visual imagery (described in the next section).

Other verbal mnemonics include rhymes, as mentioned previously, and alphabetical searching. Warrington and Weiskrantz (1982) showed that patients with amnesia can learn rhyming associations, Gardner (1977) taught a man with Korsakoff's syndrome a rhyme to help him remember the name of the ward and hospital he was in, and Moffat (1984) suggested that rhymes could be used to help people select an appropriate strategy for a particular problem: For example, *Pegs are the key to my memory/Numbers make sounds and/Names I can see/I can PQRST stories/And say my ABC* (p. 81).

The PQRST method is covered in the next chapter in the discussion of study techniques. The ABC method Moffat (1984) used is the alphabetical searching strategy. This involves working through the alphabet in the hope that a particular letter will act as a retrieval cue for an elusive word or name. It is probably helpful only when considerable information about the word is already available, such as the number of syllables, or when the searcher is aware that the word is particularly common or unusual. It is an erratic method, however, and not likely to be highly used in rehabilitation. Nevertheless, some memory-impaired people do report using this method (Wilson & Watson, 1996).

## Visual Mnemonics

Visual mnemonics can be defined as remembering by pictures. These may be mental images or actual pictures. For example, one can transform a name into a visual image and remember the image in order to recall the name. I once visited a beautiful Dutch Island off the Friesan coast and had difficulty remembering its name: 'Schiemonnikoog.' In English this sounds rather like "Sheer monarch oak," so I made an image of a sheer (very tall and steep) monarch (a king size) oak. I always remember the name of this island now even though I do not always remember the correct Dutch spelling. For people who find images difficult, a real picture can be used instead. One of my patients who could not remember the names of his therapists or neighbors learned them by practicing with drawings. The name "Julian" was captured by drawing a "jewel on a lion." The man was shown the drawing and the mnemonic was explained to him. The drawing was removed and after a few minutes he was asked to recall the name of this neighbor. He thought for a while and pointed to the place on the table where the drawing had been. He then said, "A dog? No. A bull? No. It was a … a … a lion. On the side was a stone? No, not a stone it was … a … a … a jewel! Jewel lion—Julian!" Over time he became quicker at recalling Julian. A few weeks later, I asked the patient to describe how he learned names: "Can you tell me how you learned the name of your neighbor?" He replied, "Julian?" "Yes," I said. "Oh, I've always known that," he responded.

A more sophisticated version of imagery is the face–name association. Suppose we want to remember the name of "Mrs. Crossley." The first step is to find a prominent feature of Mrs. Crossley's face. If her ears are particularly noticeable, we could select this as the prominent feature. The next step is to transform her name into something meaningful, so "Crossley" could be transformed into a "cross" (as in "angry") "lea-"f, or a leaf in the shape of a cross. The final step is to link the distinctive feature with the transformed name, so a cross leaf could be imagined growing out of her ears. The next time one meets Mrs. Crossley one would scan her face, notice her ears, and then recapture the image of the cross leaf. Although both verbal and visual mnemonics are described and evaluated in some detail in Wilson (1987), it has become clear that some of these are more likely to be used in memory rehabilitation than others. Visual imagery for remembering names is certainly still used and has had some success (Thoene & Glisky, 1995). The method of loci, on the other hand, appears to be used rarely; no published studies can be found using this strategy with survivors of brain injury. Yet another variation on visual imagery is interactive visual imagery whereby one creates an image of the first word or object to be remembered (e.g., a box of matches) and links this with the second object to be remembered (e.g., a yacht). Then the second object (yacht) is linked with the third, the third with the fourth, and so on. In Wilson (1987), this method proved superior to the no-strategy method but not significantly different from the method of loci method or the first-letter mnemonic method and significantly poorer than the story method.

Yet another kind of visual mnemonic is the visual peg method. In peg systems, a standard set of peg words are learned and items to be remembered are linked to the pegs by means of visual imagery. The best known peg system is the rhyming peg method whereby the numbers one to 10 are associated with rhymes such as "one is a bun; two is a shoe; three is a tree; four is a door; five is a hive; six is sticks; seven is heaven; eight is a gate; nine is a line, and 10 is a hen." The first item to be remembered is then linked with a bun, the second with a shoe, and so on. This memory aid is useful when writing a list is impractical (e.g., while driving). So, for example, if I want to give something to my secretary, I imagine her sitting on top of a giant bun holding the paper I want to give her. If I then need to mail a videotape to a patient, I imagine the video tape stuffed into a shoe, and so on. This works well for me, and I retain the images until the tasks are completed or until I need to start again with new tasks. It would be difficult for people with severe memory problems to complete these steps, however, and the method is probably of little value in real-life situations for the majority of those with organic memory deficits (Tate, 1997). Nevertheless, Kaschel et al. (2002; Kaschel, 2003) suggested that people with severe memory deficits can be successfully treated with simple mnemonics such as visual imagery, so success is not limited to those with mild problems.

One of the oldest mnemonic strategies is the method of loci (or remembering by place). This was used by the ancient Greeks. Yates (1966) described how Simonides of Thessaly was able to recall the names of many people crushed at a banquet by remembering where each guest was sitting or, in other words, remembering by location or place. The famous mnemonist Shereshevski studied by Luria (1968) sometimes used this method. For example, he would form images of items to be remembered placed at various points along a well-known street such as a window sill, a doorway, and by the curb. Although this method did not lead to significantly better recall than the first-letter mnemonics and visual imagery conditions in the Wilson (1987) study, some individuals did respond well to the method of loci. Even for these individuals, however, it was less effective than the story method.

## Motor Movements as a Memory Aid

There is considerable evidence that people with severe memory difficulties can learn some tasks with little difficulty (e.g., Brooks & Baddeley, 1976; Corkin, 1996; Wilson et al., 1996; Cavaco et al., 2004). These are tasks involving implicit memory where no conscious recollection is required. Some of these tasks are procedural tasks that involve motor memory such as tracking a target on a computer screen or mirror drawing. This intact motor memory in people with amnesia has led to speculation about the effectiveness of motor movements as a memory aid. Powell (1981) suggested that certain names like Mr. Potter and Mr. Hatter could be learned by a pattern of movements. Moffat (1984) described an experiment with a man who had sustained a severe TBI: Two lists of words were taught, one using movement (e.g., the word *baby* was represented by an arm-rocking action) and the other using rehearsal. The mean number of words recalled following the motor condition was 7.58 compared with only 3.17 words in the rehearsal condition.

Wilson (1987) compared motor movements as an aid to learning names with visual imagery. This single-case study involved a 27-year-old man with dense amnesia as well as unilateral neglect and prosopagnosia. Twenty names of staff and patients at the rehabilitation center were selected and randomly allocated to the motor movement condition or the visual imagery condition. The man was encouraged to think of a sign (motor condition) or a drawing (visual imagery condition) to help him recall the name. For the name of his physiotherapist, "Sue," he chose "soup" and pretended to eat soup. For his nurse, "Mike," he chose "microphone." The drawing was of a man holding a mike (microphone). The picture was removed and later he was shown the sign (eating soup) or the drawing (microphone) and asked for the name of the person this represented. Two new names were introduced each session. After 11 training sessions, the patient recalled significantly more names when shown the sign compared with drawing. However, this did not help a great deal in real life because he never reliably learned the names of three therapists despite a further 85 training sessions.

There is convincing evidence that people with a severe amnesia can learn motor skills. Cavaco et al. (2004), for example, taught five new skills (each analogous to real-life tasks) to 10 people with severe amnesia. Nine had survived herpes simplex viral encephalitis and one had sustained a thalamic stroke. The participants had impaired episodic recall of the tasks, yet their acquisition and retention of the skills were comparable to those of a group of 25 control participants. Thus, although new motor learning is certainly possible for people with severe memory deficits, there is little evidence that this ability can be harnessed as a mnemonic aid.

## How Successful Are Mnemonics in Memory Rehabilitation?

Visual imagery has probably been investigated more than other strategies. Although there are conflicting reports as to the value of visual imagery with people with brain damage, the weight of the evidence appears to support them as aids to learning certain kinds of material. Thus, Jones (1974) found that two patients with global amnesia were not helped by visual imagery when trying to remember groups of words, whereas two patients who had undergone a left temporal lobectomy did benefit from this procedure. Cermak (1975) found that patients with Korsakoff's syndrome performed better under imagery than no-imagery conditions. Downes et al. (1997) provided further evidence for the value of visual imagery. They found that imagery significantly enhanced face–name learning compared with nonspecific instructions, with even further enhancement occurring with preexposure (exposing the faces to be learned for 6 seconds before training began). During the preexposure phase, participants had to make judgments about the person being portrayed, such as whether the person was honest. None of these studies, however, used material relevant to the person's real life.

Wilson (1987) reported on several studies using visual imagery to help people learn names of real people known to the patients and names they wanted to remember. This could have improved motivation, which in turn could have improved learning. Another difference in the Wilson (1987) studies was that the learning took place over several trials, whereas in the earlier experimental studies participants were typically given one to three learning trials. The teaching methods were also different. A more recent randomized controlled trial by Kaschel et al. (2002) found that visual imagery was superior to pragmatic memory training. After a 4-week baseline period, patients were randomly allocated to imagery training ($n = 9$) or the usual training provided in the patient's rehabilitation center ($n = 12$). All patients received 30 single sessions of therapy in 10 weeks. The results suggested that imagery training significantly improved delayed recall of everyday relevant verbal materials (stories and appointments). Furthermore, the frequency of memory problems observed by relatives was reduced and the improvements were still found at 3-month follow-up.

Wilson (1987) suggested that, to help memory-impaired people retain information, learning should take place one step at a time rather than presenting several items of information at once. Clare et al. (1999, 2000; Clare, Wilson, Carter, Hodges, & Adams, 2001) and others have also taught new information in this way. The method of EL learning (learning without errors) addressed in Chapter 6 is also advocated. Thus, visual imagery appears to be of benefit in improving learning of some information under certain circumstances. This may also be true for other mnemonics such as first-letter mnemonics and the story method. Ponds and Hendriks (2006) suggested that, although mnemonics can solve some everyday memory problems of people with memory difficulties, generalization is often poor. This emphasizes the fact that generalization is an important part of memory rehabilitation and must be built in to any treatment programs. Generalization is addressed in more detail in Chapter 10.

## Advice When Using Mnemonics

Not all people with memory impairments will be able to use mnemonics spontaneously to learn new information (although there is no doubt that some can and do). Nevertheless, therapists and others can provide mnemonics to teach particular pieces of information, such as names of a few people or a new address. Mnemonics lead to faster learning. In addition, it may help to use two or three strategies to improve learning of one piece of information such as visual imagery, VC, and spaced retrieval/expanding rehearsal (described in Chapter 6). Although Hodder and Haslam (2006) found that combining two methods conferred no extra advantage on learning, this could have been because of the methodology used.

It is also important to remember that new things should be taught one step at a time. We need to take into account individual preferences and styles because different people may prefer different strategies, and, as far as possible, we should focus on things that the person with memory impairments wants and needs to learn. This means we should work on material that will be useful in everyday life. Finally, generalization or the transfer to real life must be built in to the training program.

## What Do We Mean by Rehearsal Strategies?

*Rehearsal* simply means to practice or repeat something until it is remembered. Rote rehearsal, or simply repeating material, is widely used by the general population, but it is not a particularly good learning strategy for people with memory deficits. We can hear or read something many times over and still not remember it, and this may be a question of "going in one ear and out the other." Take, for example, the British Shipping Forecast, which gives the weather for the 31 sea areas around the United Kingdom (e.g., Forth, Tyne, Cromarty). I have heard this forecast thousands of times since I was a small child. I like it, it is soothing and somewhat like a mantra, but despite the thousands of repetitions of information, I would find it difficult to recall more than 10 of the 31 areas. I have not processed the material, and it has no real significance for me. On the other hand, I could repeat the 50 United States in alphabetical order because I have thought about them, processed them, visualized them, and made them personally meaningful.

As long ago as 1973, it was clear that there was no relationship between rehearsal time (number of repetitions) and amount learned (Craik & Watkins, 1973). Even in circumstances in which repeated practice does lead to improvement, there may be no generalization. A famous experiment carried out by Ericcson, Chase, and Falcon (1980) involved training a student to increase his forward digit span from the norm of seven plus or minus two (Miller, 1956). After 20 months of practice, the student's span increased from seven to a phenomenal 80 digits; that is, having heard the 80 digits *once* only, he could repeat them back correctly in the same order as originally presented! To do this, however, he had to convert them into something meaningful. He was an athlete, so he imagined the digits as representing running times or distances or other athletic information. As impressive as this performance was, the improvement did not generalize to other memory tasks, not even to remembering consonants, his span here at the end of the 20 months training was about six.

Rote rehearsal or repeated practice, then, is of limited value by itself, but there are other rehearsal methods that do improve recall. Indeed, we discuss spaced retrieval or expanded rehearsal at some length in Chapter 6. Verbal mnemonics, as discussed in this chapter, can also be seen as types of rehearsal techniques.

Apart from the method of expanded rehearsal/spaced retrieval (see Chapter 6) and verbal mnemonics, the most commonly used rehearsal strategies in memory rehabilitation are the PQRST (**P**review, **Q**uestion, **R**ead, **S**tate, and **T**est) method, first described by Robinson (1970), and the similar method of SQR3 (**S**urvey, **Q**uestion, **R**ead, **R**ecall, and

Review; Rowntree, 1982). In practice, the stages followed are virtually identical. The procedure for PQRST is:

1. *Preview*: Preview the material to be recalled (i.e., get a general idea of the passage or text).
2. *Question*: Ask key questions about the text (e.g., What is the main point to be conveyed? In what year did the action take place? How many people were involved?).
3. *Read*: Read the material carefully to answer the questions.
4. *State*: State the answers and if necessary read the text again until it is possible to state the answers.
5. *Test*: Test regularly for retention of the information.

## Studies Evaluating PQRST

Glasgow et al. (1977) was one of the first to evaluate this rehearsal strategy in a nonexperimental situation with a survivor of brain injury. A 22-year-old undergraduate had sustained a TBI in a motor vehicle accident more than 3 years earlier. She had difficulty remembering lectures and what she had read. During baseline assessments, her immediate recall of prose passages was about 88%, but at the end of a session she retained only 54%, and 1 week later this had dropped to only 8%. She was better with multiple-choice questions, and when presented with these she answered 60% of the questions correctly. Two treatment conditions were compared. One involved repeated practice of the material she was able to remember and the other was a modified PQRST procedure. The modifications included combining the first two steps (preview and question) and providing the young woman with four standard questions for each passage rather than asking her to provide her own questions. The PQRST procedure was superior to the rehearsal strategy, although this, in turn, was better than the baseline performance.

The next step was to generalize by applying the strategy outside the clinic. The student was asked to read articles from a newspaper and to rate her recall performance. After 10 days, she was asked to apply the PQRST procedure to newspaper articles and again rate her performance. She felt she was retaining more, but the procedure took about twice as long, so not only was this self-rating hard to quantify but it was also possible that the extra time led to improved performance.

The largest number of PQRST case studies were reported by Wilson (1987), who compared rote rehearsal and PQRST. The first case study involved a man who had sustained a subarachnoid hemorrhage followed by a right frontal craniotomy. In addition to a number of cognitive deficits, including a severe memory impairment, the man asked two questions repeatedly: "Will I always have a memory problem?" and "Why have I got a memory problem?" Such repetition may *sound* trivial, but it is very irritating for those who have to listen to the same questions many times a day for weeks, months, or even years on end.

Baselines assessments were conducted over 6 weeks during the man's attendance at a daily memory group. During 30 sessions, the first question was asked at least once each session, and the second question was asked 17 times during the same 30 sessions. The PQRST strategy was then applied in the man's individual sessions. First, the patient was asked to write a summary of what had happened to him, what was likely to happen in the future, and what factors were hindering his progress. He used his notebook to find the information because it was all written there. He was also asked to write the summary as a list of questions and answers so Question 1 was (1a) What happened to me, (1b) when, and (1c) what was the result? The answers were (1a) I had a hemorrhage, (1b) in April, and (1c) I was left with a poor memory and impaired concentration. There were five main questions, most in three parts. The following day, the patient was asked to apply the PQRST procedure to his written summary. Once he had read through the summary, it was removed and he was asked the questions he had selected himself the day before. After this, the RST stages of the strategy were followed. The next day, this process was repeated, but from then on the patient was tested without reading the summary first. He did, however, read the summary at the end of each session to remind himself of the answers he had forgotten. The man learned 90% of the answers correctly; thus, when he was asked one of his self-selected questions, he could usually provide the correct answer. The method was experimentally successful, but not clinically because he continued to ask the same questions of the staff as frequently as he did before the introduction of the PQRST method. The patient seemed to be unable to use the information he had learned. Like other frontal lobe patients, he was unable to use the recall strategies to utilize the information he had learned (Walsh, 1978).

A second patient reported by Wilson (1987) was a man with a pure amnesic syndrome described by Wilson and Baddeley (1988). Like the Glasgow et al. (1977) study, newspaper articles were used to compare PQRST with repeated practice but, unlike the Glasgow et al. investigation, an equal amount of time was spent on the two methods. For a period of 8 days over 2 weeks, two short paragraphs were selected from a daily newspaper. One was allocated to each of the two methods; the order of presentation was changed each day. The PQRST paragraphs were read to him (the preview) and then the remaining four steps were followed. This took between 7 and 10 minutes. For the repeated practice paragraphs, each was read to him four times. After each reading, he was asked to recall as much as possible. Finally, questions were asked about the paragraph. Thus, in each condition, there were five stages, with approximately equal amounts of time allocated to both methods. Thirty minutes later, the man was again asked questions about each of the newspaper articles. An analysis of the percentage of questions answered successfully in immediate and delayed conditions (a Wilcoxon matched-pairs signed ranks test) showed no difference between the two methods for immediate recall, but there was a statistically significant difference in favor of PQRST at delayed recall ($T = 2.5$, $p < .05$). This difference was only for responding to questions, however, because on free recall the man could remember nothing from either method because of his severe amnesia. The results can be seen in Figure 5.1.

This procedure was replicated with three patients (one with a closed head injury, one with Korsakoff's syndrome, and one with a penetrating brain injury from a gunshot wound). The PQRST strategy resulted in superior performance for each of the three men ($T = 6$, $p = .032$). Once again, this was for questions only, because none of the three could recall anything from any of the passages after a delay. All were, of course, very amnesic.

The final study by Wilson (1987) sought to determine whether people with less severe memory deficits would also show better performance with the PQRST strategy compared with repeated practice and whether there would be a difference in free recall between the two methods. The criteria adopted for less severe memory impairment were based on

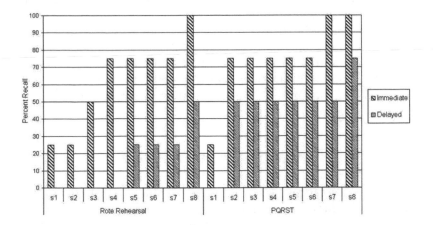

**FIGURE 5.1.** A comparison between PQRST and rote rehearsal for recall of passages in a single case study. S, session.

delayed recall of the passages from the WMS (Wechsler, 1945). Delayed recall had to be less than 51% of immediate recall but above "floor" (the delayed recall score of the Wechsler passages ranged from 33 to 50%). All the previous patients described in Wilson (1987) scored zero after a delay. Five men and three women were included. All had sustained a TBI and were between 6 and 58 months postinjury. Twelve short stories were selected. Each patient was seen individually on six occasions. Two stories were presented on each occasion, with the two methods balanced across patients and across sessions. The questions were selected by the experimenter. One modification was made to the repeated practice condition: Questions were introduced early on instead of at the end. This was done to see whether presenting questions early (as occurs in the PQRST method) could account for improved performance in the earlier studies. Comparisons were made between the two methods for (1) immediate free recall, (2) delayed free recall, (3) immediate questions, (4) delayed questions, and (5) delayed recall as a percentage of free recall. Again, a Wilcoxon matched-pairs test was used to analyze the results. There was no significant difference between PQRST and repeated practice for immediate free recall, but for each of the other comparisons PQRST was statistically superior to repeated practice. For the delayed-recall comparison, $p < .05$; for the immediate questions, $p < .01$); for the delayed questions, $p < .02$); and for the percentage retained, again, $p < .01$. Thus, PQRST was superior to repeated practice for all but one of the comparisons.

Two more recent studies have looked at PQRST as a way to enhance verbal recall. Franzen, Roberts, Schmits, Verduyn, and Manshadi (1996) used PQRST with two boys who had sustained a TBI and compared this with a metacognitive training strategy. The latter had no effect, but the PQRST led to similar performance in a boy without a brain injury and matched for age. A German study by Bussman-Mork, Hildberandt, Giesselmann, and Sachsenheimer (2000) compared spaced retrieval with PQRST and a no-treatment control method. They suggested that the PQRST was superior to the no-treatment control but that spaced retrieval led to better generalization.

## Why Does PQRST Work?

There are at least three reasons why PQRST might lead to better recall than repeated practice: It might provide better retrieval cues, it might be due to encoding specificity, and it might be due to deeper levels of encoding. First, let us consider retrieval cues. Does PQRST provide better retrieval cues than repeated practice? Maybe the questions themselves provide retrieval cues, and there is something about the questions that aids retrieval. Perhaps that is why the severely amnesic people did reasonably well at delayed questions even though they could remember nothing in the free-recall condition. This is unlikely to be the explanation, however, because there were questions provided in the repeated practice condition, yet none of the participants did as well here as they did with the PQRST procedure.

What about encoding specificity? Encoding specificity is a principle that refers to the fact that retrieval is enhanced when the original encoding or learning situation is reinstated at the time of recall (Tulving, 1983). If the test situation is similar to the original learning situation, then more information will be retrieved. In the PQRST situation, questions are part of the original learning situation *and* part of the test situation, so that could be why people do better with this strategy than with repeated practice. Although this looks promising as an explanation, it does not explain why less severely impaired people do better with delayed recall and percentage retained, because they are not asked for delayed free recall in the original learning situation. Original learning and testing do not match; thus, encoding specificity cannot be the whole explanation.

This leaves us with the levels of processing explanation. Is this sufficient? Craik and Lockhart (1972) proposed the levels of processing idea that material processed at a deep level is retained better than information processed at a shallow level. Remember that I could not recall the British shipping areas. This was because I did not process them deeply, whereas the 50 United States were processed and thus could be remembered. It is not simply a question of hearing or seeing material: If one wants to remember, one has to think about the material to be learned, question it, and relate it to something else, or, in other words, process it. The PQRST method appears to lead to deeper processing than repeated practice because people have to think about the passage and what they are listening to or reading in order to complete each of the stages.

## Using PQRST in Clinical Practice

Psychologists and therapists can use this technique with memory-impaired people to aid recall of verbal material. It is typically used as part of study skills for people wishing to return to education. The method is flexible, so, for example, when working with very impaired people, one can join with them in the assignment by reading the passage with them or to them, help them devise the questions, and follow the procedure in a way that is nonthreatening. At the other extreme, one can write

the steps down on a card and have the memory-impaired people work
through the stages by themselves. The PQRST method can be applied
to newspaper articles, short stories, journal articles, textbooks, scientific
material, or whatever needs to be retained. Whatever it is applied to, it
is probably better to work on a paragraph or short piece at a time rather
than a whole chapter or scientific article. It is not used spontaneously by
many memory-impaired people. In a survey of memory aids and strategies used by survivors of brain injury, Evans et al. (2003) found that not
one of nearly 100 people interviewed mentioned it. It is used, however,
in some rehabilitation centers and a few people use it alone or with therapists to learn some information. It appears to be better suited to people
with less severe memory problems; if they have at least some recall after
a delay, then PQRST may enhance the amount retained.

CHAPTER 6

# New Learning in Rehabilitation

*Errorless Learning, Spaced Retrieval*
*(Expanded Rehearsal), and Vanishing Cues*

## What Is Errorless Learning?

One of the main procedures in memory rehabilitation is helping memory-impaired people learn more effectively. Those of us with sufficient memory functioning to remember our earlier mistakes can benefit from trial-and-error learning, but for those who cannot remember incorrect responses it is not a good method. Indeed, the very fact of making an incorrect response may strengthen or reinforce that response. This is the underlying assumption behind *errorless* (EL) *learning*. EL learning is a teaching technique whereby people are prevented, as far as possible, from making mistakes while they are learning a new skill or acquiring new information. This can be carried out in a number of ways, such as providing spoken or written instructions or guiding the person through a task. The principle is to avoid mistakes being made during learning and to minimize the possibility of erroneous responses. There is some suggestion that monkeys also learn better with EL learning. Brasted, Bussey, Murray, and Wise (2005) found that errors made before the first correct response in control monkeys retarded one-trial learning.

## Theoretical Underpinnings of EL Learning

Two theoretical backgrounds underlie EL learning. First is the work of Terrace (1963, 1966) from the field of behavioral psychology. He taught pigeons to discriminate a red key from a green key with a teaching technique whereby the pigeons made no (or very few) errors during learning. Furthermore, the pigeons conditioned with EL learning were reported to show less emotional behavior than those that learned with trial-and-error learning. The EL learning principle was soon applied to children with developmental learning difficulties (Sidman & Stoddard, 1967). They used EL learning principles to teach children to discriminate ellipses from circles. Cullen (1976), Jones and Eayrs (1992), and Walsh and Lamberts (1979) followed suit, teaching children with developmental delays tasks, including weight and size discriminations.

Cullen (1976) believed that if errors were made during learning, it was harder to remember what had been taught. He also pointed out that more reinforcement occurred during EL learning because only successes occurred, never failures. To this day, EL learning is a frequently used teaching technique for people with developmental learning difficulties.

The second theoretical impetus came from studies of implicit memory and implicit learning from cognitive psychology and cognitive neuropsychology (e.g., Brooks & Baddeley, 1976; Graf & Schacter, 1985; Tulving & Schacter, 1990). Although it has been known for decades that memory-impaired people can learn some skills and information normally through their intact (or relatively intact) implicit learning abilities, it has been difficult to apply this knowledge to reduce the real-life problems encountered by people with organic memory deficits.

Glisky et al. (Glisky & Schacter, 1988; Glisky et al., 1986) tried to capitalize on intact implicit abilities to teach people with amnesia computer terminology using a technique they called the "method of vanishing cues (VC)." Despite some successes, the method of VC involved considerable time and effort both from the experimenters and the people with amnesia. Implicit memory or learning, on the other hand, does not involve effort because it occurs without conscious recollection. This, together with certain other anomalies seen during implicit learning (e.g., the observation that in a fragmented picture/perceptual priming procedure, if an amnesic patient mislabels a fragment during an early presentation, the error may "stick" and be repeated on successive presentations), led Baddeley and Wilson (1994) to pose the question, "Do amnesic patients learn better if prevented from making mistakes during the learning process?" In a study with 16 young and 16 elderly control participants and 16 densely amnesic people, using a stem completion procedure, it was found that every one of the amnesic people learned better if prevented from making mistakes during learning (see Figure 6.1).

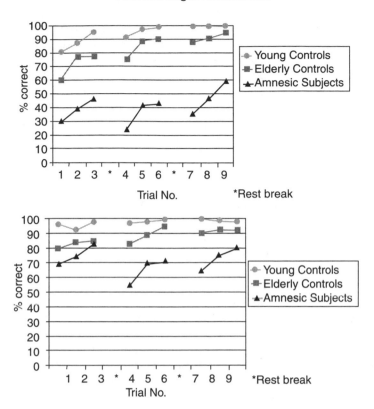

**FIGURE 6.1.** Results from errorful (top graph) and errorless (bottom graph) learning study (Baddeley & Wilson, 1994).

Baddeley and Wilson (1994) believed EL learning was superior to trial-and-error learning because it depended on implicit memory. Because the amnesic people could not use explicit memory effectively, they were forced to rely on implicit memory. This system is not able to discriminate between correct responses and errors, so it is better to prevent the errors in the first place. In the absence of an efficient episodic memory, the very fact of making an incorrect response may strengthen or reinforce the error. This view is discussed further later. A similar rationale provided by Hodder and Haslam (2006) suggests that error elimination reduces competing memory traces and thus facilitates memory performance.

Another way of understanding EL learning is to use the principle of Hebbian plasticity and learning (Hebb, 1949). At a synaptic level, Hebbian plasticity refers to increases in synaptic strength between neurons that fire together ("Neurons that fire together wire together"). Hebbian learning refers to the detection of temporally correlated inputs. If an input elicits a pattern of neural activity, then, according to the Hebbian learning rule, the tendency to activate the same pattern on subsequent occasions is strengthened. This means that the likelihood of making the same response in the future, whether correct or incorrect, is strengthened (McClelland, Thomas, McCandliss, & Fiez, 1999). Like implicit memory, Hebbian learning has no mechanism for filtering out errors.

## EL Learning Studies with Memory-Impaired People

Following Baddeley and Wilson (1994), EL learning principles were quickly adopted in the rehabilitation of memory-impaired people. Wilson, Baddeley, Evans, and Shiel (1994) described a number of single-case studies in which amnesic people were taught several tasks such as learning therapists' names, learning to program an electronic organizer and learning to recognize objects. Each participant was taught two similar tasks in an errorful or an errorless way. In each case, EL learning was superior to errorful (EF) learning. Wilson and Evans (1996) provided further support for these findings. Squires, Hunkin, and Parkin (1996) taught a man with amnesia to use a notebook with an EL learning procedure. Parkin, Hunkin, and Squires (1998) taught a man with encephalitis the names of politicians, and the same group (Squires, Aldrich, Parkin, & Hunkin, 1998; Squires, Hunkin, & Parkin, 1997) found that EL learning procedures enabled amnesic people to learn novel associations and to acquire word-processing skills. O'Carroll, Russell, Lawrie, and Johnstone (1999) also found that people with schizophrenia benefited from EL learning procedures. For Evans et al. (2000), more severely amnesic patients benefited to a greater extent from EL learning methods than did those who were less severely impaired, although this may only apply when the interval between learning and recall is relatively short (i.e., within an hour or so), which was the length of the individual experimental session.

How long the EL learning advantage is maintained is a question that is open to debate. One patient, Jason (Wilson, 1999, Chapter 9), maintained the information taught through EL learning for at least 3 months. Clare et al. (1999, 2000, 2001; Clare, Wilson, Carter, Roth & Hodges, 2002), described in more detail next, found considerable maintenance of learning after 2 years in one patient (Clare et al., 2001). On the other hand, Ruis and Kessels (2005) suggested that the effect of EL learning is short lived. One of the implications from this finding is that EL learning should be combined with expanding rehearsal to enhance its effectiveness.

Clare et al. (1999, 2000, 2001, 2002) have used EL learning techniques with people with AD. In the first study, Clare et al. (1999) were able to teach V. J., a 74-year-old man in the early stages of AD, the names of his colleagues at a social club. Following the EL learning principle, preventing guessing and errors as far as possible, they used a combination of strategies that included finding a distinctive facial feature, backward chaining, and expanding rehearsal. For example, one of the patient's colleagues was named Gloria, and this name was learned using a combination of all methods described previously. The distinctive feature selected was her gleaming smile, which V. J. was asked to associate with the name ("Gloria with the gleaming smile"). At the same time, backward chaining was used: The patient was given written versions of his colleague's name with progressively more letters omitted, as in the following example: GLORIA, GLORI__, GLOR____, and so on. V. J. completed the missing letters and eventually learned the name without any cues. These two strategies were combined with expanding rehearsal, otherwise known as spaced retrieval, in which the information to be remembered is first presented, tested immediately, tested again after a very brief delay, tested again after a slightly longer delay, and so on. (This procedure is covered further later). V. J. learned the names of his colleagues using photographs in his memory therapy sessions and demonstrated generalization by greeting his colleagues by name at a social club. A similar study with another man with AD showed comparable results (Clare et al., 2003).

Metzler-Baddeley and Snowden (2005) conducted a somewhat similar study but looked at the learning of novel and familiar material (V. J. had relearned familiar material but was not taught new material) with four patients with AD. Although they found that there was a significant advantage of EL over EF learning for the group, this was not at an individual level, because certain patients also learned under EF learning conditions. They argued that EL learning may be more beneficial for people with a profound amnesia. Evans et al. (2000) also suggested this in the case of people with nonprogressive memory impairment. A study with non-brain-injured older and younger people (Kessels & de Haan, 2003) found, however, that the prevention of errors during learning resulted in better performance for both groups.

There is now considerable evidence that EL is superior to EF learning for people with severe memory deficits. In a meta-analysis of EL learning, Kessels and de Haan (2003) found a large and statistically

significant effect size of EL learning treatment. However, there are conflicting views about the benefits of EL for people with less severe memory impairments. We return to this in the next section. There is also
some debate about the benefits of EL learning for problems other than
episodic memory deficits.

McKenna and Gerhand (2002) showed that EL learning was helpful in the relearning of visual and verbal semantic concepts for an amnesic patient and also that his retention of this information after several
months with no treatment was as good as that of his wife, who acted as a
control. Several studies have looked at EL learning for people with language difficulties and, in particular, word-finding problems, or anomia.
One study found a significant benefit from EL learning for the treatment of anomia in a patient with dementia (Frattali & LaPointe, 2004).
However, results of a series of studies by Fillingham et al. (Fillingham,
Hodgson, Sage, & Lambon-Ralph, 2003; Fillingham, Sage, & Lambon-
Ralph, 2005a, 2005b, 2006) appear to suggest no difference between
EL and EF learning as applied to the treatment of anomia. Given that
both types of learning result in equal amounts of success and that EL
learning is typically preferred by the patients because there are fewer
failures, perhaps EL learning should be the method of choice.

Wilson and Manly (2003) tentatively suggested that a combination
of sustained-attention training and EL learning may improve self-care
in people with unilateral neglect, and a few studies have also looked at
EL versus EF learning for motor task training. For example, Masters and
Maxwell (2004) taught a motor task to patients with Parkinson's disease
under EL and EF learning conditions. They found that more robust
learning occurred after EL than EF learning.

## Does EL Learning
## Depend on Implicit or Explicit Memory?

Baddeley and Wilson (1994) believed that the efficacy of EL learning as a
teaching technique for memory-impaired people was beneficial because
amnesic patients had to rely on implicit memory, a system that is poor
at eliminating errors (this is not to say that EL learning is a *measure* of
implicit memory). Nevertheless, there are alternative explanations. For
example, the EL learning advantage could be due to residual explicit
memory processes or to a combination of both implicit and explicit systems. There has been a lively debate over this issue. Hunkin, Squires,
Parkin, and Tidy (1998) have argued that it is due entirely to the effects
of error prevention on the residual explicit memory capacities and not

to implicit memory at all. Tailby and Haslam (2003) also indicated that the benefits of EL learning are due to residual explicit concurrent memory processes, although they did not rule out implicit memory processes altogether. According to these authors, the issue is complex and different individuals may rely on different processes. Support for this view can also be found in Kessels, Boekhorst, and Postma (2005). See Table 6.1.

A study by Page, Wilson, Shiel, Carter, and Norris (2006) claims, however, that preserved implicit memory in the absence of explicit memory is sufficient for EL learning to occur. They challenged Hunkin et al.'s (1998) conclusions, because the design of their implicit task was such that it was unlikely to be sensitive to implicit memory for prior errors. Furthermore, there was an element of EF learning in both the EL and EF explicit memory conditions. They also challenged Tailby and Haslam (2003) because the latter study conflates two separate questions: Is the *advantage* of EL learning due to the contribution of implicit memory? Is *learning* under EL conditions due to implicit memory? Perhaps some people do use both implicit and explicit systems when *learning* material, but this does not negate the argument that the *advantage* of EL is due to implicit memory, particularly implicit memory for prior errors after EF learning.

Tailby and Haslam looked at three groups of patients with different degrees of memory impairment under EL and EF conditions. They argued that if implicit memory was responsible for the EL learning advantage, then all three groups should perform equally well. There was a highly significant difference, with the less severely impaired people performing better. This means undoubtedly that the less impaired

**TABLE 6.1. Studies Claiming Errorless Learning Is Dependent on Implicit Memory and Those Claiming It Is Dependent on Residual Explicit Memory**

Implicit

Baddeley & Wilson (1994)
Page, Wilson, Shiel, Sarter, & Norris (2006)

Explicit

Hunkin, Squires, Parkin, & Tidy (1998)
Tailby & Haslam (2003) {but possibly both}

Both

Kessels, Boekhorst, & Postma (2005)

group with better implicit memory was using both systems, but it does not provide evidence for the source of the benefit of EL over EF learning. When they looked at the *size* of the benefit of EL over EF learning, the most severely impaired group did as well as the others. Given that the severely impaired group had little, if any, explicit memory function, this finding is difficult to reconcile with the claim that the results were due to residual explicit memory.

In an attempt to clarify the issue, Page et al. (2006) gave stem completion tasks presented in an EF or EL way to people with moderate and severe memory deficits. Instructions encouraged either explicit or implicit recall. They also administered recognition tasks and a source memory task to elucidate the contributions of explicit and implicit memory under the two conditions. They wanted to demonstrate that EL learning is robust even in people with no explicit memory functioning as measured by tests of memory, thus supporting the view that implicit memory is sufficient for the EL learning advantage to occur or, in other words, that residual explicit memory functioning is not necessary for this advantage.

Page et al. (2006) found that people with severe deficits and those with moderate deficits were good at the recognition tasks provided their own errors were not included. When asked to distinguish between their own mistakes and genuine target words, they were unable to do so. Source memory was absent for those with severe deficits and poor for those with moderate deficits. Thus, memory-impaired people showed an advantage of EL over EF learning that did not depend on whether they were asked for implicit or explicit recall; they could not distinguish their own errors from genuine targets, and they could not tell from which source the information had been obtained. All this suggests that implicit memory can explain why people with no or very little explicit recall can learn under certain conditions such as EL learning.

It should be remembered that EL learning is not a program of treatment. Instead, it is a description or an approach whereby the task is manipulated to eliminate or reduce errors (Fillingham et al., 2003). There are many different ways to reduce the likelihood of errors, such as providing written instructions, guiding someone through a particular task, or modeling the steps of a procedure little by little.

## What Is Spaced Retrieval (Expanded Rehearsal)?

*Spaced retrieval*, also known as expanded or expanding rehearsal, involves the presentation of material to be remembered (e.g., a new extension number) followed by immediate testing and then a gradual building up of the retention interval. So if the number 355294 is presented, the patient immediately repeats this number. People with a normal digit span (and this includes most memory-impaired people) will be able to do this without much difficulty. The tester then waits for 1 or 2 seconds and requests (but does not repeat) the number again. The test interval is very gradually increased until the number is learned. In case of failure, the correct information is supplied, and the retention interval shortened and gradually built up again. New names, short addresses, and items of general knowledge can also be taught in this way. An alternative way of using this technique is to increase the number of items between the target and the test or recall situation (Grandmaison & Simard, 2003). Camp and Foss (1997) also described a fixed interval (e.g., requesting the correct information every 2 minutes) rather than the expanding interval, which is more commonly used. Bjork (1988) showed that the longer the distracting interval between the first and second recall, the greater the chance of success at the third recall attempt.

## Why Does Spaced Retrieval Work?

Bjork (1988) suggested that spaced retrieval is a shaping procedure. Shaping is a well-established technique from behavioral psychology whereby there is a gradual approximation to the final goal. Although spaced retrieval has some similarities to shaping in that the long-term goal of recalling a piece of information is gradually achieved through increasing the retention interval, it differs from traditional shaping as used in behavior programs. The difference is that, in shaping, the actual behavior selected for shaping is close to but different from the final goal. Carr (personal communication, 1975), for example, used shaping with a developmentally delayed child who would drink from a cup but not from a spoon. The shape of the original cup was gradually changed and made smaller until it turned into a spoon. This is a classic example of shaping. The recall of a new name or telephone number is not changed over time it is just strengthened so that it is less likely to be forgotten.

Fridriksson, Holland, Beeson, and Morrow (2005) and Turkstra and Bourgeois (2005) claimed that spaced retrieval is essentially an EL learning procedure, but, although spaced retrieval restricts the likelihood of errors, it is not in and of itself an EL learning procedure because errors can always be made after an interval.

Hochhalter, Overmier, Gasper, Bakke, and Holub (2004) found that learning with spaced retrieval was superior to learning after a uniform delay *even though more errors* were made under spaced retrieval. Nevertheless, the two methods are often combined, as we see in the following section. As early as 1997 Vanhalle et al. suggested that spaced retrieval and EL learning should be combined to optimize acquisition of new information.

My view is that spaced retrieval works because it is a form of distributed practice: Distributing the learning trials over a period of time rather than massing them together in one block increases the likelihood of learning. Massed practice is a less efficient learning strategy than distributed practice (Baddeley, 1999), a phenomenon that has been known since the 1930s (Baddeley & Longman, 1978; Lorge, 1930). Lorge gave three groups of nonimpaired individuals a mirror tracing task. One group had 20 consecutive trials, one group had 20 trials interspersed with rests between each trial, and one group had 20 trials spread over 20 days. The group with the longest breaks between trials performed best and those with no breaks performed worst. Baddeley and Longman (1978) wanted to see how best to teach mail carriers to type. All participants had 12 hours of instruction. One group had 6 hours a day for 2 days, another 4 hours a day for 3 days, and the third group 1 hour a day for 12 days. This last group learned more and forgot less. Landauer and Bjork (1978) showed that name learning proceeds faster with expanded rehearsal/spaced retrieval and from that time the procedure has been used in memory rehabilitation (Camp, 1989; McKitrick & Camp, 1993; Moffat, 1989; Schacter, Rich, & Stampp, 1985). Camp, in particular, has used the method extensively in helping people with dementia learn new information. Camp, Bird, and Cherry (2000) also showed how spaced retrieval could be used to reduce distress in a woman who believed her belongings had been stolen. A list was drawn up of those to whom she had given her belongings. This list was kept in her wardrobe and a spaced retrieval program used to teach her to go to the wardrobe to check what had happened. She was initially taken to the wardrobe and shown the list at gradually increasing intervals. If she asked where her belongings were or who had taken them, she was asked how to find out and then taken to the wardrobe to see the list. Her distress decreased and was maintained at a low level over a period of months.

## Spaced Retrieval Combined with EL Learning

Clare et al. (1999, 2000, 2001) used a combination of EL learning, spaced retrieval, and VC to teach information to people with AD. Arkin (2000) also used EL learning and spaced retrieval to teach autobiographical facts to people with AD, and Kixmiller (2002) used the two strategies together to teach prospective memory tasks such as writing down appointments, taking medication, and remembering future dates. At the end of training, the experimental group was significantly better than the control group at these tasks. In a review of memory stimulation programs in AD, Grandmaison and Simard (2003) said, "In summary, the 17 subjects trained with the errorless learning approach combined with the spaced retrieval technique all showed a significant improvement in the percentage of information recalled after the training sessions." (p. 138). Lekeu et al. (2002) used both spaced retrieval and EL learning to teach two patients with AD to use a mobile telephone. The spaced retrieval method was used first to teach the patients to consult a card pasted onto the telephone. The card contained details of how to use the telephone. In the second stage, repetitive exercises in making calls was implemented, following EL learning principles. The authors believed that learning resulted from the fact that the patients had relatively preserved procedural memory, which is similar to the implicit memory learning hypothesis for the effectiveness of EL learning.

## Spaced Retrieval Alone

Although spaced retrieval is often combined with other methods, it can also be used alone. Camp et al. are perhaps the best known proponents of spaced retrieval, particularly for people with dementia (Camp, Foss, Stevens, & O'Hanlon, 1996; Camp et al., 2000; Brush & Camp, 1998). McKitrick, Camp, and Black (1992) used spaced retrieval to teach patients with AD to remember prospective memory tasks. Although all four patients in the study learned the tasks with 100% success, the long-term effects of the training were not reported.

Hodder and Haslam (2006) compared EL learning alone with spaced retrieval alone and then the two methods combined. Their sample of healthy controls were given a dual task to reduce their explicit memory performance while leaving implicit memory intact. In this way, the ability of the control participants did not differ significantly from that of people with mild to moderate memory impairments. They found that spaced retrieval alone led to better recall than EL learning alone, and there was no significant improvement when the two methods were combined. Thus, spaced retrieval was the better method to use. There are methodological problems with this study, however, because the EL learning procedure required participants to simply listen to the correct answer. They did not have to process it in any way, and we know from the work of Clare et al. (1999, 2000, 2001) and Riley and Heaton (2000) that it is important for participants to be engaged and active in the learning task. Furthermore, in the Baddeley and Wilson (1994) study, all of the 16 densely amnesic people involved benefited from EL learning, making it hard to argue that EL learning is ineffective for people with amnesia.

## Using Spaced Retrieval in Clinical Practice

On the basis of 15 published studies, Hopper et al. (2005) recommended spaced retrieval training for people with dementia. The person who has probably completed the most work in this area is Camp. With his colleagues, Camp demonstrated the efficacy of spaced retrieval for a variety of problems in a number of situations. For example, in speech and language therapy, spaced retrieval can be used to help with anomia and dysarthria. In occupational therapy, people with dementia can be taught to use wheelchairs, walking frames and other adaptive equipment, and activities of daily living. All therapists and nurses can use it to teach names, orientation items such as the number of a patient's room, and telephone numbers. It can also be used to reduce behavior problems (Bird, 2001; Camp et al., 2000). Brush and Camp (1998) produced a manual to help those working in the field. They provided tips for spaced retrieval training, such as "Face the client, making eye contact at all times. Monitor your tone of voice and body language so that you are always conveying a positive attitude and message" (p. 23) and "If the [spaced retrieval] training upsets the client, STOP. This experience should be fun and rewarding. The individual should look forward to participating with you" (p. 23). The authors pointed out that learning should be relatively effortless because it is building on implicit memory. They also recommended combining spaced retrieval with EL learning.

Clare et al. (1999, 2000, 2001) used EL learning and spaced retrieval together and included VC as well. We have already seen that Hodder and Haslam (2006) argued that the two together did not increase benefits, but Hodder and Haslam's work was not with people with dementia so it is possible the findings might be different with a different population.

Although most studies of space retrieval have focused on people with dementia, the technique has been used with other groups. Sohlberg (2005) discussed work with people who have developmental learning disabilities. In rehabilitation it has been used with people with nonprogressive memory difficulties (Moffat, 1989; Wilson, 1999). Hillary et al. (2003) showed that spacing of repetitions leads to improved recall in people with moderate and severe TBI. However, it should be taken into account that this was a list-learning experiment and not a rehabilitation study. There appears to be less research with brain-injured patients, and I suggest more is required.

## What Do We Mean by Vanishing Cues?

*Vanishing cues* (VC) is a method whereby prompts are provided and then gradually faded out. For example, someone learning a new name might be expected first to copy the whole name, then the last letter would be deleted, the name would be copied again and the last letter inserted, then the last two letters would be deleted, and the process repeated until all letters were completed by the person learning the name. This is similar to the method of backward chaining used to teach new skills to people with learning disabilities (Yule & Carr, 1987). In backward chaining, the patient is prompted or guided through a complete task (e.g., putting on a coat) and then guided through all steps of the chain except for the last one, which he or she is required to complete without help; then the last two steps of the chain are omitted and so forth. In forward chaining, which is also used, the first step of the chain is the first to be omitted instead of the last.

## Studies Evaluating VC

Glisky et al. (1986), the first to report VC with memory-impaired people, used a mixture of forward and backward chaining to teach computer vocabulary to four amnesic patients. Initially, patients were presented with a definition and asked to produce the word being defined. They were given increasing cues: Thus, if the target word was "Delete" they were presented first with *D*, then with *De*, *Del*, and so on (forward chaining). On subsequent trials, the letters were reduced one at a time (backward chaining or VC). Initially, the four patients in the study were very dependent on the first letter of each of the computer-related terms. Nevertheless, all acquired some computer vocabulary and were eventually able to produce the target words in the absence of the first letter. Furthermore, they retained the vocabulary over a 6-week period. The VC procedure was superior to a condition in which the correct answer was provided each time there was an error. Despite this success, the patients learned much slower than control participants and could not generalize to minor changes of wording; thus, the learning was said to be "hyperspecific." In a later study, Glisky and Shacter (1989) taught a severely amnesic woman, a survivor of encephalitis, more than 250 discrete pieces of new information concerning the rules and procedures for performing a task involving computer data entry. The woman was then able to obtain work using this skill. Not only was she able to work, but "she was able to perform the job in the real-world work environment as quickly and as accurately as experienced data-entry employees"

(p. 893). The researchers believed that the success was due to three factors: the VC training strategy, extensive repetition of all the procedures required, and the explicit and direct training of all components of the job. Glisky et al. were trying to capitalize on the relatively intact implicit learning abilities of their amnesic patients. However, they did not acknowledge the link with backward and forward chaining from the field of learning disability.

Breuning, Van Loon-Vervoorn, and Van Dieren (1989), Van der Linden, Meulemans, and Lorrain (1994), and Komatsu, Mimura, Kato, Wakamatsu, and Kashima (2000) all used VC with Korsakoff's syndrome patients and all had some, albeit limited, success. Leng and Copello (1990) successfully used a similar procedure to that of Glisky et al. (1986) to teach computer terminology to a brain-injured patient. Indeed, Glisky (1992) also worked with TBI patients, including patients in PTA; these, too, benefited from VC (Glisky & Delaney, 1996). Thoene and Glisky (1995) saw 12 patients with different etiologies and compared three different memory strategies, including VC. Visual mnemonics were found to be of most use in the 1995 study, although VC also resulted in some benefit. The VC procedure has been used not only with nonprogressive patients but also with those with dementia (Diesfeldt & Smits, 1991; Clare et al., 1999; Dunn & Clare, 2007). In the Diesfeldt and Smits study, patients in an experimental condition using VC learned the names of staff members more successfully than a control group. VC was, however, used in conjunction with other methods such as organization, directed attention, and rehearsal and is, therefore, similar to the Clare et al. 1999 study, which used a combination of strategies, as described in the previous chapter.

One group of patients who may not benefit from VC are those with aphasia (Abel, Schultz, Radermacher, Willmes, & Huber, 2005). In this study, patients were given VC or increasing cues or both. None of the aphasic patients benefited from VC alone, although some benefited from increasing cues and some benefited from both kinds of cue. The authors believed this was because VC was an EL learning procedure and aphasic patients are less sensitive to errors than amnesic patients. We return to this point in the next section.

## How Does VC Work?

Although Kessels and de Haan (2003), in a meta-analysis of EL learning and VC, found that VC did not produce a statistically significant effect size in comparison with control treatments, we have seen that some studies do indeed show an effect. Why? With the method of VC,

Glisky et al. (1986, 1989) were trying to capitalize on the intact implicit abilities of people with amnesia. Despite some successes, the method of VC involved considerable time and effort from both the experimenters and the people with amnesia. Implicit memory or learning, on the other hand, does not involve effort because it occurs without conscious recollection. So does it depend on implicit memory? Is the method of VC enhancing implicit memory processes?

Hunkin and Parkin (1995) suggested that implicit memory is responsible. They tried to teach computer-related vocabulary to a group of memory-impaired individuals with TBI or encephalitis (the same task used in the original Glisky et al., 1986, study) and compared VC with a standard rote learning (repetition) procedure. No significant differences were found between the two methods. However, when the VC procedure was modified to facilitate the use of implicit memory, the VC procedure led to superior performance *after a 6-week delay*. The modification involved the presentation of word stems even when they were not required. Thus, if the term sought was *mouse*, the letters *mous-* were shown even if they were not needed. This was thought to enhance the likelihood of the utilization of implicit memory. Hunkin and Parkin raised the possibility that mildly impaired people were more likely to benefit from the standard anticipation procedure, whereas those with more severe impairment (and thus more dependent on implicit memory) were more likely to benefit from VC.

Despite the fact that stem completion is a well-established implicit memory task, Hunkin and Parkin also questioned whether VC is truly tapping implicit memory. They argued that in the typical VC procedure the word stem (or the initial letter) functions as a cued-recall task and will thus benefit explicit rather than implicit memory. So VC is tapping implicit memory, but this is of little help when the task requires explicit memory. The benefit of VC after a 6-week delay is because by then explicit memory will be much reduced and implicit memory will more likely, of necessity, be used. Riley, Sotiriou, and Jaspal (2004) also suggested that the method of VC is more successful when explicit learning is required. This means that it is more beneficial for people with mild or moderate memory impairments and at least some explicit memory functioning. Indeed, in 1995 Thoene and Glisky found that the most severely impaired of their patients as well as those with milder deficits did not benefit from VC. Komatsu et al. (2000) also found that VC was ineffective for some patients.

Does the VC method work because it is basically using the EL learning principle? There is no doubt that VC reduces the number of errors during learning and this, in turn, reduces interference. According to Baddeley and Wilson (1994) and Wilson et al. (1994), implicit memory is sensitive to interference, produces the strongest response, and cannot be used for error elimination. Thus, we should minimize interference through EL learning. This is in part achieved by VC, because people using this method are encouraged to guess the correct answer when cued. We have already seen that people with dysphasia may not benefit from EL learning because they are less sensitive to errors than people with amnesia (Abel et al., 2005). Baddeley and Wilson (1984), Hunkin and Parkin (1995), and Selzer, Clarke, Cohen, Duncan, and Gage (2006) believe that the method works through the minimization of interference.

## VC in Clinical Practice

The main problem with VC is that it may only work when there is at least one letter left. Even though the original Glisky et al. (1986) study found that all their patients eventually learned computer terminology without the initial letter, the learning was slow and took many trials (unlike implicit memory, as I have argued earlier). If VC is the method selected to teach new information, then it should be combined with EL learning principles (Clare et al., 1999, 2000, 2001; Eslinger, 2002).

Riley and Heaton (2000) recommended avoiding errors while encouraging effortful recall. Clinically, it soon becomes clear that if patients are too passive during learning, they fail to learn. Thus, instead of telling them the correct answer, they need to engage in the process. Of course, VC encourages this by asking patients to complete the last letters of the target item. EL learning procedures also need to encourage active participation. In the words of Riley and Heaton (2000):

> We must take into account the circumstances of application, including the difficulty of the item to be learnt and the memory abilities of the learner. More difficult items and poorer memories may require more gradual fading to avoid an excess of errors and omissions; easier items and better memories may require more rapid fading to encourage effortful recall. To test this prediction, two methods of fading were compared in teaching general knowledge items to 12 individuals with a history of head injury. Consistent with the prediction, Increasing Assistance (that permits more rapid fading) was more effective for those with better memories and for easier items, and Decreasing Assistance (in which fading is more gradual) was more effective for those with poorer memories and more difficult items. (p. 133)

Finally, as ever in rehabilitation, generalization needs to be considered. If we do not plan for generalization, then treatment is likely to fail.

Clare et al. (1999) taught their patient the names of the people at his social club through the use of photographs. Generalization was tested by taking the man to his club with the photographs. He was required to look at each photograph, find the right person, and introduce that person by name to the senior investigator. Glisky and Schacter (1989) taught their patient how to perform the data entry tasks and then made sure she could carry out the tasks in the workplace. We sometimes see studies that contain no evidence of generalization (e.g., Thoene, 1996; Stark, Stark, & Gordon, 2005), and, although this may be acceptable for some of the published research studies, any good clinician should automatically include generalization as part of routine practice.

## Teaching Procedures or New Information through EL Learning, Spaced Retrieval, or VC

Ehlhardt et al. (2008) were concerned with teaching procedures or information to people with acquired memory impairments after TBI, stroke, anoxia, neurological infections, dementia, and schizophrenia. They searched the literature to find evidence for the effectiveness of different instructional procedures. Research from special education proved to be particularly helpful. Two main forms of instruction emerged from the review, called by the authors *systematic instructional* and *conventional methods*. Systematic methods included EL learning, the method of VC, and spaced retrieval. These emphasize explicit and carefully controlled prompts or models. Conventional methods comprised trial-and-error or EF learning. These emphasize recall of the targeted information or skill without prior models or prompts. Trainers only provide prompts after the learner has attempted the task and made errors.

Although the study found convincing evidence for the effectiveness of systematic instruction, it found that details with regard to the design and execution of the instruction lacked clarity. Nevertheless, the authors were able to make recommendations to assist clinicians in their design and evaluation of any instruction provided for memory-impaired people:

1. The intervention targets should be clearly delineated and/or task analyses should be used when training for any multistep procedures.
2. Errors should be constrained and the output of clients should be controlled when they are acquiring new or relearning information and procedures.

3. Sufficient practice should be provided.
4. Practice should be distributed.
5. Variation in the form of multiple examples should be provided to avoid hyperspecificity of learning and enhance generalization (generalization is covered in greater detail in Chapter 10).
6. Strategies to promote more effortful processing (e.g., verbal elaboration; imagery) should be used.
7. New learning should focus on ecologically valid targets.

# CHAPTER 7

# Memory Groups

## Why Run Memory Groups?

In human society, people are members of groups, including family, work, social, political, religious, and leisure. Groups provide us with a shared identity, roles, and peer support. After brain injury many people experience a loss of role and purpose and a sense of isolation (Malley, Bateman, & Gracey, in press). There are several reasons why one might choose to treat people in groups. Therapists are invariably short on time, and one way of dealing with this is to treat people in groups rather than individually. Group treatment is also more cost-efficient. More importantly, memory-impaired people may benefit from interaction with others with similar problems. Sometimes those with memory impairment fear they are losing their sanity, and this fear can be alleviated by observing others with similar problems. Groups can, therefore, reduce anxiety and distress. Patients can be instilled with hope and know that they are not alone. It is often easier to accept advice from peers than from therapists or to use strategies as peers rather than strategies recommended by professional staff, so groups may lead to better learning of appropriate behavior and may even lead to altruism. I have observed group members support less able people within the group and form friendships with people who are socially isolated. Staff running groups can ensure success by making the tasks appropriate to the person's ability level. This can further enhance self-esteem. "Nothing succeeds like success," so building it among peers is reinforcing. Groups also have face validity; that is, patients and relatives can see the point of groups and *believe* they are a good thing; this, in turn, can improve motivation to participate. Finally, groups are educative for therapists running them. Considerable information can be gained by noting each patient's responses to different strategies and observing which tasks are enjoyed or not. Particular problems that arise can be observed and dealt with accordingly. In short, groups are a valuable treatment resource, they are important for people in distressing or demanding circumstances, and group acceptance and mutual support may bring about important clinical changes.

## How Should a Memory Group Be Structured?

When setting up a memory group, certain decisions need to be made, including (1) whether the group should be open or closed, (2) how homogeneous the group should be, (3) how many participants should be in the group, (4) how many sessions and for how long the group should run, and (5) how much involvement there should be from the therapists in charge.

In an open group, participants can join or leave while the group is running; in a closed group, the same participants are present throughout. There are advantages and disadvantages to both. In the open group, there are always experienced people to help the newcomers, and one does not have to wait for a suitable cohort to be identified in order to start the group. However, group cohesion may be disrupted with people entering and leaving the group, and newcomers may feel overwhelmed by joining a group where they do not know people, many of whom already know each other. In practice, whether or not a group is open or closed may depend on the nature of the place where the groups are held. In centers where patients are admitted and discharged every week open groups may be the only realistic option, whereas in centers that admit patients in cohorts for a program that lasts for weeks or months closed groups make the most sense.

The homogeneity of the group may also depend on the nature of the working environment. If one is in a setting where all the patients have a similar diagnosis and level of functioning—say patients with TBI who had severe cognitive deficits—then this may lead to more homogeneous groups than a setting catering to a large variety of diagnostic groups and ability levels. Ideally, there should be some degree of homogeneity, so, for example, people with severe dysphasia or severe behavior problems may be unsuitable for memory group admission because their difficulties may preclude them from benefiting from the strategies being offered and they may disrupt the proceedings for the other members. On the other hand, some differences may be a good thing. Mixing stroke patients with survivors of TBI and encephalitis may have advantages because the stroke patients are older and may be good role models for the younger ones. The TBI patients may have more widespread problems, but the actual memory deficits may be less severe and thus they can help others (e.g., with "homework.") Some people with encephalitis may have severe amnesia, but their other cognitive problems may be less affected, making them better able to benefit from external aids. So, once again, there is not a right or a wrong decision with regard to homogeneity; it depends on the circumstances.

How many participants are needed to make a group? Between four and six participants seems to be the most common number, but, of course, this can be larger or smaller. If there are more than eight in a group, it may be difficult to give everyone the right amount of attention, and fewer than three people may be considered too small for a group; however, I have run memory group activities with as few as two people. This may not be ideal but could have some of the advantages outlined previously.

As for the number of sessions and their duration, 45 to 60 minutes once a week for 6 to 8 weeks seems a typical model, particularly for outpatients. This may not be sufficient, however, for building group cohesion. At the Oliver Zangwill Centre in Ely, where all patients are day patients and attend several days a week, the memory group may run two or three times a week for 6 to 8 weeks, 40 minutes per session. I have also run groups for inpatients 5 days a week, 45 minutes a day, for 6 weeks, and on one occasion one outpatient group ran for 2 hours a week for 11 months (Evans & Wilson, 1992). It is probably true that the timing and frequency of group meetings will depend on the circumstances the organizers find themselves in, the composition of a particular group, and the goals they are aiming for.

Therapist involvement is also an issue for consideration. Groups can, of course, run without a group leader. At the Oliver Zangwill Centre, there is a user's group of ex-clients who meet monthly without a staff member as leader. This is perhaps unusual because most memory groups do have a leader, typically a clinical psychologist, an occupational therapist, or a rehabilitation assistant. Speech and language therapists and physiotherapists can also be group leaders either alone or in partnership with one of the other professions. Nichols and Jenkinson (1990) pointed out that without a group leader the group may slide into confusion or adopt unhelpful patterns. I know of no memory groups that run without a leader unless they are groups for families and caregivers of people with brain injury. In such self-help and support groups (discussed later) memory-impaired people themselves may also attend. In a group that ran for several years in London, memory-impaired people and their families would meet together first before splitting up for an hour, during which time the families would discuss their concerns and offer help, support, and advice to each other while the memory-impaired people would gather in another room with a psychologist to engage in a project relating to their everyday problems. In one such group of memory-impaired people, the activity involved each member attempting a drawing illustrating a particular problem they experienced. The next time they met, although the members might not recognize each other or recall the previous meeting, they nevertheless recognized their own drawings, and this helped them recapture the mood of the last discussion (Wearing, 1992).

## Studies Evaluating Memory Groups

The earliest account of memory groups seems to be that of Folsom (1968), who described groups of long-stay psychogeriatric patients who met to receive *reality orientation* (RO) *therapy*, a treatment that has also been used for confused elderly people. According to Spector, Orrell, Davies, and Woods (2007), RO originates from attempts to rehabilitate severely impaired war veterans. Sessions may be held for half an hour a day, 5 days a week, with a group leader and between three and six patients. A Cochrane review (Spector et al., 2007) identified six randomized control trials with 125 patients, of whom 67 were in treatment groups and 58 in control groups. The authors concluded that RO has benefits for cognition and behavior for people with dementia, although it is unclear how far the benefits extend beyond the end of treatment. Although RO is often a part of the program for memory groups run for people with nonprogressive conditions, these group programs include more than RO (see Memory Groups in Clinical Practice section), and we must now consider their effectiveness in totality.

What evidence is there for the effectiveness of memory groups for this population? On the whole, evidence for improvement in *memory skills* is very limited (Wilson & Moffat, 1992). However, other benefits have been observed. Berg, Koning-Haanstra, and Deelman (1991), in a well-designed study, randomly assigned 39 survivors of TBI to one of three groups: (1) a memory strategy training, (2) a pseudorehabilitation (drill and practice), and (3) a no-treatment control. Those patients in the memory strategy training group did better on an objective memory score (a combination of several memory tests) compared with the pseudorehabilitation and the control groups. The assessments were carried out 2 weeks and 4 months after group treatment finished. The effects were most marked at the 4-month follow-up. Both control groups, however, rated the *effects* of therapy on their memory functioning as beneficial. Of the original participants, 31 were followed up 4 years later (Milders, Berg, & Deelman, 1995) and given the same tests. On this occasion, there was no difference between the three groups. The authors believed this was due to two reasons: First, a number of the original participants did not attend the follow-up sessions, and the majority of these were those with relatively poor memories who had been in the pseudorehabilitation group and who were, therefore, mostly responsible for the original differences between the two treatment groups. Second, improved memory functioning was seen in patients in the pseudorehabilitation and no-treatment groups. This suggests that the memory strategy training led to faster recovery of compensatory techniques for this set of participants; the other participants, however, developed these compensatory behaviors given extra time. This is reminiscent of the findings in the Wilson (1991) follow-up study of 50 severely memory-impaired people seen several years after attending a memory rehabilitation program. Most were using more memory aids and strategies when seen at follow-up than they were during or at the end of the memory rehabilitation program despite the fact that the program emphasized use of such aids. It was suggested that these aids were not used a great deal earlier because their relevance to the perceived daily needs of the memory-impaired people was not appreciated at the time. Once in a less protected environment, the relevance and need for such compensations became apparent.

One group study (Evans & Wilson, 1992) found no evidence of memory improvement as measured by tests in the group members, although use of compensations increased. The main improvement was in terms of anxiety and depression, both of which decreased as a result of memory group attendance. In a 1988 study, Ryan and Ruff provided a 6-week structured memory training program or a psychosocial support group (control group) to people with brain injury. Both groups improved on neuropsychological test measures, but only those with mild impairment benefited from the memory rehabilitation training. Jennett and Lincoln (1991) found that people attending a memory group were more likely to use external memory aids in everyday life.

One of the few studies showing improvement on memory tests as well as self- and significant other reports of improvement in real life was by Thickpenny-Davis and Barker-Collo (2007). The improvements in the experimental group followed a structured memory group program lasting eight sessions, and these were greater than those in the wait-list control group. They were also maintained at a 1-month follow up.

In sum, it seems that evidence is limited in terms of actual improvements in memory functioning, although emotional benefits may accrue and people are more likely to use memory aids to compensate for their memory difficulties. As with any memory rehabilitation program, we do not expect to restore or retrain lost memory functioning, so improving compensatory behavior and emotional well-being are both good outcomes.

## Self-Help and Support Groups

In 1946 the Association of Parents with Backward children was established in the United Kingdom. This society, later to become the Royal Society for Mentally Handicapped Children and Adults, was one of the earliest of self-help organizations. It now has several hundred local groups around the United Kingdom and has many committed members. The inauguration of other organizations followed, slowly at first and then in the 1970s with a flourish, as Headway, once the National Head Injuries Group and now the National Brain Injuries Association, was established. Many memory-impaired people belong to national organizations associated with their particular diagnosis, such as Headway (*www.headway.org.uk*), Encephalitis Society (*www.encephalitis.info*), Alzheimer's Society (*www.alzheimers.org.uk*), and The Stroke Association (*www.stroke.org.uk*). (See the Appendix for a list of worldwide organizations.)

The majority of people referred for help with memory problems will have sustained a TBI. In my own practice, the second most common group consists of people with encephalitis. Many survivors of this rare illness will have difficulties with memory. For this reason, the Encephalitis Society (Figure 7.1) as well as Headway are described in more detail next.

Headway began in 1979, when Sir Neville Butterworth, the father of a brain-injured son, placed an advertisement in a national newspaper to try to find holiday accommodations for his son. The parents of another young man who had sustained a TBI, Dinah and Barry Minton, made contact with Sir Neville, and they set out to discover what support networks, if any, existed. Because of their subsequent actions in the face of sparsity, there are now Headway branches throughout the United Kingdom delivering a range of services, including rehabilitation, respite care, and a network of local support groups, which typically meet once a month to provide support for people with brain injury and their families and caregivers. The national office provides support to local branches; offers a helpline (Headway UK Helpline); publishes many booklets, including one on memory problems; promotes under-

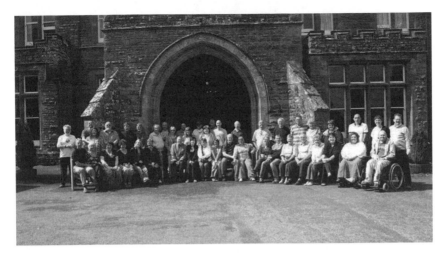

**FIGURE 7.1.** The Encephalitis Society. Copyright by the Encephalitis Society. Reprinted by permission.

standing of brain injury and its effects; and campaigns for better services. At about the same time as the founding of Headway, in the United States, Marilyn Price Spivak, the mother of a young girl who survived a TBI, set up the National Head Injury Foundation. Both the British and American organizations are alliances of families, brain-injured people, and professional staff.

Some of the services of the Encephalitis Society are similar to those offered by Headway, particularly regarding information about memory problems. Their society website declares: *"The Society's stated aim is to improve the quality of life of all people affected directly and indirectly by encephalitis"* (*www.encephalitis.org*). The society was started in 1994 by Elaine Dowell, the mother of a boy who had survived encephalitis. At that time, it was called the Encephalitis Support Group. For many years, Elaine was the main spokesperson, and she has seen it grow from a small association of parents of children who survived this illness to a flourishing society encompassing parents, neurologists, neuropsychologists, psychiatrists, occupational therapists, speech and language therapists, and, of course, encephalitis survivors. A few years ago, Ava Easton joined the society as development officer, and since then the society has become a very important resource for families, patients, and professionals. Five support meetings are held each year, usually on Saturdays. Their website explains that "support meetings have three main functions for members:

- *To gain information. Experts on various aspects of the condition are invited to speak, enabling those attending to obtain further information and insight into the condition. It is probable that significant numbers of those affected will become more expert on encephalitis than many health professionals: This empowers them and gives them confidence in making the case for the services and therapies that they require.*
- *To provide an opportunity to meet others affected by encephalitis. Such opportunities are vitally important in reducing the feelings of isolation which many people have when trying to cope with a rare condition that few if any of their friends and relatives have heard of and whose implications they are unable to understand.*
- *To give members and staff of the Group the opportunity to meet together. It is essential that members are able to offer constructive feedback as to their views on the services of the Group and contribute to its developing in ways that are as fully responsive as possible to the expressed needs of its members."*

The meetings are essentially constructive opportunities to focus on both the illness itself and the skills and strategies needed to move forward. Some members have negative feelings about these occasions because of the focus on the illness, but the overall feeling is positive, with the emphasis on maximizing recovery and utilizing remaining strengths to compensate for any losses (*www.encephalitis.info*).

For those readers working with patients with dementia, there are, of course, other societies, of which the best known and largest is the Alzheimer's Society. In the United Kingdom there are groups in more than 250 locations around the country. Their website (*www.alzheimers. org.uk*) states that *"Alzheimer's Society staff and volunteers work together to provide help and information to people affected by dementia in their communities. Our branch services include day care and home care for people with dementia, as well as support and befriending services to help partners and families cope with the demands of caring. From Alzheimer's Café's and innovative 'singing for the brain' sessions, to memory-book projects and group outings, our branches provide both practical support and an essential point of human contact".*

According to Wearing (1992), a self-help group advocate, "Most of all (a self-help group) is a platform where members have a voice" (p. 275). She believed that one of the key responsibilities of such groups is to coordinate the dissemination of information "from professionals to families, from families to professionals, from the group to health and social services, from the group to other groups and local bodies, to employers, to schools, and broadly to the general public through the media and through events" (p. 284).

In the early days after brain injury, the prospect of what lies ahead may be too appalling to contemplate and for this reason may be denied. As Caplan (1987) once said, quoting a patient, "Denial is one of the ways we get through hell" (p. 136). Families may be extremely reluctant to believe that their loved one's problems resemble in any way those experienced by the disabled brain-injured patients they have seen or read about. If written information from support groups is provided to families for them to read in their own time, the process of demystification can begin, and there may be a gradual acceptance of the situation in which they now find themselves. Such information is rarely sufficient, and at some point they are likely to benefit from meeting others in the same predicament. There is usually great value in sharing experiences with others who have been through the same kind of nightmare. Family members feel less alone and the people affected feel less vulnerable, stupid, or odd when they are with others facing the same kinds of problems. This might be one of the very few places where they can experience involvement and success.

For Wearing (1992), all self-help groups have the same broad aims: (1) provide support for patients and families in a social network of people who understand the problem, (2) inform patients and families about the particular problem they were set up to help with and how to deal with this problem, (3) access services in the community, (4) lobby for better care and support services, (5) increase public awareness of the problem, (6) are able to educate themselves about the condition through long-term liaison with professionals and families, and (7) promote research to advance knowledge.

## Memory Groups in Clinical Practice

### An Inpatient Group

Most memory groups consist of an educational component together with components addressing external and internal strategies (Berg et al., 1991). Wilson and Moffat (1984) provided a detailed day-by-day account of the Rivermead Memory Group for inpatients, which ran for 45 minutes a day, 5 days a week, for 3 weeks. Each day started with a welcome from the group leader and a reminder of the purposes of the group, which included finding ways of bypassing memory problems through the use of external aids and techniques to make remembering easier; practice in using these aids and techniques; and finding the best ways for each person to learn. Some reality orientation then took place in which group members were asked for the year, month, day and date, and the names of the people present. The most impaired people were asked the easiest questions and people were encouraged to find ways to answer the questions if they did not know (e.g., looking at the daily newspaper). Then each member was asked for a personal belonging, which was then hidden from view; each person paid particular attention to where his or her belonging was placed. The members were told that at the end of the session they had to remember their own belonging and where it was hidden. Homework from the previous session would be presented and more would be set to be completed before the next session. The homework might be easy (e.g., remembering to bring a newspaper the following day), or more difficult (e.g., remembering to listen to a radio program over the weekend and then discuss it at the next group meeting). As the homework was set, people were asked how they would remember to do the things asked of them. If one person said "I will just remember," the others were asked if they thought that was a good idea or not, and subsequently the person may or may not decide to change his or her plan. If the reply was "I will ask my occupational therapist to remind me," the patient might be asked, "How will you remember to ask your occupational therapist?" Thus, there was regular discussion on ways to remember. After homework, there was practice in using an external aid, a mnemonic, or a learning strategy. For example, the group leader might bring in an electronic aid to show to the group. This would be passed around and messages entered to remind the group to do things, such as closing the window or watering the plants. Group members would be asked to think about the advantages and disadvantages of the particular aid and why it might be of use. The session usually ended with a memory game such as pelmanism (also known as concentration), usually enjoyed by nearly everybody in the group, before retrieval of belongings. If anyone forgot what they were supposed to do at any time, cues were provided.

### An Outpatient Group

Wilson and Moffat (1992) presented details of the Dorset Group (of outpatients), which ran for an hour once a week for 10 weeks with three follow-up sessions at monthly intervals. In the first session—"How my memory works"—exercises were carried out to illustrate the various kinds of memory (e.g., short term, long term, implicit). Group members were asked to judge their own performance on various memory tasks. In session 2—"Making the best use of my memory"—attention was paid to the relationship between mood and memory, including anxiety and depression, good days and bad days, and confidence. Training in relaxation and self-instruction was provided to help people cope with memory lapses. In session 3—"Making remembering easier"—four main types of external memory aids were discussed: aids for temporary storage such as notebooks and shopping lists; aids for long-term storage such as encyclopedias and address books; forward planners such as diaries and calendars; and environmental changes such as keeping things in special places. Session 4—"Concentrating"—discussed the ways in which concentration might be disrupted and ways to improve concentration, such as incorporating brief rest periods, working in a quiet room, and using self-instruction to deal with intrusive thoughts. Session 5—"Practice makes perfect"—required group members to identify some information they needed to learn and then to practice this using a spaced retrieval/expanded rehearsal method (see Chapter 6). In session 6—"Remembering to do things"—members were asked to identify ways they found to improve or disrupt remembering and were given home assignments to implement strategies to help remembering to do things. The PQRST method (see Chapter 5) was described and practiced in session 7—"Remembering information"—and, once more, members were asked to practice this at home with newspaper articles and television news. In session 8—"Active listening and expressing an idea"—written guidelines, incorporating the strategies described the previous week, were provided on cards. Each member of the group presented a short talk to the other members using the cards and the guidelines. In session 9—"Tackling other problems"—members were asked about other difficulties, including cognitive, emotional, financial, legal, and family problems. Possible solutions were discussed and, if necessary, individual sessions were provided. Session 10 addressed "Continuing to use memory therapy techniques." Ways were sought to help members maintain and increase the application of strategies learned in earlier sessions. Sometimes this was through revision or through specific reminders of particular strategies, such as writing the PQRST steps on a bookmark.

## The Groningen Group

This group was referred to earlier as an example of a randomized control trial. All participants had sustained a closed head injury more than 9 months earlier, had both subjective memory complaints and objective evidence as measured by memory tests, and had no pre- or postmorbid evidence of severe intellectual deficits or severe language, motor, perceptual, or personality disorders. None had evidence of previous neurological or psychiatric disturbance, all were living independently, and all were between 18 and 60 years old. About half of the participants were in paid employment. Those allocated to the memory strategy training group met for 1 hour at a time, 3 days a week, for 6 weeks and had daily homework.

The patients themselves chose the problems they wished to work on, selecting those causing most distress in real life. Most patients chose three problems during the 6-week program. The most frequently reported difficulties were (1) forgetting people's names and (2) forgetting as a result of distractibility, although some had specific and personal problems such as needing to remember how to compose samples for chemical analyses or the route from the railway station to the hospital.

Patients were provided with a book containing some simple rules, as follows:

- Try to accept that a deficient memory cannot be cured.
- Make more efficient use of remaining capacities.
- Use external aids when possible.
- Pay more attention.
- Spend more time.
- Repeat.
- Make associations.
- Organize.
- Link input and retrieval situations.

Each session began with a discussion and a demonstration of the rules. For the first homework assignment, participants were asked to study the rules and to think up examples of and experiences with each principle. This was to ensure that the principles became more concrete and familiar. The next stage involved the application of the principles to the particular problems selected by the patients. In general, the same principles were applicable to all problems whether remembering names or composing a chemical sample, even though the *emphasis* might be different for each patient and problem depending on individual strengths and weaknesses. Every time a new situation arose, the rule book was referred to. In addition to the rule book, each patient was given a workbook to write down experiences with each rule. If necessary, the group leader added remarks and suggestions. As mentioned earlier, the greatest effect of this training appeared after 4 months. The authors believed this was because the participants continued to practice the strategies after they finished attending the group, and this led to them performing even better on the tasks after time had passed. Of course, we should not forget that at a 4-year follow-up, the patients in the sham treatment and no-treatment groups were performing as well as those who had received the strategy training. Thus, the treated group may have learned to compensate earlier and, even if this was the only effect, it may still be desirable to move people faster in the early days of rehabilitation.

## A Day-Patient Group

Evans (in press-a) described the memory group at the Oliver Zangwill Centre for Neuropsychological Rehabilitation. Patients at this center are usually at least 2 years postinsult, most of them have had earlier rehabilitation, and most have at least a chance of returning to work or further education. This means they are less severely impaired than members of the inpatient group described previously. The Oliver Zangwill Centre group typically runs once a week for up to 2 hours, for 6 weeks, although this can be shortened or lengthened if circumstances dictate. One difference between this group and the others described is that each member has at least one additional individual 40-minute session each week to review materials from the group, develop an understanding of how topics discussed in the group are of relevance to him or her, and identify how to apply strategies discussed in the group in everyday life. The members are told about the purposes of the group and how the group will be run. This structure is provided in Table 7.1.

**TABLE 7.1. Introductory session to the Oliver Zangwill Memory Group**

Objectives

1. To learn about memory and develop an understanding of your own memory problems.
2. To understand the purpose behind some of the assessments you may have done.
3. To discuss different memory strategies.
4. To practice memory strategies.
5. To apply and evaluate memory strategies in relation to your problems.

How the group will be run

It will be split into three sections:

- Education (providing information on memory, models of memory, and possible consequences to memory after a brain injury).
- Internal strategies (introducing internal memory strategies and the opportunity to use them).
- External strategies (introducing different external memory strategies and how they can be incorporated into a memory system).

At the end of each group, a volunteer will agree to give a brief summary of the material covered at the start of the next group. You will be provided with handouts, with space to make additional notes if you wish.

In the educational part of the syllabus, different aspects of memory are discussed: working memory, long-term memory, semantic and episodic memory, retrospective and prospective memory, and implicit and explicit memory. In addition, the various modalities of memory (visual, verbal, olfactory, gustatory, kinesthetic) are covered. Explanations are provided about other terms and aspects of memory (e.g., encoding, storage, and retrieval), the areas of the brain involved in memory, and the terminology (e.g., amnesia, RA, AA).

Over the next few sessions, the group members cover assessment of memory and the causes of memory impairment. They consider how TBI, stroke, encephalitis, and anoxia can lead to memory difficulties and use their own histories to provide examples of specific memory problems. They are also taught about other cognitive and emotional difficulties that may impair memory functioning. The final part of the educational component of the group is to consider common, everyday problems resulting from memory impairment and whether or not members of the group face these difficulties. The second half of the syllabus is more concerned with solutions to memory problems. They are given handouts with general guidelines such as:

- Understand your own memory problems through education and effective monitoring.
- Capitalize on strengths within your memory system to overcome any weaknesses.
- Find and use strategies that work for you and use them consistently.
- Adapt the environment.
- Be planful and use routines.
- Pace yourself to avoid fatigue (Evans, in press-a).

Internal strategies and external aids are covered much the same way as mentioned for the other groups.

Although memory groups do not appear to result in improved memory functioning, they do appear to be beneficial as ways of providing education about memory, particularly memory aids and strategies to help people compensate for their problems. They provide the opportunity for memory-impaired people to develop an awareness of their problems. Hearing other patients talk about their own problems may enable certain individuals to think about their own difficulties, and hearing others accept the fact that they have problems may make it easier to acknowledge their own. Similarly, with regard to use of strategies, hearing another person say how useful a particular strategy or aid is may convince others to try it, which they may be more reluctant to do just on the recommendation of a professional (Evans, in press-a). Finally, memory groups can reduce emotional distress (Evans & Wilson, 1992).

## Groups for People with Dementia

The RO groups described earlier are not the only groups for people with progressive conditions. Scott and Clare (2003) described four different forms of group therapy offered to people with dementia: the RO groups, groups that attempted to improve memory and cognition, groups offering psychotherapy, and groups providing support similar to the self-help and support groups described previously. Scott and Clare (2003) reviewed the literature on this topic and found plenty of evidence of creativity and support but little formal evaluation, so it was difficult to judge which kind of group was most beneficial.

Like memory groups for people with nonprogressive conditions, some are for families and patients together while others are only for the patients, and some are for people in residential homes while others are based in the community. Clare (2008) described some of the studies that have been carried out. Bernhardt, Maurer, and Frolich (2002) ran a residential home group for people with mild to moderate dementia twice a week for 6 weeks. Each session lasted for 1 hour. Although no statistical differences were found between this group and a control group, raters felt that the patients in the training group had improved and those in the control group had declined. Berger et al. (2004) evaluated a group offering support for caregivers, together with memory training and music therapy for patients, and compared this to a control group. The treatment groups were conducted once a week for 1 hour. Measures were taken at 6, 12, and 24 months. The authors found no differences between the two groups in terms of perceived burden of care, functional status of the patients, or patients' behavioral and psychological symptoms at any of the three time periods. They suggested this might be due to the normal standard of care patients were receiving.

Clare (2008) discussed a study comparing individual and group treatment (Koltai, Welsh-Bohmer, & Schmechel, 2000). This study, too, found no differences in either individual or group treatment compared with a control group. One of the earliest studies of memory group therapy was by Zarit, Zarit, and Reever (1982). They offered group intervention for patients living in the community and for their caregivers. Three groups were compared: In one, patients were taught to form visual images and make associations; a second involved problem-solving training whereby participants discussed practical steps that could be taken to manage everyday problems; the third was a wait-list control group. At the end of training, patients in the treatment groups did better than the controls on tests of recall, but caregivers in both treatment groups felt more depressed at the end of the training, and their feelings of burden, perceived severity of memory impairment, and behavior problems were unchanged. This led Small et al. (1997) to suggest that such therapy was not to be recommended. A number of subsequent reviews were more positive (Gatz et al., 1998). Several studies showing neutral or more positive findings are described by Clare (2008). For example, she cited a study by Arkin (2001) in which patients were given memory training, language activities, physical exercise, group activities, and outings. Mood and physical fitness improved as did scores on certain tests. Despite some evidence in favor of the beneficial effects of groups on patients and caregivers, the evidence is thin. One problem highlighted by Scott and Clare (2003) is the reluctance of many people with early AD to attend groups focusing on memory deficits, preferring instead to have individual sessions. This problem is also seen occasionally in people with nonprogressive conditions but is probably less likely for these people.

## Groups for Elderly People without Dementia

A number of studies have reported groups for elderly people with no neurological impairment and, although a full review is beyond the scope of this book, it is worth mentioning two recent studies, one by Craik et al. (2007) and one by Troyer, Murphy, Anderson, Moscovitch, and Craik (2008). The former describes a group for cognitive rehabilitation in older people. The rehabilitation comprised several modules, including goal management, psychosocial training, and memory. Five or six people attended these groups. In the memory module, participants learned strategies and techniques to improve their organizational and memory abilities. Participants learned about different forms of memory and about factors affecting remembering and forgetting. They were taught to notice individual memory slips and were introduced to a variety of external aids and internal strategies. Homework tasks were used to ensure practice of the use of strategies and aids. The study showed evidence of improvement in some aspects of memory and strategic processing.

The second study, by Troyer et al. (2008), described a group for older people with mild cognitive impairment (MCI) particularly affecting memory. People with MCI are at high risk for dementia, with the majority developing this within 3 to 6 years (Fisk & Rookwood, 2005), but when diagnosed with MCI many are still independent in everyday life. In this randomized controlled trial, 54 people were allocated to a multidisciplinary group-based intervention program or to a wait-list control condition (these were later given the group treatment). Treatment consisted of evidence-based memory training and lifestyle education to optimize memory behavior. The 10-week 2-hour sessions covered a number of topics, including information, intervention, and homework. For example, in session 2, information included an overview of memory strategies, the intervention covered memory for future events and the rationale for a memory book, and the homework task was to create a memory book. Those in the treatment group showed an increase in knowledge and use of memory strategies between pre- and posttest compared with the control group, and they maintained this improvement at 3-month follow-up.

## A Group for Families and Caregivers

Sander (2002, 2008) described a group for families and caregivers of people with brain injury, many of whom had memory impairments). The group contains six to eight participants and runs for six sessions, each lasting 2 hours. It is led by a psychologist, counselor, social worker, or post doctoral fellow with expertise in TBI. The group follows a cognitive-behavioral model with a mixture of didactic presentation and interactive problem solving, with frequent opportunities to interact with other group members. The first session serves as an introduction and general overview. The second provides education about TBI. The third examines changes in roles and relationships. The fourth and fifth sessions cover stress management, with part 1 focusing on relaxation and coping and part 2 on problem solving and positive thinking. The sixth, and final, session considers local and national resources and the "wrap-up." After completing the group sessions, members report a significant reduction in anxiety and escape-avoidance behavior. Members expressed overall satisfaction with the group (89% were very satisfied and 11% were somewhat satisfied). In terms of satisfaction with specific aspects (e.g., learning new ways to manage family members and feeling more confident about your ability to care), almost everyone was satisfied. In response to the question "What do you feel is the most important thing that you learned?," some of the comments were "Not feeling guilty at having time to myself," "I don't think my husband is doing this on purpose," and "How to handle stress."

In conclusion, the main benefit of memory groups is the opportunity to meet with others with similar problems. This is true for both patients and their families or caregivers. Meeting others is likely to provide emotional support. It also enables people to exchange information about strategies that work and sources of information. These groups are themselves a source of education for professionals as well as for patients and families. There is no one correct way to run a group; this depends on the level of functioning of the patients as well as the practicalities of the environment in which the professional is working and in which the memory-impaired people, together with those around them, are living.

CHAPTER 8

# Treating the Emotional and Mood Disorders Associated with Memory Impairment

## Why Is It Important to Treat the Emotional and Mood Disorders Associated with Memory Impairment?

Neuropsychological rehabilitation is concerned with the amelioration of cognitive, emotional, psychosocial, and behavioral deficits caused by an insult to the brain (Wilson, 2008). Most memory-impaired people will not only have cognitive deficits (possibly memory problems as well as other cognitive problems such as slowed information processing, executive difficulties, and word-finding problems) but also noncognitive problems, including, perhaps, anxiety, depression, mood swings, anger, and fear. Although cognitive deficits are likely to be the main focus of neuropsychological rehabilitation, it has been recognized for a number of years that the emotional and psychosocial consequences of brain injury need to be addressed in rehabilitation programs (Prigatano, 1994, 1999). Furthermore, it is not always easy to separate cognitive, emotional, and psychosocial problems from one another. Obviously, emotion affects how we think and how we behave, and cognitive deficits can be exacerbated by emotional distress (Dalgleish & Cox, 2002). They can also cause apparent behavior problems (Wilson, 1999). Psychosocial difficulties can also result in increased emotional and behavioral problems, and anxiety can reduce the effectiveness of intervention programs. There is clearly an interaction between all these aspects of human functioning, and, indeed, this is the core assumption of the holistic approach to brain injury rehabilitation pioneered by

125

Diller (1976), Ben-Yishay (1978), and Prigatano (1986). This approach is founded on the belief that the cognitive, psychiatric, and functional aspects of brain injury should not be separated from emotions, feelings, and self-esteem. Holistic programs include group and individual therapy in which patients are (1) encouraged to be more aware of their strengths and weaknesses, (2) helped to understand and accept these, (3) given strategies to compensate for cognitive difficulties, and (4) offered vocational guidance and support. Prigatano (1994) suggested that such programs appear to result in less emotional distress, increased self-esteem, and greater productivity.

Gainotti (1993, 2003) suggested three main reasons why emotional problems occur after brain injury: neurological issues resulting directly from the injury, psychological reasons, or psychosocial factors. An example of neurological issues is a severe apathetic syndrome with lack of any emotional reaction because of frontal lobe damage. An example of psychological issues is loss of self-esteem caused by inability to read because of a stroke. Psychosocial factors could be due to social isolation resulting from the brain injury. Gainotti (2003) also discussed the anatomical lesions involved in emotional disorders.

## How Prevalent Are Emotional and Mood Disorders after Brain Injury?

Williams (2003) suggested that survivors of brain injury are at particular risk for mood and emotional disorders. He referred to Brooks, Campsie, Symington, Beattie, and McKinlay (1987), one of the first studies to show that the emotional and behavioral consequences of brain injury were more common and distressing for caregivers than cognitive problems and, incidentally, more likely to worsen over time. Caregivers in this survey reported that 73% of their brain-injured relatives had mood problems and personality change, 67% had anger outbursts, and 63% were depressed. The cognitive problems most often reported were memory (73%), with 67% misplacing objects and 58% repeating themselves. Even earlier, Tyerman and Humphrey (1984) found that of 25 TBI survivors 60% were depressed and 44% were anxious. Garske and Thomas (1992) found that 55% of TBI survivors (from a sample of 47) were depressed. Jorge et al. (1993) had slightly lower numbers; 26% reported major depression at 1 month postinjury and 42% showed signs of depression sometime during the following year. Like the Brooks et al. (1987) study suggesting that emotional and mood problems are likely to worsen over time, Varney, Martzke, and Roberts (1987) found that major depression occurred in 77% of their brain-injured sample 3 years postinjury. Bowen, Neumann, Conner, Tennant, and Chamberlain (1998), using the Wimbledon Self Report Scale for Mood Disorders, found that 38% of their sample of 77 TBI survivors were in the clinically impaired range at 6 months postinjury.

In a more mixed sample, Kopelman and Crawford (1996) found that more than 40% of consecutive referrals to a memory clinic were in the clinically depressed range. Another study of people with TBI (Hibbard, Uysal, Kepler, Bogdany, & Silver, 1998) found that depression and anxiety were the most frequently reported emotional problems and that 44% of the sample had two or more diagnoses. Kreutzer, Seel, and Gourley (2001) in a large sample of 722 outpatients, found that 42% had a major depression. The variation in rate is, at least in part, due to the time postinjury when the studies were carried out, with the first year resulting in lower rates. What is clear, however, is that a substantial proportion of TBI survivors are likely to suffer from depression. Fleminger, Oliver, Williams, and Evans (2003) suggested that the prevalence of depression after both head injury and stroke is 20 to 40% in the first year and that 50% will experience it at some stage.

It appears that generalized anxiety disorder is less common than depression, although, as we have seen, comorbidity may well occur (Hibbard et al., 1998). Evans and Wilson (1992) reported that anxiety was frequently observed among people attending a memory group. Brown (2004) described some studies showing a rate of emotional difficulties between 9 and 25% following TBI and 30% after stroke. He also discussed the prevalence of emotional and mood disorders among people with progressive conditions. Williams (2003) believed that anxiety disorders may be underdiagnosed because of the difficulty in identifying symptoms in the context of other issues; that is, the symptoms of anxiety may be attributed to the organic consequences of brain injury.

Other kinds of anxiety include phobias, panic disorder, obsessive–compulsive disorder (OCD), and PTSD (Williams, 2003). It has been acknowledged that these are common after TBI (Hibbard et al., 1998). According to Williams, Evans, Needham, and Wilson (2002), OCD was once considered rare after brain injury, but now there is increasing evidence of its occurrence (Lishman, 1998). The stroke patient reported by Evans, Emslie, and Wilson (1998) showed strong OCD behavior (she had to wash parts of her body in a certain prespecified order in the bath and count the cars going past her window) but, when prevented from doing this, she lacked the emotional distress that typically accompanies OCD. True OCD is not uncommon. Berthier, Kulisevsky, Gironell, and López (2001) reported 10 TBI patients with OCD, including contamination obsessions and the need for symmetry and compulsions such as checking and cleaning. They suggested that "posttraumatic OCD has a relatively specific pattern of symptoms even in patients with mild TBI and is associated with a variety of other psychiatric disorders, particularly non-OCD anxiety" (p. 23).

Scheutznow and Wiercisiewski (1999) reported a single-case study of a man with phobia and panic attacks. The man avoided situations and feared having a heart attack. According to Brown (2004), however, there is little useful epidemiological or even good clinical data on the prevalence of phobias and panic disorders after brain injury. There are a few studies on PTSD, which is characterized by intrusive experiences, hypervigilance, anxiety, fear, and avoidance of activities (Williams, 2003). It is worth pointing out that PTSD is often found together with panic disorder, phobic reactions, OCD, and substance abuse (McMillan, Williams, & Bryant, 2003).

Although it was once believed that TBI patients in coma could not have PTSD because they were unable to recall the incident surrounding the trauma (Sbordone & Liter, 1995), research has since shown this to be untrue. McMillan (1996) found that just over 3% of his sample showed PTSD symptoms, whereas Bryant, Marosszeky, Crooks, and Gurka (2000) reported a high of 27% and Williams, Evans, Wilson, and Needham (2002) 18%. Some survivors have "islands of memory." One patient reported by Williams, Evans, and Wilson (2003), for example, remembers regaining consciousness for a short period following a car accident. He described smoke and blood, the fact that he could not see and felt he was going to die, and when he reached for his girlfriend's hand and realized she was dead. According to McMillan, later secondary experiences can fuel intrusive ruminations. King (1997) believed that confabulated memories of the event can traumatize people.

Several researchers have expressed the belief that traumatic experiences can be processed independently of higher cortical functions (Brewin, Dalgleish, & Joseph, 1996; Bryant, 2001a, 2001b; Williams et al., 2002). In some cases, of course, there is no loss of consciousness. The second case reported by Williams et al. (2003) and described in further detail by Evans (in press-b) is a young woman who, at the age of 24, was attacked by a man with a hunting knife while on a train. The knife entered the right parietal area, but the victim did not lose consciousness and recalled the entire event. Not surprisingly, she developed PTSD along with cognitive problems (memory and visuospatial difficulties). This case is described in more detail later in this chapter and in Chapter 9.

Psychoses seem relatively rare after brain injury. Achté, Hillbom, and Aalberg (1969) found that only 3% of a sample of 3,552 soldiers from World War II had signs of psychotic illness, and similar low rates have been found for stroke patients (Robinson, 1997; Chemerinski &

Levine, 2006). Fleminger (2008) suggested that psychosis in the form of schizophrenia is not unusual after TBI, although it has been difficult to confirm that the schizophrenia was actually caused by the brain injury.

Personality change is frequently reported after brain injury; Hibbard et al. (2000) suggested that 66% of 438 TBI patients had a diagnosis of personality disorder. Tate (2003), studying the effects of preinjury factors on personality change, found that changes occurring as a result of TBI are largely independent of the premorbid personality structure. There is also an increased risk of suicide after brain injury (Fleminger et al., 2003). Teasdale and Engberg (2001a) looked at *all* stroke patients discharged from hospitals in Denmark between 1979 and 1993 ($n$ = 114,098) and concluded that the risk of suicide was doubled for this group; younger patients and those hospitalized for a relatively shorter time were at greater risk. The risk appeared to decrease over time, with suicide more likely in the first 5 years. Teasdale and Engberg (2001b) carried out a similar study with TBI patients. Covering the same time period. They included patients who had a concussion ($n$ = 126,114), a cranial fracture ($n$ = 7,560), or a traumatic intercranial hemorrhage ($n$ = 11,766). The increased risk of suicide compared with that in the general population was 3.0 for the first group, 2.7 for the second group, and 4.1 for the third group. The ratios were higher for females than males and lower for those injured before the age of 21 or after 60. According to Fleminger et al. (2003), the overall increased risk is three times that seen in the general population.

A summary of anxiety and depression, apathy, and lack of emotional control in stroke, TBI, and AD is provided by Gainotti (2003), who observed that, after stroke, anxiety and depression are very frequent, being seen in 40–50% of hospitalized patients and less common (20–30%) in community patients. In TBI patients, anxiety and depression are less common in the earliest periods but tend to develop with increased awareness. In AD, about 40% of patients show depression or anxiety in the initial stages; the rate declines as the disease progresses. About 20 to 25% of right-hemisphere stroke patients demonstrate apathy compared with 10 to 15% of left-hemisphere stroke patients. Apathy is seen frequently after TBI as a result of neurological causes in the early stages and psychosocial causes in late periods. Apathy is also seen in 30 to 80% of AD patients. Loss of emotional control is uncommon in stroke patients, very common in the early stages after TBI, and "rather common" in the most advanced stages of AD. Selassie, Lineberry, Ferguson, and Labbate (2008) in a population-based study in South Carolina, conducted telephone interviews of 1,560 adults who had sustained a TBI approximately 1 year earlier. Of these, 40% had clinically significant mood and anxiety disorders, a further 12.6% had probable disorders, and 27.5% had possible disorders. Thus, the vast majority of the sample reported some mood and anxiety problems.

The majority of studies just discussed involved TBI or stroke patients, but a substantial proportion of people referred for memory rehabilitation will have survived one of the many kinds of encephalitis. A special issue of *Neuropsychological Rehabilitation* (Dewar & Williams, 2007) is devoted to encephalitis, and some of the studies address the issue of prevalence. In particular, Pewter, Williams, Haslam, and Kay (2007) considered the long-term psychiatric outcome in acute encephalitis. They cited two studies reporting that between 45 and 66% of patients show personality change or emotional disability. In their own study of 37 patients with encephalitis, the Symptom Checklist—90 (Derogatis, Lipman, & Covi, 1973) showed elevated levels of interpersonal sensitivity, depression, phobic anxiety, and obsessive–compulsive behaviors.

All these figures relate, of course, to brain injury in general and not specifically to people with memory impairment. Nevertheless, many brain-injured people will experience memory difficulties, so the risk of emotional and mood disorders may be similar. There is some evidence that people with a pure amnesic syndrome (i.e., with no other cognitive problems apart from the memory deficit) may be at less risk of emotional disorders. Tate (2004), for example, examined published studies of three well-known amnesic patients: H. M. (Scoville & Milner, 1957; Ogden, 1996), N. A. (Kauschal, Zetin, & Squire, 1981), and S. S. (O'Connor et al., 1995). Investigations suggested that they did not admit to emotional difficulties and, if anything, showed reduced emotionality. Tate commented, however, that although they did not *admit* to problems, other assessments did indeed show there was some emotional distress. She also cited the three patients with a pure amnesic syndrome reported in Wilson (1999). The lifestyles of all three were changed irrevocably by the memory impairment, and although there was variability in their emotional responses to the handicap, all found life difficult.

## Assessment of Emotional and Mood Disorders in People with Brain Injury

Much of what was written about assessment in Chapter 3 also applies here; assessments are performed to answer questions, and the nature of the question will determine the assessment procedure to be used. When simply asking people about their memory problems, we need to be aware that they may have forgotten their symptoms or their typical difficulties. For this reason, the assessment of memory can be a large problem in circumstances where one depends on the use of questionnaires and rating scales for an objective account of the frequency and intensity of certain symptoms. If, however, the concern is with immediate *perception* of the feelings about oneself, then the memory component is less of an issue. In the former case, one may need to ask a caregiver or close relative to ensure reasonably accurate information, but for subjective experiences and self-perception (e.g., "Do you feel sad, worthless, fearful?") the memory-impaired person's responses are valid.

Brown (2004) suggested that, for the diagnosis of psychological problems in people with neurological impairments, there is no substitute for the clinical interview, observation, and standard diagnostic criteria. Code and Herrmann (2003), citing Starkstein and Robinson (1988), argued that the most reliable method of gaining information about someone's emotional state is to ask them. Thus, the clinical interview will play a large part in identifying whether or not a brain-injured person has emotional difficulties. Brown (2004) recommended a checklist to act as an aide-mémoire when carrying out an interview. Even though standardized assessments are considered less relevant for emotional than for cognitive problems (Gainotti, 2003), there will be times when we need to use certain psychometrically validated instruments to know how people perform in comparison to others of the same age or with the same diagnosis. Therefore, certain standardized tools for measuring emotion and mood will also be part of our comprehensive assessment.

The most common depression and anxiety scales used among neuropsychologists appear to be the Beck Depression Inventory (Beck, 1987), Hospital Anxiety and Depression Scale (HADS; Zigmond & Snaith, 1983), Wakefield Self Assessment Depression Scale (Snaith, Ahmed, Mehta, & Hamilton, 1971), Hamilton Depression Rating Scale (Hamilton, 1960), Wimbledon Self Report Scale (Coughlan & Storey, 1988), Post Stroke Depression Rating Scale (Gainotti, Azzoni, Razzano, Lanzillotta, & Gasparini, 1997), and the Zung Self Rating Depression Scale (Zung, 1965). All have been designed for psychiatric patients except for the HADS, which has been used for neurological patients, the Wimbledon Self Report Scale, designed to assess mood in brain-injured patients, and the Post Stroke Depression Scale, designed for use with stroke patients. All have their own strengths and weaknesses (see Brown, 2004, for a partial summary), with perhaps the major problem being that the effects of the brain injury may be confused with the effects of depression (e.g., a response of "I am much slower now" could be due to brain injury *or* to depression).

The most commonly used tool for PTSD appears to be the Clinician-Administered PTSD Scale (CAPS; Turner & Lee, 1998). This 30-item structured interview covers 17 PTSD symptoms. According to Blake et al. (1995), it is the gold standard of PTSD assessment tools. It provides a comprehensive scaling of the frequency and intensity of each of the key symptom areas associated with PTSD. There are also questions regarding the impact of symptoms on social and occupational functioning. For each item, standardized questions and probes are provided. The Life Events Scale (Holmes & Rahe, 1967) may also be administered along with the CAPS to identify traumatic stressors. The Profile of Mood States (McNair, Lorr, & Droppleman, 1992) is a measure of six mood states and their fluctuations. Although it was not originally designed for people with brain injury, several studies have used it with brain injury survivors (Moore, Stambrook, & Peters, 1993; Perlesz, Kinsella, & Crowe, 1999).

A number of tools measure OCD (see Steketee & Nziroglu, 2003, for a summary). The Yale–Brown Obsessive Compulsive Scale (Goodman et al., 1989) includes a symptom checklist and a scale to assess the severity of OCD symptoms. The 60-item Padua Inventory (Sanavio, 1988) is reported to show good reliability and validity. There are also two briefer versions of this measure. The Obsessive–Compulsive Inventory (Foa et al., 2002) has both a long form and a short form. It is psychometrically good and is steadily increasing in popularity. Table 8.1 lists the most widely used measures for assessing mood and emotion, with a brief description of each, at the Oliver Zangwill Centre in Ely, England.

Another area that should be assessed is facial expression recognition. People with brain damage often have difficulty determining emotion from facial expressions. Sprengelmeyer, Rausch, Eysel, and Przuntek (1998) showed that people with Huntington's disease and with OCD had difficulty identifying disgust; people with lesions restricted to the amygdala had particular problems understanding fear. Diehl-Schmid et al. (2007) found that patients with frontotemporal dementia had difficulty recognizing basic emotions. Radice-Neumann, Zupan, Babbage, and Willer (2007) found this with survivors of TBI, as have Evans, Wilson, Calder, and Bateman (2007). Such findings raise the possibility that emotional perception deficits may contribute to the psychosocial (i.e., social communication) difficulties that are common after brain injury.

The six basic emotions common to all cultures are *happiness, anger, sadness, fear, disgust,* and *surprise* (Ekman & Friesen, 1971), and the Ekman Faces (1976) are most often used to assess the ability of people to recognize such expressions. Evans et al. (2007) studied recognition of these expressions in 104 patients with nonprogressive brain injury and 90 matched control subjects. More than 50% of patients had difficulty with at least one emotion. Perception of fear appeared to be the most

**TABLE 8.1. The Most Widely Used Measures for Assessing Mood and Emotion at the Oliver Zangwill Centre**

Beck Anxiety Inventory (BAI)

A validated 21-item measure that assesses anxiety symptoms. Both physiological and cognitive components are addressed describing subjective, somatic, and panic-related symptoms.

Beck Depression Inventory (BDI)

A 21-item multiple-choice self-report instrument designed to assess the severity of depression in adolescents and adults. This validated measure is composed of items relating to depression symptoms such as hopelessness and irritability, cognitions such as guilt or feelings of being punished, as well as physical symptoms such as fatigue, weight loss, and lack of interest in sex.

Beck Hopelessness Scale (BHS)

A 20-item self-report inventory designed to measure three major aspects of hopelessness: feelings about the future, loss of motivation, and expectations. The BHS is one of the most widely used measures of hopelessness. Several studies support its validity.

Coping Inventory for Stressful Situations (CISS)

A 48-item Likert scale questionnaire that measures three major coping styles: task-oriented, emotion-oriented, and avoidance coping (which consists of two patterns: distraction and social diversion) in adolescents and adults.

Generalized Anxiety Disorder Scale (GADS)

A multicomponent rating scale for assessment of dimensions of worry. This clinical rating scale, which measures distress, positive and negative beliefs, behaviors and control strategies, is considered important in treating generalized anxiety disorder.

Hospital Anxiety and Depression Scale (HADS)

A validated brief measure designed to detect the presence and severity of anxiety and depression in individuals with physical health problems. The items are designed to be sensitive to anxiety and depression without being confounded by physical symptoms that may be associated with health problems.

Posttraumatic Cognition Inventory (PTCI)

A 33-item questionnaire measuring negative and dysfunctional posttrauma cognitions, which are thought to maintain PTSD. The measure consists of three subscales (Negative Cognitions About the Self, Negative Cognitions About the World, Self-Blame).

Posttraumatic Stress Diagnostic Scale (PDS)

A validated and efficient 17-item self-report measure that assesses the presence and severity of symptoms of PTSD. Each item addresses how often a particular PTSD symptom has bothered the respondent in the past month. The symptom severity score ranges from 0 to 51.

*(continued)*

**TABLE 8.1.** *(continued)*

Response Styles Questionnaire (RSQ)

A validated 71-item questionnaire that measures how participants react to feelings and symptoms of dysphoria.

Robson Self-Concept Questionnaire (Robson SCQ)

A 30-item questionnaire that measures seven components of self-esteem: sense of significance, worthiness, appearance and social acceptability, competence, resilience and determination, control over personal destiny, and the value of existence.

State–Trait Anger Expression Inventory—2 (STAXI-2)

A validated questionnaire that provides an objective measure of the experience, expression, and control of anger. The State Anger scale assesses the intensity of anger at a particular time. The Trait Anger scale measures the frequency of angry feelings over time. The Anger Expression and Anger Control scales assess four relatively independent anger-related traits: expression of anger toward others or objects (Anger-Expression Out); suppressing angry feeling (Anger-Expression In); controlling anger by preventing anger expression toward others or objects (Anger-Control Out); controlling suppressed angry feeling by calming down (Anger-Control In).

Symptom Checklist—90—Revised (SCL-90-R)

A 90-item screening instrument for psychiatric symptoms that helps evaluate a broad range of psychological problems. The scale measures nine primary symptom dimensions and is designed to provide an overview of a patient's symptoms and their intensity at a specific point in time. The nine symptom dimensions are Somatization, Obsessive–Compulsive, Interpersonal Sensitivity, Depression, Anxiety, Hostility, Phobic Anxiety, Paranoid Ideation, Psychoticism.

Well-Being Questionnaire

An 18-item questionnaire that measures perceived current self and ideal self on six aspects of well-being: self-acceptance, positive relations with others, autonomy, environmental mastery, purpose in life, and personal growth.

vulnerable to brain injury. For some patients, this might result from damage to fear-specific systems, but for others it may be that more general cognitive impairments are responsible, because fear is less readily perceived by controls, suggesting that it might require greater cognitive resources than other emotions for successful perception.

Other tests to measure the ability to interpret facial expressions include the Facial Expressions of Emotions: Stimuli and Tests (Young, Perrett, Calder, Sprengelmeyer, & Ekman, 2002), a test in which faces are morphed so that they gradually change from one expression to another or change in intensity (see Figure 8.1).

Another clinically useful test for identifying emotions is the The Awareness of Social Inference Test (McDonald, Flanagan, & Rollins,

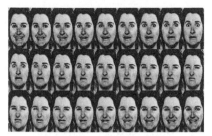

- Examples of continua or morphed
  facial expressions for three basic
  emotions (happiness, fear, and disgust.)
- The top row shows the happiness—
  fear continuum, the center row fear—
  disgust, and the bottom row disgust—
  happiness.

FIGURE 8.1. An example of morphed faces from the Facial Expressions of Emotions: Stimuli and Tests. From Young, Perrett, Calder, Sprengelmeyer, and Ekman (2002). Copyright 2002 by Paul Ekman, www.ekmangroup.com. Reprinted by permission.

2002), which assesses recognition of emotions from audiovisual displays. In part 1, videotaped vignettes of people interacting are shown, with four examples of neutral expressions and expressions of the six basic emotions. After each vignette, patients are asked which of the seven emotions was displayed. Because the scripts are ambiguous, the judgments have to be made on the basis of facial and vocal expressions. In Part 2, patients are required to make social inferences from videotaped conversations on the basis of emotional expressions and other nonverbal cues. They have to distinguish between sarcasm and sincerity or sarcasm and lies. All these tests are useful additions for clinicians to evaluate their patients' ability to understand emotional expressions and social inference.

## Group Treatments for Emotional and Mood Disorders in People with Memory Impairments

A number of methods exist for treating emotional and mood difficulties, including educational and psychotherapeutic group treatments, behavioral management techniques, pharmacological interventions, and holistic rehabilitation programs (Gainotti, 2003). Pharmacological interventions are not covered here. For those readers interested in this topic, see Turner-Stokes and Hassan (2002) for a good review of antidepressant medication use after stroke; Williams et al. (2003) for a short discussion of drug treatment for anxiety; Gainotti (2003) for a brief summary; and Thase and Denko (2008) for an up-to-date review of pharmacotherapy for mood disorders (but not for people with brain injury). We return to behavior management strategies later. We now consider group therapies, followed by individual therapies.

Interaction within groups increases participants' level of awareness of defects and capabilities and allows people to check the adequacy of their current behavior (Williams et al., 2003). In Chapter 7 we discussed some reasons why group treatments are beneficial. In groups for emotional and mood disorders, patients may benefit from one another's support; they are in a protected setting, which can enable them to put into practice any strategies learned in individual sessions; and feedback from peers may facilitate awareness of one's difficulties.

Of course, when working with memory-impaired people, certain procedures will be necessary to compensate for memory difficulties. For example, a summary of the group session will need to be written down. It may be necessary for one of the leaders or rehabilitation assistants to accompany or provide special assistance to some of those with severe memory impairments to remind them (e.g., to make a note of any memory lapses or to check the memory notebook when an alarm sounds). In some cases, an external memory aid such as a pager may be required to remind people to engage in a relaxation procedure. Tyerman and King (2004) discussed psychotherapy with people with different cognitive deficits and provided suggestions on how to circumvent problems. For those experiencing memory difficulties, for example, they suggested notes, audio- and videotapes of sessions, frequent repetitions, minireviews, telephone reminders to complete homework tasks, and use of family members as cotherapists.

Psaila and Gracey (in press) and Gracey, Yeates, Palmer, and Psaila (in press) described two groups in detail: a mood management group and a psychological support group. Both are included as part of a holistic rehabilitation program. The former focuses on education and strategy development; the latter is less structured. Relevant topics relating to the stresses of life after brain injury are introduced for discussion and mutual support (Klonoff, 1997). The mood management group runs for 1 hour a week for 12 weeks and aims to provide patients "with an opportunity to develop an awareness of problems they may have in mood and behavior and for developing skills and strategies for coping with such problems." The psychological support group runs for 6 months with no more than about eight clients and two facilitators. It provides the opportunity to gain support through shared experiences and enables clients to discuss their emotional response to their present situation, helping them to adjust to changed circumstances. Other groups, including an anger and stress management group, are run as necessary.

The mood management group tries to fulfill its aim by providing information and support in helping clients make sense of what is happening to them as well as helping them to develop skills to deal with changes in their experience and expression of emotion. The group starts with a 10-minute review of the previous week and any homework. This is followed by a presentation of a key topic such as "The Adjustment Process" or "Why Brain Damage Causes Emotional Difficulties." The group continues with further discussion and practice of certain exercises such as relaxation techniques, mindfulness meditation, attention control, and emotional problem solving. The group also considers how these strategies can be applied in real life. This key topic discussion and exercises last for about 40 minutes; the final 10 minutes are used to review and summarize the main points of the session. The group interaction is based on a general cognitive-behavioral model. Although there are a number of educational points the facilitators aim to cover in each session, the group has a strong discussion component to encourage clients to learn from one another. All will have individual psychological therapy sessions in addition to attending the group and are encouraged to make links between individual and group work. This applies not only to the mood group but to all the other groups they attend. All clients are provided with handouts and copies of any slides used during the discussion. For a more detailed discussion of other groups, see Wilson, Gracey, Evans, and Bateman (in press).

The syllabus is in three parts. Part I is the introduction to the group and a discussion about the aims together with a group exercise to find out what clients hope to gain from the group. Part II (weeks 2–5) addresses the question, "What affects mood and emotion?" This covers neurological damage, personality pre- and postinjury, adjustment to changes and losses, and the environment. Part III (weeks 6–12) covers strategies to help manage emotional and behavior changes, including awareness, managing frustration, irritability and anger, managing anxiety-related problems, and low mood, sadness, and depression.

The psychological support group aims to provide opportunities to identify, discuss, and practice strategies for managing the emotional consequences of brain injury. The cognitive impairments of the clients are considered, so structure and repetition are required. At the same time, it is important to ensure that clients can use their own knowledge and experience to support one another (Gracey et al., in press). The authors draw on a number of different models, including Bion's (1961) model of group process, Goldstein and Denny-Brown's (1942) and Ben-Yishay's (1996, 2000) therapeutic milieu model, and Foulkes's (1965) and Yalom's (1975) theories of group psychotherapy.

Although the clients attending this psychological support group are heterogeneous, individuals with significant communication or behavior problems may need to be excluded for the benefit of the group as a whole. Those with less disruptive behaviors may benefit from group feedback and responsibility. Executive deficits are the most frequent cognitive problem faced by group members, although sometimes memory problems dominate. In the latter case, the facilitator may need to be more proactive in suggesting strategies such as note taking, recapping from last week, or setting topics for discussion (Gracey et al., in press). The main purposes of the group are to instill hope, show patients they are not alone with their struggles, provide knowledge and information, provide support, help develop socialization techniques, provide opportunities for interpersonal learning, encourage group cohesiveness, and allow patients to express any pent-up feelings.

Sometimes more practical issues including advice on medicolegal cases, welfare benefits, and additional sources of support are addressed by group members. Further details on how the group is managed and topics covered can be found in Gracey et al. (in press). The authors conclude by saying that the psychological support group is one of the most challenging groups to run and can be difficult for some patients. Indeed, some people with brain injury may find the work of such a group too demanding.

## Individual Psychological Therapy
## for Emotional and Mood Disorders

We now turn to treatments for individuals with emotional and mood deficits alongside memory impairments. Khan-Bourne and Brown (2003) pointed out that traditionally psychological interventions in neurorehabilitation have adopted a learning theory or behavioral approach. Behavior therapy techniques and behavioral experiments are included in cognitive-behavioral therapy (CBT), which is derived from both the cognitive model of depression (Beck, 1970) and learning behavior therapy (Khan-Bourne & Brown, 2003). These authors summarize some of the positive findings of the behavioral approach to the treatment of emotional disorders. Wilson, Herbert, and Shiel (2003) provided further discussion, including emotional disorders directly resulting from cognitive deficits. For example, they reported on a stroke patient who became very anxious when she had to walk because she had lost the ability to judge depth and distance; thus, the anxiety was a direct result of the cognitive impairment. The treatment in this case involved a compensatory approach in the form of providing a rope for her to hold or a shopping cart for her to push when moving. Tyerman and King (2004) also addressed neuropsychological counseling for individuals to help them understand and cope with the complex effects of brain injury. They cited Prigatano (1994, 1995), whose ideas on the treatment of emotional disorders have been so influential in neuropsychological rehabilitation. According to Prigatano, many of the questions faced by survivors deal with the meaning of life such as "Will I be normal?" and "Is life worth living after brain injury?" Tyerman and King (2004) listed the therapeutic components that they believe to be important in working with individuals:

1. Establish the person's life history as well as his or her hopes and plans before the injury. This is achieved through an in-depth interview with the brain-injured person and other family members as appropriate.
2. With the help of medical records, neuropsychological assessments, and personal accounts, review the nature of the brain injury and its effects in order to establish a framework for understanding.
3. Track the course of recovery as experienced by the person and professionals in order to place the current difficulties in context.
4. Explain the recovery process and chart this or use analogies that are personally meaningful.
5. Evaluate changes in life circumstances and chart changes in personal and social circumstances pre- and postinjury.
6. Explore changes in self-concept and personal values arising since the brain injury.
7. Guide and support the person as he or she searches for and evaluates new experiences.
8. Establish a clear and balanced view of how the injury has impacted upon the survivor of brain injury and then build and reinforce a positive image of a person seeking to cope and rebuild his or her life.
9. Reevaluate current problems, identify priorities, and formulate appropriate action plans.
10. Guide the person as he or she addresses high-priority, achievable goals and help evaluate the costs and benefits in order to achieve a more positive life that is sustainable without undue pressure.

The main theoretical approach to the treatment of emotional and mood disorders after brain injury, at least in the United Kingdom, is CBT (Wilson, Rous, & Sopena, 2008). CBT has been shown to be highly effective in a range of disorders and has at its center a "process of guided discovery that enables a person to share in an examination of [his or her] cognitive, emotional and behavioural experiences" (Williams, 2003, p. 127). Both cognitive rehabilitation and CBT share much in common. Both are goal directed; involve problem solving; are client centered; collaborative, and educative; test hypotheses; include measures of outcome and skills training; ensure the person is ready to change; and are structured and time limited (Gracey, 2002). Khan-Bourne and Brown (2003) characterized CBT as an approach that accommodates and seeks to tackle the many personal and social consequences contributing to psychological difficulties; it provides the therapist with a range of working tools and is flexible with the potential to allow for differences in individual circumstances, strengths, and weaknesses. These authors also addressed the problem of providing CBT to people with memory problems and, like Tyerman and King (2004), offered suggestions, including how to use memory aids (written notes, cue cards, and audiotapes); shorten the length of individual sessions; increase the frequency of sessions, involve a family member or friend to remind/reinforce strategies; and assist with homework and use techniques such as summarizing.

CBT has been used for many emotional and mood difficulties, including depression, anxiety, OCD, and PTSD. Mohr, Boudewyn, Goodkin, Bostrom, and Epstein (2001) found that people with multiple sclerosis and depression benefited from CBT; Macniven, Poz, Bainbridge, Gracey, and Wilson (2003) used a number of approaches, including CBT, with a survivor of encephalitis to improve her emotional distress; Williams (2003), Williams et al. (2003), Dewar and Gracey (2007), and Arco (2008) are just some of the investigators who have reported single-case studies of CBT with survivors of brain injury.

Some of these cases have more than one emotional problem because, as stated previously, comorbidity is common. K. E., a survivor of TBI reported by Williams (2003), had a number of cognitive and emotional problems, and in the formulation of his situation he was noted to have executive, memory, and attentional difficulties. He also had severe PTSD, including intrusive reexperiences, avoidance behaviors and emotional blunting. The PTSD symptoms were thought to be due to survivor guilt stemming from his experience in a car crash in which his girl friend had been killed. In addition, he had mild generalized anxiety and moderate to severe depression with moderate alcohol dependency. He had some degree of insight into his mood disturbance. The symptoms were thought to be maintained because he lacked opportunities to develop adaptive responses. Without appropriate support, he was believed to be at risk for even more severe depression and for continued PTSD.

In addition to individual psychological support, K. E. attended several groups, including the psychological support and mood groups described previously. In the cognitive groups, he developed systems for dealing with his planning, memory, and attentional difficulties, which included use of a palmtop computer to plan and monitor home activities. The palmtop also reminded him to take essential breaks and spend time with family members. In the mood group, CBT helped K. E. become aware of factors influencing his mood. He also learned relaxation techniques and how to check for evidence to support his views. In his twice weekly individual sessions, he focused both on triggers and environmental influences that affected his mood and on coping strategies. With the palmtop, he recorded his alcohol intake, sleep problems, arguments with others (including antecedents, behavior, and consequences), and nightmares and flashbacks. Alcohol misuse and anger management techniques were addressed in both group and individual sessions.

In the next stage of the program, K. E. progressed to dealing with the intrusive experiences. Although the nightmares did not disappear completely, they now occurred occasionally rather than nightly. The relaxation techniques helped him to sleep so he drank less and thus functioned better during the day. He felt much more able to control his PTSD symptoms.

Dewar and Gracey (2007) reported on the anxiety case of V. O., a mother of four and a school nurse who survived herpes simplex viral encephalitis at the age of 43. She was left with a number of cognitive deficits, including prosopaganosia (an inability to recognize faces) and a severe retrograde memory loss. She described her mood as being low, with a loss of interest and hopelessness about the future. V. O. was not severely depressed but she did have a generalized anxiety disorder. She said she felt she was a "was" and wanted to become an "am." Specific trigger situations were identified, which led to feelings of anxiety and loss of identity, including failure to recognize someone, people doing things for her that she felt she should do herself, and her family not "getting along."

V. O. was introduced to the CBT model and the therapeutic alliance developed. She was taught relaxation exercises, and began to monitor her emotional responses and identify negative automatic thoughts (Padesky & Greenberger, 1995). The main approach, thereafter, was the use of behavioral experiments. One of V. O.'s beliefs, because of her inability to recognize people, was that "it is unfriendly or rude to ask people who they are; they will be offended." For one day, staff and clients in the rehabilitation center did not wear their badges, and because of her prosopagnosia, V. O. had no way of identifying them. V. O. agreed to ask people their names if she was unsure of their identities. She did this and noted that people did not take offense. When asked to reflect on this, V. O. said, "It's okay to ask people who they are if I am not sure."

The behavioral experiments provided new positive learning experiences for V. O., and once she felt comfortable compensating for her face recognition deficits (she was also taught to recognize a few faces and was one of the people described in the semantic relearning study in Chapter 1), her sense that she lost her self became less of a problem. The feeling that she was a bad mother and her family was not "getting along," associated with the change in her family role, was helped by encouraging the family to understand V. O.'s difficulties.

Mateer, Sira, and O'Connell (2008) described a simple treatment for a man with Korsakoff's syndrome who experienced severe anxiety. A page was inserted into his memory book with the heading "What to Do When I Feel Anxious," followed by a list of statements such as "I have had an illness," "It is not my fault," "I am not a burden to my parents," etc. Judd (1999) used a similar approach, including a four-stage chart to help people manage anger, as follows: (1) "My anger risks," which includes statements like "Being tired" or "In a noisy environment"; (2) "My anger signs," which includes such examples as "Tight muscles" and "Clenched teeth"; (3) "What to do," including "Remove myself from the situation"; and (4) "Preparing to return," including "When I can smile I am ready to go back."

Arco (2008) described successful treatment for a 24-year-old man with OCD after a TBI sustained 1 year earlier. Although this man did not have severe memory problems, his memory scores on standardized tests were below average. He presented with compulsive counting and the need to empty his bladder frequently. Baseline measurements showed that he was counting in 80% of daily hourly intervals and emptying his bladder 12 times a day. The intervention consisted of home-based consultations, self-regulation procedures (including self-recording of compulsive behavior), stress coping strategies, EL remediation, social reinforcement, and gradual fading of interventions. At the end of treatment, he was no longer counting and was emptying his bladder eight times a day. This was further reduced to seven times a day at follow-up (6 months), and the counting was still absent.

Several cases of treatment for PTSD have been reported including C. M., otherwise known as Caroline (Williams et al., 2003; Evans & Williams, in press). This was the young woman who had been attacked by a man with a knife mentioned previously. Evans and Williams's (in press-b) formulation summarizes the problems:

> As a result of experiencing a traumatic assault that was out of her ordinary experience and involved a threat to her life, Caroline was suffering severe PTSD, with intrusions (flashbacks, intrusive images and nightmares) and avoidance (of reminders of the injury). She had some cognitive impairment including some reduction in speed of information processing, attention/concentration and memory. It was hypothesized that Caroline's mood disorder contributed to cognitive difficulties. For example, it seemed likely that intrusive thoughts/images and hypervigilance to perceived threat would further affect concentration and also memory and planning skills. With regard to the functional consequences of her difficulties, it was concluded the PTSD was primarily responsible for limitations in social, leisure, domestic and occupational activities, but that brain injury related problems with speed of information processing, attention, and memory would also make addressing these problems more difficult.

There were three parts to Caroline's program: (1) to understand more about her brain injury and its consequences both for the cognitive impairments and for the PTSD; (2) to develop strategies for managing the cognitive and emotional consequences of her injury; (3) to apply these strategies in everyday situations in order to achieve her personal goals. (We return to the actual goals in Chapter 9.) Caroline attended a group for understanding brain injury to achieve the first part of the program and also completed her own personal portfolio about her brain injury and its consequences. To achieve control over her PTSD, a CBT approach was used with four main elements: psychoeducation, exposure, cognitive restructuring, and anxiety management training. Each of these elements was incorporated into Caroline's broader neuropsychological rehabilitation program. In addition, she attended the cognitive group to help with her cognitive problems, and the mood management and psychological support groups to help her develop and put into practice strategies for dealing with the cognitive and emotional problems. Further work on developing and implementing strategies was carried out in her individual sessions. These strategies were gradually applied in everyday situations, including traveling on public transportation and returning to work.

This section ends with a brief note about the treatment of disorders of emotional perception after brain injury. Bornhofen and McDonald (2008) reminded us that although many studies have targeted social skills deficits in survivors of brain injury using a behavioral approach, there has been very limited success possibly because of difficulty with the appreciation and monitoring of social cues such as facial expression, vocal prosody, and body posture. This led Bornhofen and McDonald (2008) to try to remediate deficits of emotional perception. Patients were randomly allocated to treatment first or wait list first. The treatment lasted 25 hours over an 8-week period. The program was hierarchically structured so that at first people worked on the semantic aspects of emotion: For example, how would people feel on their birthdays or the first day at school? This semantic knowledge was, by and large, intact. In stage 2, people practiced judging static visual emotion cues, first from line drawings and then from photographs. The next stage involved judgment of emotion from dynamic cues (through, e.g., videotapes or role-plays) first in one modality (visual or verbal) and then with a combination of modalities. In the final stage, participants practiced making social inferences on the basis of emotional demeanor and situational cues. Although the numbers were small, with only five in the treatment group and six in the wait-list group, there was significant improvement in the treatment group, suggesting that it is possible to improve recognition of emotion and social inference.

## Treatment of Emotional and Mood Disorders in Clinical Practice

Ylvisaker and Feeney (2000) stated that "rehabilitation needs to involve personally meaningful themes, activities, settings and interactions." This means that the emotional as well as the cognitive and psychosocial problems have to be dealt with in rehabilitation. Interviews with each client and possibly family members will need to establish the history as well as the hopes and aspirations of the individual. This will be supplemented with medical records and information from previous assessments and treatments. The nature of the brain injury and its effects will need to be clarified.

In addition to the interviews, assessments will provide further information. These are likely to include neuropsychological assessments plus mood and emotional measures and self- and observer ratings. The formulation is crucial because it uses theories and models to understand the development and maintenance of problems and can be used to make predictions about treatment. It is constantly under revision as situations change and evolve. The factors to be considered in a formulation are given in Figure 8.2.

We addressed the formulations of K. E. and Caroline. Williams et al. (2003) also report the formulation of D. C., a survivor of TBI with OCD

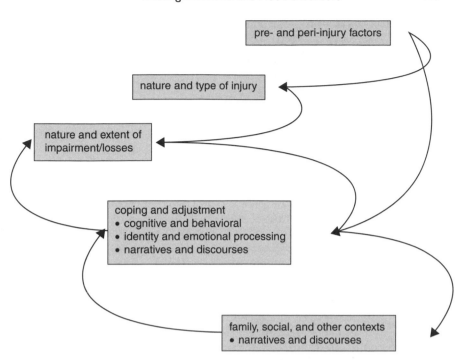

**FIGURE 8.2.** Factors to be considered in formulation.

and anxiety. D. C. had severe amnesia with attentional deficits associated with his TBI and OCD as an indirect consequence of his injury.

> DC's OCD symptoms appeared to be related to the following: (1) cognitive disorders triggering self doubt and rumination with checking as an overcompensation for poor memory; (2) checking and tidying providing a means of controlling aspects of his immediate environment and sense of safety in the absence of other, more meaningful activities; (3) behaviors being negatively reinforced by avoidance (the behavior "saved" him from social demands); (4) distorted self image being maintained, and exacerbated, by avoidance of activities, with core negative self-beliefs, leading to negative automatic thoughts; (5) health fears contributing to general avoidance behavior pattern; and (6) problems being maintained and exacerbated by a lack of opportunity developing adaptive responses. (pp. 141–142).

Once assessments and formulation have been completed, the rehabilitation program will probably include some or all of the following

**TABLE 8.2. Coping Strategies for Stress, Anxiety, and Panic**

- Identifying triggers and reactions.
- Relaxation and anxiety management.
- Stopping avoidance.
- Challenging negative thoughts.
- Increasing independence step by step.
- Establishing realistic targets—not too much at once!!
- Understanding and self-instruction.
- Obtaining professional help.

steps. The long-term and short-term goals will be set (goals are addressed in Chapter 9); all the therapists and psychologists involved will ensure they are working together to facilitate patients' understanding of the intervention and goals; intervention for the cognitive and emotional difficulties; attendance at groups for support and encouragement of awareness and acceptance of the use of strategies; and supported social reintegration to facilitate the transfer of the use of strategies to other situations. Some coping stategies for managing stress, anxiety, and panic are presented in Table 8.2. Issues relating to putting theory into practice are further discussed in Chapter 10.

CHAPTER 9

# Goal Setting to Plan and Evaluate Memory Rehabilitation

## What Are Goals?

The *Concise Oxford English Dictionary* (1999) defines a *goal* as "the object of a person's ambition or effort; a destination; an aim" (p. 505). Ylvisaker and Feeney (2000) suggested that "rehabilitation needs to involve personally meaningful themes, activities, settings and interactions." Wade (1999), discussing rehabilitation goals in particular, indicated that "a goal is the state or change in state that is hoped or intended for an intervention or course of action to achieve" (p. 2). In practice, for our purposes, a goal is something the individual in receipt of and participating in rehabilitation wants to achieve, and subsequent actions will be relevant and meaningful to this person when they reflect his or her longer term aims. Although other people, who may be family members or therapists involved in the particular therapy program, may help in the achievement of goals by their efforts and support, their *actions* in this process are not regarded as goals.

Houts and Scott (1975) and McMillan and Sparkes (1999) proposed several principles of the goal-planning approach to rehabilitation. First, the patient should be involved in setting goals. Second, the goals set should be reasonable and client centered. Third, they should describe the patient's behavior when a goal is reached. Fourth, the method to be used in achieving the goals should be presented in such detail that anyone reading the plan would know what to do. McMillan and Sparks summarized the principles of Houts and Scott and added to them, suggesting that goals should (1) be client centered, (2) be realistic and potentially attainable during admission, (3) be clear and specific, (4) have a definite time deadline, and (5) be measurable.

In most rehabilitation centers, long-term goals are those the patient or client is expected to achieve by the time of discharge from the program, whereas short-term goals are the steps set each week or two to achieve them. Long-term goals target disabilities and handicaps in order to improve day-to-day functioning, and they should be achievable by the time of discharge from the center. Collicut-McGrath (2008) captured the essence of goal-planning philosophy by stating that ideally rehabilitation should be "patient centered *not* profession centered; participation/role based *not* impairment or activities based; interdisciplinary *not* multidisciplinary; goal directed *not* problem focused; individualized *not* programmatic" (p. 41). Regarding Collicut-McGrath's third stipulation, Nair and Wade (2003) suggested that in interdisciplinary rehabilitation professionals work toward common goals, whereas in multidisciplinary rehabilitation the different disciplines individually set goals appropriate to their profession.

## Why Use Goal Setting in Memory Rehabilitation?

Nair and Wade (2003) argued that incorporating people's life goals into treatment leads to better outcomes. The main purposes of rehabilitation are to enable people with disabilities to achieve their optimum level of well-being, to reduce the impact of their problems on everyday life, and to help them return to their own most appropriate environments. In other words, rehabilitation is ultimately concerned with enabling people to participate effectively in valued activities (Hart & Evans, 2006). Memory rehabilitation is no different. Its purpose is not to teach people to do better at memory exercises, to improve performance on memory tests, or to learn lists of words but rather to enable them to achieve personal goals. These goals, therefore, should be the main focus of memory rehabilitation, and if they are pursued then, whether or not they are achieved, they represent one of the best channels for evaluating the success of memory rehabilitation.

Some studies use standardized test scores as the main or only outcome measure (see, e.g., the studies reviewed by Carney et al., 1999). This is inappropriate not only because memory rehabilitation is not about improving test scores but also because the relationship between test performance and real-life skills is at best modest and at worst nonexistent (Sbordone & Long, 1996). For the same reason, it is wrong to use test scores to determine those memory problems that should be tackled in rehabilitation. Although tests provide a profile of a person's cognitive strengths and weaknesses, they do not tell us a great deal about how people with neuropsychological deficits cope in everyday life. Nor do they tell us what brain-injured people and their families hope to achieve and what is important for them.

As an illustration, take the example of an amnesic patient who was able to live on his own, hold a job, and complete his own tax forms. He could do all of these things because he used compensatory strategies very efficiently and because of excellent organization and planning abilities. Almost anyone working in rehabilitation would describe him as a rehabilitation success, but if standardized tests were used to measure this success, then he would be a failure because he scored zero on any test of delayed memory (Wilson, 1999; Wilson, Gracey, Evans, Bateman, in press).

There are several advantages to a goal-setting approach. First, it makes certain the aims of the admission are clearly documented. Second, patients, relatives, and caregivers are all involved as well as the rehabilitation team. Third, such an approach promotes team work. Fourth, it incorporates a measure of outcome. Fifth, it removes the artificial distinction between outcome and client-centered activity. Goal setting as a measure of outcome is further addressed later in this chapter. Among the disadvantages of goal setting are:

1. It does not provide systematic data on all problems. To address this issue, one can, of course, include additional data such as questionnaires, rating scales, and demographic data.
2. It depends on a good and experienced chairperson. This can be overcome by having new members of staff shadow experienced members before they take on the position of chair.
3. It is possible to set goals that are too easy.

McMillan and Sparks (1999) believed this latter point can be resolved with staff training and experience; in addition, one could make the case that some easy goals are a good thing because they may increase motivation and self-esteem. Although, according to Wade (1999), "good rehabilitation practice should set meaningful and challenging but achievable goals" (p. 41), there is surely a place for a few easy goals to improve patients' morale. Furthermore, one can always use goal attainment scaling (GAS; Kiresuk & Sherman, 1968) to weight the goals and thus make them more comparable. GAS also allows for the comparison between patients. Once goals have been negotiated, weights can be applied to each of them to reflect their relative importance.

GAS was developed in 1968 by Kiresuk and Sherman for use in mental health settings. Ottenbacher and Cusick (1990), recommending it for occupational therapists, suggested that GAS provides a framework for goals that is "measurable, attainable, desired by all, and socially, functionally and contextually relevant" (p. 520). Malec (1999) described the steps involved in GAS.

1. The initial goals are agreed.
2. The goals are weighted, with high-priority goals rated 1 (if all goals are of high priority, they can all be given a rating of 1). (Malec also stated that in rehabilitation settings weighted goals are not typically used.)
3. The time by which the goal is to be achieved is specified.

So far, GAS appears to be much like goal setting described elsewhere in this chapter. The fourth and fifth steps are what sets GAS apart.

4. Articulate the "expected" level of outcome in specific behavioral terms (Malec, 1999, p. 256). The expected outcome is scored 0.
5. Articulate other possible outcomes.

A better than expected outcome is scored +1 and an even better outcome scored +2. Next, determine a worse outcome, which is scored -1 and an even worse outcome scored -2. So, for example, if the goal is for Jim to remember to take his medication four times a day for 2 weeks (i.e., 56 times over the specified time period) and all parties involved in the negotiation believe Jim will manage to do this approximately half the time (26–30 occasions), this score will be 0; if he does better (e.g., managing 31–38 times), he will score +1; if he remembers more than 38 times, he will score +2. On the other hand, if he remembers fewer than 26 times but more than 18, he will score -1, and if he does worse than this he will score -2. The final step is to score the patient on the goals before treatment and at the time when it is expected he or she will achieve the goal.

Zweber and Malec (1990) were probably the first to describe GAS for people with brain injury. They suggested using GAS in addition to, and not in place of, more traditional goal setting. Malec, Smigielski, and DePompolo (1991) followed this up with a further study looking at outcome after a brain injury rehabilitation program. They found that GAS was "a quantifiable individualized measure that is useful for (1) monitoring patient progress, (2) structuring team conferences, (3) ongoing rehabilitation planning and decision-making, (4) concise, relevant communication to family, referral sources, and funding sources, and (5) overall program evaluation when used in the context of other objective outcome measures" (p. 138).

Rockwood, Joyce, and Stolee (1997) studied 44 people with brain injury. They reported a range of correlations between GAS and other outcome measures such as the Disability Rating Scale and Daily Living Scales. Malec et al. have published several papers on GAS in brain injury rehabilitation (e.g., Malec, Smigielski, DePompolo, & Thompson, 1993; Malec, 1999). Although Tennant (2007) believes GAS has serious flaws, the 1999 paper is a useful review of GAS and includes a discussion on strengths and weaknesses. A 2006 appraisal of GAS studies by Hurn, Kneebone, and Cropley also suggested strong evidence for the reliability, validity, and sensitivity of GAS.

## Theories of Goal Setting

Hart and Evans (2006) observed that theories of treatment try to explain the process by which received treatment results in improved health. They found that social cognitive theory is a useful source for rehabilitation because it proposes that "human behavior is self regulated to meet personal standards or goals" (p. 143). People attempt to reduce the discrepancy between the actual state of affairs and the desired state of affairs or, in other words, they are trying to achieve personal goals. Other sources that have value for brain injury rehabilitation include commerce, education, and sport. Locke and Latham (2002) carried out a meta-analysis of more than 30 studies of goal setting and concluded that there is strong evidence that goal setting improves performance. They suggested that there are a number of mechanisms by which goal setting influences behavior. Goals serve a directive function, directing attention toward goal-relevant activities and away from goal-irrelevant activities. They have an energizing effect, with more demanding goals leading to greater effort than less demanding goals. They also affect persistence, with hard goals leading to more prolonged effort. Finally, goals are thought to lead to the arousal, discovery, and use of task-relevant knowledge and strategies.

Gauggel and Fischer (2001) found that specific goals are better than vague or general goals, such as "do your best." In one study, 45 people with brain injury were randomly divided into two groups. Each group was assessed on the Purdue Pegboard Test. One group was given a general goal to "do your best." The other group was set a specific goal: "Try to increase your speed by 20 seconds." Those given the specific goal performed significantly better than the group set the general goal. Gauggel et al. have found similar results with other tasks, including mental arithmetic (Gauggel & Billino, 2002) and reaction times (Gauggel, Leinberger, & Richardt, 2001).

Latham and Seijts (1999) also found that setting long-term goals alone resulted in poorer performance than when long-term and short-term goals were combined. As stated by Wilson, Gracey, Evans, and Bateman (in press), feedback is likely to be critical in brain injury rehabilitation and achievement of short-term goals provides feedback in the quest to achieve long-term goals because they serve as markers of the progress attained. Carver and Scheier (1990) also argued that reducing the discrepancy between current state and goal state is critical in reducing emotional distress. A study of 82 brain injury rehabilitation patients by McGrath and Adams (1999) suggested that progress in rehabilitation (through goal setting and achievement) was associated with reductions in anxiety. Young, Manmathan, and Ward (2008) also found that goal setting reduced anxiety in caregivers and provided psychological benefits to patients and to caregivers in the form of increasing motivation and providing reassurance.

## Identifying and Setting Goals: The Art of Negotiation

Some patients may seem to want to achieve the impossible. A patient with a spinal injury may say "My goal is to walk again." A patient with severe and widespread cognitive deficits may say "I want to return to my former employment as a lawyer." An amnesic patient may say "I want to get my memory back." This is where the art of negotiation comes in. In the case of the amnesic patient, the answer may be along the lines of "We don't think it is possible for you to restore your memory to what it was before your accident/illness/injury, but we can find a way to help you remember what you have to do each day. How do you feel about having that as one of your goals?" This may be sufficient to get the first memory goal set. If not, we could try to persuade the patient to accept a simpler goal first: "Let's try this first and we can look again at other possible goals in a few weeks." Sometimes it is necessary to accept an unrealistic goal if the patient and/or family will not compromise; in these situations, however, staff may feel uncomfortable agreeing to goals they firmly believe are unattainable. After all, one of the main principles of goal setting is that goals should be potentially achievable. If the goals are to do with return to work, it is more realistic to have as a goal "Identify the tasks you need to do in order to be able to return to work." The reason for this is that it is difficult to predict, in most cases, how achievable the return to work goal is, depending, as it does, on so many other factors such as community support, whether or not the person was employed at the time of the injury, the economic situation of the country or town where the person lives, and so forth. In the end, however, the patient has the last word because he or she "owns" the goal.

The first step in goal setting is to discuss with the patient, family, and members of the rehabilitation team just what it is they would like to achieve in the long term and short term. All parties need to consider what changes would be required for any goals to be achieved: Does the person need to learn a new skill or do something more frequently or for a longer duration, or does he or she need more support in order to carry out the task or behavior? Negotiation, as discussed earlier, is important. It is also necessary to decide how one will know whether or not any goal has been achieved. Sometimes this is easy, when, for example, behavior leading to and attaining the goal can be observed. Checking a memory book after each meal would fit this category. However, a goal involving, for example, the development of more confidence would probably have to be rated through a rating scale or questionnaire or through the number and nature of self-critical statements made, and this would be more difficult to observe and evaluate.

Once goals have been set, intervention can begin. After a period of time, goals should be reviewed. If the goal has been achieved, then a new goal can be set; if it has not been achieved, reasons for failure need to be examined. Was the goal inappropriate? Is more time required? Do other people need to be recruited to ensure consistency throughout the day? The next step in the process will depend on answers to these questions.

Typical goals for memory-impaired people include setting up a memory system to remind one of the day's activities; remembering to take medication; remembering to carry out self-care activities; learning the way to the shops or around the neighborhood, hospital, school, or workplace; learning the names of one's work colleagues; and other everyday, functionally relevant and meaningful activities. Each of these behaviors or attainments will need to be scaled down into short-term goals. (We return to this later.) Of course, memory problems are not usually observed or treated in isolation. People with memory difficulties may well have other cognitive problems such as attention deficits, poor planning, and slowed thinking as well as noncognitive problems such as anxiety, social isolation, and fatigue. Goals may need to be set for each of these problems. In addition, goals for people with severe and widespread cognitive problems or who are still in PTA will differ from those set for people who have less severe problems or who have a pure amnesic syndrome. A goal for someone in the first category might be to find his or her bed on the ward or learn the location of the toilet. Environmental modifications may be the treatment of choice here. Goals for someone who is hoping to return to work or who has no other cognitive deficits apart from problems associated with impaired memory may be more focused on external memory aids and learning important pieces of information. As people recover, change, or develop better awareness, goals may need to be altered to reflect changes in status.

## Goal Attainment as an Outcome Measure

As in any rehabilitation program, we need to know whether our efforts to help people with memory difficulties have been effective or worthwhile; that is, we need to know the outcome of the intervention. Outcome can be defined as the result or effect of intervention, and it is not easy to measure partly because of the heterogeneity of the patients and their aims or goals resulting from treatment. However, if we recognize the overall purpose of rehabilitation as enabling patients to achieve personal goals, then we must assess whether or not those goals are achieved.

In acute medical care, the main outcome may well be survival or death. This is obviously not appropriate for rehabilitation because the patients have certainly survived. Rehabilitation has a number of outcome measures, the main ones being the Glasgow Outcome Scale (GOS; Jennett & Bond, 1975); the Glasgow Outcome Scale—Extended (GOSE; Jennett, Snoek, Bond, & Brooks, 1981); other disability rating scales such as the Barthel Index (BI; Mahoney & Barthel, 1965), the Functional Independence Measure (FIM), the Functional Assessment Measure (FAM; Keith, Granger, Hamilton, & Sherwin, 1987); and the Mayo–Portland Adaptability Inventory (Malec, 2004). This last named is a well-documented and psychometrically sound scale and highly appropriate for measuring outcome after rehabilitation. It includes measures of physical, cognitive, emotional, behavioral, and social problems that people with brain injury may encounter.

The GOS is a 5-point scale and the GOSE an 8-point scale ranging from *death* to *good recovery*, so neither is useful for determining the effects of cognitive rehabilitation because the categories are too broad. The BI is a 20-point scale covering bowels, bladder, feeding, stairs, dressing, and so on. The upper score equals independence. Although this scale has its uses in physical rehabilitation, it does not capture changes in cognitive functioning. The 18-item FIM has items similar to the BI, whereas the FAM includes 12 items assessing cognitive, behavioral, communication, and community functioning. Again, the scales are too broad and insensitive to measure such changes as better use of an external memory aid or whether someone remembers to take medication. The Mayo-Portland is a useful measure; it is predictive of employment and independent living (Testa, Malec, Moessner, & Brown, 2005). The participation index can be used to measure the amount people engage socially, and a brief eight-item version exists.

Other scales such as the European Brain Injury Questionnaire (EBIQ; Teasdale et al., 1997) and the Brain Injury Community Rehabilitation Outcomes (Powell, Beckers, & Greenwood, 1998) capture some aspects of rehabilitation. In addition to these standardized scales, measures such as return to work or return to independent living may be used. As far as memory is concerned, however, if we accept that the essence of rehabilitation is to help people achieve personally relevant goals and participate in personally valued activities, then goal achievement is the obvious way to measure success. Goals are what patients want to achieve; they may be at "floor" or "ceiling" on other measures, yet may still become more independent, learn to use a memory system, and gain a better understanding of the nature of their problems. Randall and McEwen (2000) considered that the more specific the goals in terms of the patient's personal context, the better the outcome will be.

In summary, memory rehabilitation should be centered around goals: Goal setting is the focus of current rehabilitation and achievement of goals is a straightforward outcome measure that does not preclude the use of other measures such as rating scales, questionnaires, and measures of independence. We can even use standardized tests to determine whether people have, incidentally, improved on these, although we should always be aware that the purpose of rehabilitation is not solely to improve test scores. Finally, we need to be very sure that any change is not the result of a practice effect (Wilson, Watson, Baddeley, Enslie, & Evans, 2000).

## Goal Setting in Clinical Practice

We now consider the process of goal planning, short-term versus long-term goals, and action plans. We then look at goals for day patients, inpatients, and outpatients. The stages involved in goal planning can be seen in Figure 9.1.

Following multidisciplinary assessments and observations, there will be discussions with clients, families, staff, and possibly other support services to consider the person's needs, desires, and hopes. Then there will be a formulation. As mentioned, formulation is a process of deriving hypotheses concerning the nature, causes, and factors influencing current problems or a client's present situation. Formulation takes into account the multitude of possible influences on an individual's level of functioning and psychological state. It also helps the team and the client to understand the problems. In an interdisciplinary rehabilitation

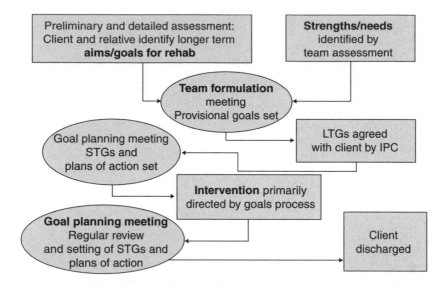

**FIGURE 9.1.** Stages involved in goal planning. STG = short-term goal; LTG = long-term goal; IPC = Individual Program Coordinator. Courtesy the Oliver Zangwill Centre.

team, where a range of assessments (and interventions) may be carried out by different professionals, formulation helps bring together results of these assessments into a single coherent whole. Presenting this visually, through a chart or graph, may help summarize the information and promote a shared understanding and team work. A good clinical formulation should lead to appropriate and relevant interventions. In a situation where multiple influences on functioning are present, it is likely that a range of interventions are required. These are most likely to be effective if they are conducted in the same time period and by people who are aware of what else is going on.

After formulation, the identification of goals can proceed. As stressed earlier, it is essential that clients be involved in the process of setting goals. Holliday, Cano, Freeman, and Playford (2007) examined the impact of increased patient participation in goal setting. The patients who had more input in the establishment of their goals perceived their goals to be more relevant and expressed more satisfaction with the goal-setting process than those who received the treatment-as-usual procedure. Goal setting should follow SMART principles: being **Specific**, **Measurable**, **Achievable**, **Realistic**, and **Time based** (*www.projectsmart. co.uk*). An example of a SMART goal involves Peter (Wilson, Gracey, et al., in press). One of Peter's long-term goals was to manage his own financial affairs. One of the short-term goals toward achieving this was to be able to sign his own checks. He had apraxia, so writing was difficult for him. The aim was for Peter to sign any check in 6 seconds, and he was to achieve this within 2 weeks (this was certainly specific). At the start, he took almost 30 seconds to sign each check (easy to measure); he could do the task but was very slow. The team felt he could achieve a goal requiring him to do the task faster (achievable). Because Peter needed to be able to sign checks in order to manage his own financial affairs, the task was realistic. The time of 2 weeks was set, so the "T" element (time based) of SMART was part of the process. Two extra letters can be added to make the acronym "SMARTER," with the last "E" and "R" standing for **Evaluate** and **Review** (MEC Services Ltd., *www.mecservices.co.uk*). Peter was evaluated (timed) on each occasion he needed to sign a check and was reviewed every 2 weeks at a goal-planning meeting. The wording of the goal should be thought through carefully, with the client having the last say to ensure he or she retains "ownership" of the goal. Short-term goals and plans of action need to be established (see following discussion). The goals must then be reviewed.

In most rehabilitation centers, there will be a lead person for each patient or client. This person will probably chair the goal review meetings and provide an update on progress, along with any issues or concerns that have arisen. This may be followed by comments and general concerns from the staff. There will probably be a review of the formulation and the goals. New short-term goals and plans of action will be set together with a date for next meeting. If the long-term goals have been achieved or are considered unachievable, then new ones may also be set.

Although the frequency of the review meetings depends on time scales for goal achievement, regular reviews are essential. Goals may be achieved, partially achieved, or not achieved. If they are not or only partially reached, the team and the client need to know why. Variance codes may be useful. Four category codes are used at the Oliver Zangwill Centre to record the reason why goals were not achieved: client/caregiver (e.g., client was unwell), staff (e.g., insufficient therapy time available), internal administration (e.g., bus to collect the patient did not arrive), and external administration (e.g., a work trial was canceled).

We now turn to examples of goals for day patients, inpatients, and outpatients. Although the goal areas are different for each group, some aspects are common to all. Collicutt-McGrath (2008) discussed nine life goal areas that are likely to affect all rehabilitation patients (see Table 9.1). These can be measured by the *Rivermead Life Goals Questionnaire* (Davis et al., 1992).

**TABLE 9.1. Life Goal Areas Likely
to Affect All Rehabilitation Patients**

1. Residential and domestic issues.
2. Personal care.
3. Leisure, hobbies, and interests.
4. Work.
5. Relationship with partner.
6. Family life.
7. Friends.
8. Religion or life philosophy.
9. Finances.

*Note.* Data from Davis et al. (1992).

This questionnaire may help us decide which areas are of particular importance to our clients. Our specific goals are likely to fit under broad domains such as mobility, communication, self-care, productivity, leisure, understanding brain injury, mood, and cognitive functioning. Memory, of course, comes under cognitive functioning, but memory-impaired people will also have a range of other goals set in addition to the specific memory ones. Bateman et al. (2005) examined 680 goals set for 95 clients at the Oliver Zangwill Centre in the United Kingdom. The most common goals ($n = 248$) were those concerned with managing activities of daily living, followed by leisure goals and goals relating to understanding the consequences of brain injury (both $ns = 154$), and then work or study skill goals ($n = 119$). This same study showed that of the 680 goals set, only 50 were not achieved. The remainder were wholly or partially achieved, and on two of the other outcome measures—the EBIQ (Teasdale et al., 1997) and the Dysexecutive Questionnaire (Burgess et al., 1998)—there was a significant improvement in scores from the beginning to the end of the program.

The Oliver Zangwill Centre in Ely provides a 6-month day rehabilitation program for people who have some chance of returning to work or further education. Before patients begin the full program, they will have received a 2-week detailed assessment. During this time, they will have undergone a neuropsychological assessment of their cognitive and emotional functioning as well as assessments from other therapists regarding, for example, activities of daily living. The latter might include shopping, cooking, road safety, communication skills, and psychosocial assessments. In addition, they will have been observed in group and individual sessions. During this two-week period, clients are asked to think about possible goals for the full program.

When clients start the 6-month program, goals are reconsidered and drawn up following meetings with other team members, the client, and family members. Most will work on seven or eight long-term goals during the program, but some will have more and some less. Many, but not all, have one or two memory goals, and most have a goal concerned with understanding the consequences of their brain injury. There will also be one or two goals relating to mood and emotion, a goal concerned with leisure, and one connected to work or education. Other frequent goal areas relate to driving, family responsibilities, self-esteem or confidence, emotional well-being, and, frequently, specific personally important goals. Peter, for example, was passionate about flying his model helicopter and, because he was no longer able to do so because of his brain injury, felt strongly that he wanted to include this as a goal (Wilson, Evans, & Keohane, 2002; Wilson, Gracey, et al., in press). Lorna, a patient with dysphasia and severe word-finding difficulties, used pictures to remind her to achieve her goals (Prince et al., in press; see Table 9.2).

Like all goals, memory goals are broken down into short-term goals and action plans. Long-term goals are those expected to be achieved

**TABLE 9.2. A Brief Description of One of the Goals Set for Lorna, a Woman with Dysphasia**

- Lorna, a 34-year-old woman, sustained a gunshot wound to her head in 1999.
- Scans showed the bullet entered through the left lateral orbital margin and exited in the left parieto-occipital region.
- She was assessed in 2004 at the Oliver Zangwill Centre.
- Residual difficulties were expressive and receptive dysphasia, memory, attention, and anger management.
- One goal selected by Lorna was to be independent in remembering appointments and other daily tasks.
- Because of her language and communication difficulties, written and spoken prompts were inappropriate.
- Lorna decided she wanted to use a filofax, or personal organizer.
- Picture stickers were used for her to put onto the relevant date to remind her what she had to do (e.g., a picture of teeth to remind her to go to the dentist, of people dancing to remind her to go to her dance class, and of tablets to remind her to collect her prescription).
- Weekly therapy helped Lorna learn to plan out her week.
- She was able to recall appointments.
- Her husband helped her to print out the stickers.
- On discharge from the center her husband helped Lorna to plan her week.

*Note.* Data from Prince et al. (in press).

by the time of discharge from the program, in this case 6 months. As mentioned, short-term goals are steps toward the long-term goal and are expected to be achieved in 1 or 2 weeks. Action plans are steps taken by someone other than the client to help achieve a short-term goal. If someone other than the patient is carrying out the activity, this is not a goal. When drawing up an action plan, it should be made clear who is to do what and *how* this will be achieved. Take, as an example, the long-term goal "Joe will learn to use a memory system to remember what he has to do each day." The first short-term goal might be "Joe will choose an aid and try it out for a week to see if he thinks it might be suitable for him." The action plans might be as follows: "1. Donna, Joe's occupational therapist, will take Joe to the memory aids resource center by car on Wednesday to look at the memory aids there. 2. Donna will discuss with Joe the pros and cons of several aids and help him select one. 3. Donna will arrange for Joe to borrow the chosen aid for a week to try out at the rehabilitation center." If Joe likes the aid, the second short-term goal for him might be "Joe will learn to put in the day, date, and time of one new appointment by himself." The action plan might be "Donna will demonstrate to Joe how to do this and, using an errorless learning approach, teach Joe how to accomplish this task." The EL learning approach might be to take Joe through each step three times and then use a backward chaining approach to see whether he can accomplish the steps himself. If he looks as if he is about to make a mistake Donna will preempt this by guiding his hand," and so the process goes on. Wilson, Gracey, et al. (in press) provided detailed examples of this approach at the Oliver Zangwill Centre. Another action plan might be that Donna will purchase the aid for Joe when the one he is trying out has to be returned to the resource center.

For inpatients the principles are the same, but the nature of the goals may be very different. For somebody in PTA, the goal maybe to teach him or her to look at the orientation board in the ward to check what day it is. The first short-term goal might be learn the location of the board ("Susan will learn the location of the orientation board"), and the action plan might be "Kate (Susan's nurse) will take Susan to the board and say, "This is the board that tells you today's day and date." Kate will follow a spaced retrieval plan so once Susan has dressed and had breakfast, Kate will take her to the board and return to the day room. She will repeat the process after 2 minutes, then 5 minutes, 10 minutes, 20 minutes, and 30 minutes. Susan will then be asked if she can find the board that tells today's day and date. She can be prompted if necessary. If Susan appears confused, Kate should return to the beginning but build up more slowly in 5-minute increments. For inpatients who are out of PTA, the goals may be focused on finding their way around the hospital to different departments or learning the names of staff and other patients plus learning to use an external memory aid.

A colleague in London, Rene Stolwyk, described a goal for an inpatient who needed to remember to go to the toilet. The long-term goal was for the patient to use the toilet independently. To maximize motivation, the patient was told there would be a number of short-term goals that would become progressively more difficult. The first short-term goal was for him to agree to go to the toilet when the nurse prompted him. Once this was achieved, the second short-term goal was to set an alarm and for the patient to ask the nurse for the toilet once the alarm sounded. This was followed by the patient setting the alarm when prompted, then for him to set the alarm without prompting, then to only use the alarm at night before achieving the final step of using the toilet independently with no alarm or prompting. This was successfully achieved within 2 weeks.

For outpatients, once again, the principles are the same but the goals will probably be different and possibly have more to do with independence in everyday life. Wilson (1999), for example, discussed the case of Jack, who became amnesic because of carbon monoxide poisoning. An outpatient seen weekly for several weeks, Jack wanted to remember where his car was parked and where he had put his belongings; he also wanted to make sure he did not double-book appointments. As discussed, Clare et al.'s (1999) patient, V. J., diagnosed with AD 6 years earlier, wanted to relearn the names of people at the club he attended once a week. He was seen weekly at home and learned 11 names, one each week from photographs of the club members. This learning generalized to the real people at the club and was maintained for 9 months.

Whether working with inpatients, day patients, or outpatients, other goals set for memory-impaired people will need to take into account their memory problems. Sometimes specific learning strategies will be required to teach the use of an electronic aid or to become familiar with a new computer program. Hart, Hawkey, and Whyte (2002) asked clients to record their goals on a voice organizer, which was used to prompt them to review their goals from time to time. There was evidence that this led to better recall of therapy goals. For emotional and mood goals, it may be helpful to use a pager or timer to remind people to perform relaxation exercises or breathing techniques to reduce anxiety.

Caroline (Evans, in press-b), described in Chapter 8, had severe PTSD plus memory problems, so using the general guidelines outlined in Chapter 1 helped her to achieve her goals. These included the following:

1. Understand the consequences of her brain injury, their impact on her daily life, and the strategies that she can use to manage them.
2. Reduce the intensity of daily intrusive thoughts/images.
3. Reduce the frequency of unpleasant dreams (from severe to moderate).
4. Rate herself as comfortable in more than 70% of interactions in personal relationships.
5. Rate herself as being hopeful more than 50% of the time.
6. Use a memory and planning system to carry out independent living activities successfully on at least 80% of occasions.
7. Use strategies to sustain attention during everyday activities in order to concentrate on them successfully on more than 70% of occasions.
8. Be able to engage comfortably in identified activities previously avoided, including (a) travel independently by train on at least one short familiar route, (b) go shopping at a moderately busy time, (c) feel comfortable in an unfamiliar pub or restaurant, and (d) feel comfortable in a cinema.
9. Engage in a physical leisure activity on a weekly basis.
10. Undertake a vocationally related course and have a clearly documented plan for returning to paid employment (Evans, in press-b).

In Chapter 10 we aim to encapsulate previously discussed knowledge by designing a program for memory rehabilitation.

# CHAPTER 10

# Putting It All Together

## Before Starting a Memory Rehabilitation Program

Anyone referred for help with memory problems should be given some general advice and memory tips—for example, that drugs and alcohol will affect memory, fatigue and poor sleep may impair functioning, and people may need to reduce their expectations. Kapur (2008) offered 10 memory tips to help cope with difficulties, and he divided these into four sections (see Table 10.1). The general guidelines on ways to improve encoding, storage, and retrieval described in Chapter 1 should also be borne in mind.

## First Steps in Planning a Memory Rehabilitation Program

When one is asked to see a memory-impaired person for help with everyday problems, there will probably be information in the referral letter about the original cause of difficulties (i.e., whether the person has sustained a TBI, a stroke, encephalitis, or anoxia or whether there has been a diagnosis of dementia). The exact nature of the problems may not be addressed, however, so an interview and an assessment may be required. If the person has already had a neuropsychological assessment, then this may suffice for a cognitive map of the individual's strengths and weaknesses. Is the person currently functioning in the average range of ability or the superior range, or is she or he below average or impaired? Is this below the expected premorbid level? Is the

**TABLE 10.1. Ten Key Memory Tips**

Take it easy

1. Try not to do too many things at once.
2. Anxiety and tiredness can affect memory, so try to avoid stressful situations. Be positive and have regular breaks.
3. If you do forget something, don't get too upset about it. Stay calm and think of connections that may jog your memory.

Be well organized

4. Keep to a fixed routine, with set things at set times of the day and on set days of the week.
5. Be systematic: Have a place for everything and put everything back in its place. Put labels on drawers and files.

Concentrate better

6. If you have to do something, do it now rather than later: "Do it or lose it."
7. Try not to let your mind wander: Keep on track.
8. If you have to remember something such as a message or a name, go over it in your mind at regular intervals.
9. Try to find meaning in things you have to remember (e.g., by making associations or linking things together).

Use memory aids

10. Use memory aids such as Whiteboards, Post-it Notes, notebooks, diaries/ calendars, mobile phones, and alarms to help you remember messages and help you remember to do things at the right time.

*Note.* Reprinted with permission from Narinder Kapur.

level of memory functioning severely impaired, moderately impaired, or mildly impaired? Does the person have memory deficits across all modalities, or is verbal memory better or worse than visual memory? Is there a significant period of RA? Is the immediate memory span in the normal range (as one would expect for most people with impaired memory functioning)? What about other cognitive abilities? Does the person have normal language and reading skills? Are their scores on tests of visuoperceptual and visuospatial functioning normal? Is there evidence of poor attention and executive skills? A good picture of intellectual functioning will help us select the right program and strategies, because we should not ask the cognitively impossible of any patient. What about emotional difficulties? Does the person suffer from extreme anxiety or depression or PTSD? A thorough emotional assessment using the procedures described in Chapter 8 should complement the cognitive assessment.

# Complementing the Neuropsychological Assessment with a Behavioral Assessment

A full neuropsychological evaluation will not tell us which problems are causing the most stress for the patient and the family; it will simply inform us of the person's strengths and weaknesses and determine whether we need to address additional cognitive and emotional difficulties as well as the memory ones. A functional or behavioral assessment will be required to determine which everyday problems should be targeted. This can be carried out through observations; interviews with staff, patients, and families; and self-report measures, such as diaries, rating scales, and questionnaires. Of course, patients with memory problems will not always be aware of the nature of their difficulties because they may not remember them, but we can at least see how they *perceive* their problems and obtain some idea about their level of insight. Family members, caregivers, and other professional staff involved may have a better understanding, and we may well want to ask these significant others to complete rating scales, checklists, or questionnaires. Is there a discrepancy between the results of the patient and the significant other or not?

Behavioral assessment procedures have provided cognitive rehabilitation with a number of techniques for measuring behavior. According to Hall (1971), there are three main types of measurement: automatic recording, measurement of permanent product, and observational recording. Automatic recording, could, for example, be used to measure how many times a patient wanders from the ward provided an alarm system could be used to monitor each time the patient went through the door leaving the ward. Measurement of permanent product refers to measurement of something that remains after a particular behavior, for example, how many lines of typing have been completed or how many crossword puzzles have been attempted? There is no doubt, though, that observational recording is the most relevant for rehabilitation. This recording can also be subdivided into the following categories:

1. *Continuous recording.* One records *everything* a person does in a given situation (i.e., each movement, word, activity, and so forth). Continuous recording is difficult to achieve over an extended period of time, although video- or audiotapes can be used to achieve a more accurate record.

2. *Event recording.* A target behavior is defined and every instance of that behavior is recorded. We might, for example, be interested in how many times a question is asked during the course of a day or how

many times a notebook is referred to. Again, although this might be difficult for some high-frequency behaviors, it can be useful for certain behaviors such as applying wheelchair brakes before transferring or remembering to take medication. In practice, event recording is usually confined to certain periods of the day or week, such as during an occupational therapy session or during lunch break. This recording method can also lead to inaccuracy if one is sampling a period when the behavior is more or less likely to occur. If people only repeat questions when a certain member of staff is present or at a particular time of the day and we are not sampling this, we will have an inaccurate record. In these cases, one would need to ensure that the periods sampled were, indeed, representative or else we need to sample a range of times to reduce the likelihood of a false picture.

   3. *Duration recording.* This is used when it is important to know for how long a certain behavior lasts. For example, if we need to know how long it takes someone to read a particular passage or how long someone can work at a task, then duration recording might be the method of choice. One disadvantage is that it is not always easy to determine when a particular behavior stops and starts. For example, if one is measuring time on task and the person stops to look at the ceiling, it may not be clear whether the person is thinking about the next step or has lost concentration.

   4. *Interval recording.* This is a convenient method of sampling behavior. The total observation period is divided into time intervals and the observer notes whether or not the target behavior occurs at all during that time interval. This method is particularly useful for certain behaviors such as repetition of a story, question, or joke. A further advantage is that is that it can indicate both the severity and duration of a behavior. A major disadvantage is that it is an *estimate* and not an accurate recording of the frequency of the target behavior. If repetition of a question occurs at all in the interval, it will be noted but the note does not distinguish between one or two repetitions and 50 repetitions. In practice, clinicians may combine interval recording and event recording, so that if one samples repetition behavior for a 15-minute interval four times a day, one could note *how many* (event recording) repetitions occur during that interval.

   5. *Time sampling.* The observer records at the end of a predetermined interval (e.g., every hour *on* the hour). The length of the interval depends on the target behavior itself and the time available to the observer. Thus, one might decide to observe whether or not a person is in the correct room at the end of every 15-minute period during the morning or whether the person is present for meals at the start of every mealtime. The advantage of this method is that it does not require con-

tinuous monitoring, although it does require precise timing to avoid biasing the results. Murphy and Goodall (1980) found that time sampling was a more accurate reflection of the true rate of occurrence of a target behavior than interval recording.

Another way of classifying behavioral assessment procedures is to divide them into self-report and behavioral observation procedures (Hay, 1982). Self-report measures include (1) interviews, (2) questionnaires, rating scales, and checklists, and (3) self-monitoring.

## Behavioral Interviews

The purpose of a behavioral interview is to gain an understanding of the antecedents of the problem behavior, to describe the behavior precisely and unambiguously, and to identify the consequences that maintain the behavior. This may, at first glance, seem strange in the case of memory-impaired people. After all, the antecedents of the problem behaviors, such as forgetting information or failure to acquire new skills, are almost certainly due to the brain injury and the organic memory deficit incurred; the problem behavior is that little or nothing is recalled after a delay; and the consequence of maintaining the behavior is that the memory structures to ensure consolidation, storage, and retrieval are not functioning. Despite this, there are situations when such interviews are helpful. For example, if someone is repeating the same question, story, or joke ad infinitum, there may well be circumstances that trigger and maintain this. Constant repetition can infuriate relatives and caregivers. A behavioral interview might elicit triggers that cause the behavior. Wilson (1999) described a young man, Martin, who was very memory impaired, physically disabled, and very friendly and sociable. To ensure he was paying attention during therapy sessions, Martin was asked, "Are you ready, Martin?" His reply was invariably, "Ready, willing, and disabled." Although amusing at first, the response quickly became irritating. This is a straightforward case. The antecedent to his repetitive "joke" was the question "Are you ready?" The problem behavior was his response, "Ready, willing, and disabled" and the consequence maintaining the behavior was that he had no memory of ever saying this before. The solution was simple: Change the question. To ensure he was paying attention, Martin was told, "We are going to start now, Martin."

Another example (Wilson, 1999) can be found in the chapter on Clive, also described in Chapter 3 of this text. Clive frequently said that his situation was like being dead. Typically, he would say, "This is the first taste I've had, the first sight I've had, it's like being dead." If people sympathized with him or repeated back to him "so it feels like being dead?," he became more and more agitated. Certain questions triggered this behavior as did memory tests. These were the antecedents. The behavior was the statement, "It's like being dead." The consequences maintaining the behavior were responses indicating sympathy or empathy. The problem reduced when caregivers or therapists changed the subject and, instead of sympathizing, asked him something he was comfortable with such as "What age should a child start to learn to play music?" or "What is the best instrument for a child to learn to play?" This calmed him down, and the same calming questions could be asked as often as necessary because Clive did not remember he had been asked the same things before. Behavioral interviewing may not lead to accurate information with the majority of memory-impaired people because they cannot remember what it is they cannot remember or, in other words, they forget what it is that they forget. Alternatively, they may have poor insight. Here one may also wish to interview the relatives, caregivers, and therapists, who may be aware of the situations and can give more accurate information.

### Questionnaires, Rating Scales, and Checklists

These have been used since the early days of psychology (e.g., Galton, 1907). With regard to memory assessment, several questionnaires, rating scales, and checklists have been developed. Questionnaires related to memory failures include the Short Inventory of Memory Experiences (Herrman & Neisser, 1978), the Subjective Memory Questionnaire (Bennett-Levy & Powell, 1980), the Cognitive Failures Questionnaire (Broadbent, Cooper, Fitzgerald, & Parks, 1982), the Everyday Memory Questionnaire (Sunderland, Harris, & Baddeley, 1983), and the Prospective and Retrospective Memory Questionnaire (Crawford, Smith, Maylor, Della Salla, & Logie, 2003). A short 13-item version of the Everyday Memory Questionnaire (originally 28 items) has been published by Royle and Lincoln (2008), who suggest that the short version is a reliable and valid measure.

Rating scales and checklists include the Everyday Memory Symptoms Questionnaire by Kapur and Pearson (1983), which is a simple, short and practical scale. Patients are asked to compare current performance on memory tasks (e.g., remembering to deliver messages or how to get somewhere new) with premorbid performance. Rating is on a 3-point scale (*no change, slightly worse,* and *a great deal worse*) As mentioned before, memory-impaired people are often unaware of their deficits and may overestimate their ability to remember, but this scale is a good measure of their insight and, of course, one can give the scale to relatives and caregivers to see whether there is a marked discrepancy. Olsson, Wik, Ostling, Johansson, and Andersson (2006), however, found a good degree of consistency between self-ratings and significant other ratings among 30 people with brain injury and their caregivers on a modified version of the Everyday Memory Questionnaire. Checklists can provide additional information to that obtained from questionnaires and rating scales. Sunderland, Harris, and Gleave's (1984) checklist has been modified for use with brain-injured people to provide information on the type and frequency of memory failures in different situations (Wilson, 1999). Checklists can, of course, also be used as memory aids, and we return to this later.

## Self-Monitoring Techniques

As far back as 1970, Kanfer said that self-monitoring techniques (i.e., observing one's own behavior) can lead to increases or decreases in that behavior. Recording the amount one eats, for example, can lead to a reduction in the amount eaten. Self-monitoring is sometimes used in memory rehabilitation, typically to try to obtain a record of memory lapses. Patients may be asked to complete a memory diary or note each occasion of a memory failure (see Wilson, 1999). Once again, the problem with using self-monitoring for memory-impaired people is that they may forget to record incidents. Sometimes this can be overcome through training. Alderman, Fry, and Youngson (1995) described how they taught a brain-injured patient to improve her self-monitoring; Kime et al. (1996) also improved self-monitoring in an amnesic patient.

## Behavioral Observations

Observations in the natural environment are important. Because the purpose of rehabilitation is to improve functioning in everyday life, we often need to observe in everyday life. Observations may reveal behavior that is not detected by assessments, interviews, questionnaires, rating scales, or checklists. Clive, the amnesic musician, suffered frequent outbursts of belching and jerking thought to be epileptic in origin. Observations by a trainee psychologist working with him, Avi Schmueli, showed that the outbursts were more frequent when there was a change of activity, such as being asked to do a different test or going from one room to another (Wilson, 1999). This finding would have been hard to detect without observation.

Through observation, one can also see the events leading up to the problem and the consequences maintaining the behavior, and this aids a functional analysis (determining the antecedents, behavior, and consequences). In addition, one can observe how a patient prefers to spend his or her time, which might include sitting doing nothing, reading, chatting with other people, or watching television. These activities can then be used as motivators. One can also observe whether or not any new strategies, skills, or information are used in other situations (i.e., is there transfer of new learning?). Certain behaviors are not amenable to direct observation because they occur in private, because observation changes the behavior, or because the concern is with attitudes, beliefs, or feelings.

Simulated observations are worth considering in some situations such as when one wants to measure an infrequent behavior (e.g., to see how the memory-impaired person explains the brain injury or memory problem to a stranger) or when the observer is short of time or can only observe in a restricted range of situations. It is always possible that simulated situations may lead to inaccurate information, but if one is reasonably confident that the simulated and naturalistic situations are close, then there is much to be said for them. In memory rehabilitation, patients can be asked to role-play in order to observe an aspect of their behavior. Thus, if one of the goals is for a patient to be able to explain to others what has happened to him or to her, this can be observed in role-play situations. If we want to know how someone copes with the telephone and whether he or she can take down messages accurately, we can use role-play to do this. Other options are to use a special room or area to construct a situation. Most occupational therapy departments have a kitchen where one can observe how well patients can cook a meal or follow a recipe, and this principle can be applied to a mock office, classroom, or shop.

There are advantages and disadvantages in all the recording and behavioral assessment techniques, but we need to have some measure of real-life difficulties to provide a baseline against which to judge the efficacy of rehabilitation interventions. When the information from the cognitive, emotional, and behavioral assessments is compiled with other assessments, such as activities of daily living, physiotherapy, and speech and language assessments, and the formulation is completed, the next steps can be taken.

## Goal Setting

As outlined in the previous chapter, rehabilitation programs are planned around goals. In many cases, the patient, family members, and staff involved will have begun thinking about goals before the formulation is completed. The goals need to be meaningful and relevant and follow the SMART principles described in Chapter 9. It is important to set short-term as well as long-term goals because, as Latham and Seijts (1999) found, setting long-term goals alone leads to poorer performance than combining long-term and short-term goals. Goals will be set after discussion with the client, family members, caregivers, and possibly other relevant support services. We need to know what the families and patients perceive as their problems, what are their priorities and needs, and what do they want to be able to do?. We may need to set provisional goals before settling on the final agreed goals. For example, for Simon, a stroke patient, Palmer, Psaila, and Yeates (in press) set the following provisional goals:

- To improve reading and writing.
- To be able to "get words out."
- To return to work as foreman and ground worker.
- To get his driver's license back.
- To feel more like his "old self."

Following assessment, formulation, and negotiation, the goals were renegotiated and agreed on as follows:

- Understanding the injury and its consequences and managing these effectively.
- Being independent in living skills such as budgeting, planning, and managing correspondence and finances.
- Identifying a realistic vocational action plan for the forthcoming 6 to 12 months.

In addition to these areas, Simon also set three goals relevant to parenting and relationships: Simon will be confident in his ability to read short stories to his two younger children as rated by the speech and language therapist and evaluations of two independent raters. Simon will undertake specified parenting roles independently (including being "planful" in arranging their day-to-day activities, supporting them in completing homework, and engaging in leisure activities). Simon will interact more successfully in identified social interactions as rated by himself, his caregiver, and staff at the Oliver Zangwill Centre.

All goals set should be realistic and at least potentially achievable in the time and with the resources available. It is important, too, to phrase the goals in a way that not only feels comfortable to the client but also allows him or her to feel ownership of the goals set. Consistent with SMART principles, it should be specified who will do what, under what conditions, and within what time frame and how success is to be determined. The short-term goals are steps toward the achievement of the long-term goal, and the plans of action state what needs to be done in order for the short-term goal to be achieved. As with the long-term goals, both short-term goals and plans of action should specify who will do what, when, etc. Examples of long-term and short-term goals as well as plans of action can be found in Chapter 9.

Kime (2006), in her practical book *Compensating for Memory Deficits Using a Systematic Approach*, used a slightly different approach to goals. Generally, she starts off with initial short-term goals for the first 4 weeks, then moves on to revised short-term goals for weeks 5 to 11, and finally moves to further revised goals for weeks 11 to 14. One of her patients was a 55-year-old woman who had survived removal of a tumor and also had an aneurysm on the left ophthalmic artery, which had been clipped. The patient's initial short-term goals were (1) Getting to appointments on time, including picking her daughter up from school; (2) tracking medical information, including details of visits to her doctor; (3) doing the laundry each week independently. The revised goals for the middle period of rehabilitation were (4) completing home management tasks and (5) developing and using an organized file system to track financial and other personal records. The final revised goal was (6) meal planning. Compensatory aids were used to achieve all of these goals successfully.

## Selecting the Best Strategies to Achieve the Goals

If possible, we should offer both group and individual therapy to memory-impaired people. We live in groups, we function in groups, and, as stated in Chapter 7, there are many advantages to treating people in groups. Groups can also be designed to help people achieve their goals. If they are expected to use memory aids, this can be done during the group session. If the goal is to gain confidence, groups may help achieve this. If the goal is to be oriented in time and place, then, again, this can be covered during the group session.

Previous chapters describe a number of strategies to help memory-impaired people achieve their goals. If people need to learn new information, then the EL learning, spaced retrieval, and VC techniques can be considered together with mnemonics and rehearsal strategies. For learning people's names, EL learning combined with visual mnemonics, VC, and spaced retrieval may be the method of choice. If the goal is to learn a new computer program (or how to use a computer in the first place), then EL learning, spaced retrieval, and VC have all proved to be useful. For improving studying skills, the PQRST technique may be of benefit.

For patients with emotional problems, Chapter 8 outlines a number of ways to deal with these. Attending groups may also reduce anxiety and stress. The purpose of mood management groups, described in Chapter 7, is to enable patients to develop skills and strategies for coping with emotional difficulties. Toward this end, clients are helped to discuss and share their experiences with other clients and are provided with a "tool box" of strategies to help them experience different ways of coping with emotional challenges.

For people whose goal is to remember more daily events, it might be worth considering using a camera to record daily happenings. Sense-Cam was briefly described in Chapter 4. This is a wearable camera developed by Microsoft Research, Cambridge, which captures several hundred images per day, to aid autobiographical memory in memory-impaired people. It can be plugged into a standard personal computer that automatically downloads the recorded images and allows them to be viewed at speed, like watching a film. Some preliminary studies evaluating this new camera have been carried out by Berry et al. (2007), and it looks promising for at least some people with memory deficits.

If the goal is to remember to do things or to use a memory system effectively, then one of the many aids described in Chapter 4 may be helpful. Kime (2006) also described a number of aids and explained how some of these can be modified and taught to memory-impaired people. For example, her structure for learning to use a personal organizer includes the following:

1. Make sure the person has the organizer in his or her possession at all times.
2. Train the support network to cue the client to keep the organizer in possession at all times.
3. Identify a prominent place to keep the organizer (this should be highly visible).
4. Place notes or placards where they cannot be overlooked (e.g., on the door leaving the house and definitely *not* in the organizer).
5. Ensure the client checks the organizer frequently.
6. Consult the alarm every hour (associating this with an hourly alarm may be necessary for some clients).
7. Consult the organizer at predefined times or at variable times depending on the nature of the tasks to be carried out.

Kime then discussed the following:

*Using the daily pages*

- Where to enter the information.
- When to enter the information.
- Writing legible and concise notes.
- Retrieving the information through scanning and marking completed tasks.

*Using the month-at-a-glance calendar*

- Determining what information belongs here.
- Entering information.
- Remembering to review the calendar.
- Transferring information to daily pages.

There is not one right or wrong way to teach this, but they are all things to be considered when helping a memory-impaired person to use a memory system.

## Checklists as Treatment Strategies

In 1993 I had the fortune to spend time with Susan Kime in Arizona and was impressed by her ability to teach memory-impaired people how to achieve even complex tasks through the use of checklists. The patient described by Kime et al. (1996) was one such patient. She was extremely amnesic, and Kime decided to teach her to use a memory book containing many sections (e.g., a map of the rehabilitation center, her daily timetable, things to do, names of staff, and several other sections). I thought this was too ambitious, but Kime succeeded brilliantly and the young woman with severe amnesia was eventually able to hold down a job through excellent use of her memory system. Much of the work was accomplished through checklists in which the individual steps to complete any task are listed for the patient to work through and check each step. Learning to set an hourly alarm is an example. A watch with a chime and an hourly alarm is provided as well as a list of steps on how to use it (see Figure 10.1.).

According to Kime (2006), most patients will need two or three sessions with a therapist on how to use the checklist. The steps for the watch alarm are fairly complex, but lists can be made for any task, however small or difficult. Kime's example of an easier task is a list for use of the toilet with a wheelchair-dependent patient:

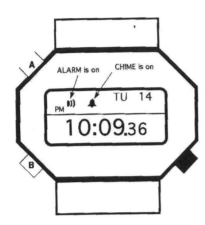

### FUNCTIONS
CHIME—goes off on the hour
ALARM—goes off for the time that is set

### CHIME INSTRUCTIONS
("chime" should always be on)
1. Press button B until the letters "AL" are displayed.
2. Press button C to rotate through "alarm" and "chime" symbols, until only the "chime" symbol is showing.
3. Press button B *once* to return to normal time mode.
4. The chime is now set.

### ALARM INSTRUCTIONS
1. Press button B until the letters "AL" are displayed.
2. Press button A to begin alarm setting procedure (hour should be flashing).
3. Press button C to advance hours. The letters PM will appear in the upper-left-hand corner if the alarm is to be set for a PM time.
4. Press button A to start next number flashing. Use button C to advance numbers.
5. Press button A once the alarm time is set.
6. Press button B to return to normal display. The alarm is now set and armed. The "alarm" symbol should be showing.

### TO TURN OFF THE ALARM
1. Press button B until the letters "AL" are displayed.
2. Press button C to rotate through "alarm" and "chime" symbols, until only the "chime" symbol is showing.
3. Press button B *once* to return to normal time mode.
4. The alarm is now turned off and the hourly chime is left on.

**FIGURE 10.1.** Instructions on using a watch alarm. Reprinted with permission from Susan Kime.

1. Lock both wheelchair brakes.
2. Put both feet on the floor.
3. Reach for the toilet arm. DO NOT USE TOWEL RACK. (p. 40)

## The Example of Jay

Jay sustained a brain hemorrhage at the age of 20 and was left with severe amnesia. With the help of his family, some rehabilitation, and his own efforts, he developed a sophisticated system over the years. This has been so successful that he is able to live alone, earn his own living, and even complete his own tax forms despite the fact that his severe memory deficits have persisted (Wilson, J. C., & Hughes, 1997; Wilson, 1999). Because of the paucity of natural histories of such systems and because Jay keeps extensive notes, his own account of the development of his system is provided here.* Of particular interest is the way Jay was able to become self-employed through use of his system.

*Stage 1.* Between October and December 1986, I used a notebook, which I kept in my shirt pocket and a watch with an alarm, which sounded every hour. Whenever the alarm sounded, I wrote down what I was doing. Later I transferred this information to a journal, but I did little in the way of forward planning.

*Stage 2.* "The Grand Plan," January 1987. I had a weekly sheet on my desk as well as a daily sheet, which I filled with details from my weekly sheet and one-time appointments from my diary. The daily card was kept in a small diary. The proposal was:

1. All appointments were to be written down.
2. There would be a daily card in my diary.
3. A written list would be on my desk of all daily and weekly tasks (the weekly sheet).
4. Tasks would be transferred to my daily card in the evening or morning. Evie [Jay's aunt] or one of my sisters would prompt me to do this.

Initially, I used the back of my appointments diary as a record of the day. Very soon, however, I used a spiral-bound notebook instead. The diary was strapped with an elastic band to the notebook, and both fitted into the top pocket of my shirt. At this stage it was important that I carried the notebook on my person at all times.

The emphasis was now focused on forward planning and not concentrating on the past.

---

*Adapted from Wilson, J. C., and Hughes (1997). Adapted by permission from Psychology Press, Taylor and Francis, and Informa-World (www.informaworld.com).

*Stage 3*. I obtained a Dictaphone to record ongoing events, which I transcribed into my journal in the evening.

*Stage 4*. April 1987. When writing the daily card, I used the pocket diary as well as the weekly sheet. This was an attempt to set up a routine whereby when the alarm goes off for an appointment, it is reset for the next appointment on the daily card. (This was never very successful, even at the time of getting my Seiko RC 4000 watch in 1989.)

*Stage 5*. In September 1987 I moved to my own flat on the same road as my parents' home. I removed the old front door key from my keyring so I would not go there by mistake.

*Stage 6*. October 1987. There was a problem of how I was to get information out of the diary since, as I read through it, I would forget what I was looking for. One of my sisters gave me a small loose-leaf diary, similar to a thin filofax, which seemed to help.

*Stage 7*. December 1987. I missed appointments because of forgetting to set my watch, so I made an extra effort to do this.

*Stage 8*. January 1988. I bought a filofax.

*Stage 9*. February 1988. In early February I missed an appointment with my youngest sister. She got cross with me to see if this would help. It seemed to have worked as I kept three extraordinary appointments during the week.

*Stage 10*. March 1988. My watch setting was better.

*Stage 11*. April 1988. Watch setting okay now. I was making notes in my filofax of the time spent on my projects.

*Stage 12*. July 1988. I started typing to see whether a computer would be useful. I worked out the framework of a computer program which would help me retrieve information from my diary.

*Stage 13*. September 1988. I started at the London College of Furniture. I had maps showing me how to get there as well as a note to get on the front of the train so I used the right exit out of the station.

*Stage 14*. 13 October 1988. I looked into the possibility of using a computer to record my diary. There were problems with the size of the database and also problems getting information out of the database.

*Stage 15*. February 1989. My diary was typed on to the computer. I was given a new watch, a Seiko RC 4000. Instructions for putting information into the watch were written on a sheet in my filofax. Six weeks later I had memorized these stages.

*Stage 16*. April 1989. When away from home I used my coat as a base. I used a Dictaphone to plan my coursework and found it best to do the planning at the end of each lesson.

My college binder had different sections for different skills. For shopping I now had different sections for different shops rather than putting everything on one list. So, for example, groceries would go in one section and meat in another.

*Stage 17*. September 1990. I started courses at the Twickenham and Richmond College. I used an A–Z map on the bus to know when to get off. After 20 journeys, I knew without checking the map when to get off. I had a map of the college grounds to get to the workshop and another map to get from Twickenham to Richmond. Finally, I had notes on bus numbers and the position of the stops.

*Stage 18.* (since 1990). In January 1991 I had a date with a girlfriend. The notes I made on my Dictaphone during the evening were written on a yellow sheet, with her name at the top, in my filofax. Later I called this a social sheet. Notes from later meetings were added to go on to the sheet. A second and third sheet followed. I then used social sheets for other people. A colleague at work holds the record, and he currently has nine social sheets. Most of these will be saved in a reserve file. Sticky-back Post-it Notes are put on to the social sheets with suggestions and ideas for future joint activities, when to make the next telephone call, and so forth. Gradually, different colored sheets were used for different aspects of my life.

Whenever anything had to be done to my flat, a green sheet was used. The pilot light on my boiler periodically gets clogged, so I need to call in the plumber. He is currently on his third social sheet. Details of what needs to be done are written on Post-it Notes so I know what to say when I phone him. Once the work has been done, I enter it on the social sheet.

If I come across a restaurant I particularly like, I note this on a red sheet. I include the name, the phone number, the address, how to get there, the kind of food served, and some idea of how much a meal would cost. I then make a note of when I've been, with whom, and how much I spent. I occasionally note a particularly good dish (e.g., "Beef with sweet basil is fab").

I began to use pink sheets in 1995 for miscellaneous information such as notes on a new swimming pool that had opened nearby or details of a holiday that required coordination of various dates and train times. I now call these "leisure sheets." The final kind of sheet is blue, and I will say more about this in the next section.

*Stage 19.* Since 1992 I have been self-employed. I French polish and recane and rerush chairs. The current system is this: A customer will phone and say he has a job for me. If it is to recane or rerush a chair, the chair is usually delivered to me but sometimes I will collect it. If it is a French polishing job, I need to go out and provide a quote.

I then open a job sheet in my filofax. A job number goes on the sheet together with the client's name, address, and telephone number. I also record the date the job began, the deadline for completion, the type of job, the price quoted, and the job details. The job number corresponds with a numbered page in an A5 duplicate book. This process is slightly modified for work with dealers.

I take the customer's details, and we agree a time when I will provide a quote. I make a note on the relevant daily sheet (e.g., "To job 455"). I also set my watch alarm so I leave in good time. I quote for the job and the customer retains the top copy from the job book as a record of what has been agreed on. We also agree on a time when I will return (or when the customer will collect). I note on my daily sheet in the filofax when I will carry out the job and also set the watch alarm. I note how long I spend on each job and log this in the job book and on the job sheet. I also note the cost of materials. When the customer pays, this is recorded in the job book, and the job sheet in the filofax is then discarded.

These colored sheets and their cross-referencing capability give a capacity to retrieve information, which is of more value than a computer program because several sheets can be viewed at the same time. It is also more portable and less prone to theft. The fact that the sheets are different colors makes them easier to find in my filofax.

Jay's aunt also kept notes about his progress and describes the different kinds of lists and alarms Jay uses. Although not absolutely foolproof, there is no doubt that Jay has developed a very effective system to cope with his memory problems, and his contribution is an admirable example of what can be achieved by someone who compensates so well.

## Generalization or Transfer of Learning

Many rehabilitation programs fail because insufficient account is taken of generalization. If we teach someone to use a compensatory aid in the rehabilitation center, this may not be used in other situations; if we can teach someone to apply the wheelchair brakes before transferring in hospital we do not know that this will happen when the person leaves hospital; and if we can stop someone asking the same question over and over again in occupational therapy, the repetitions may recur once the person goes home. Planning for generalization should be part of every program. Verfaellie, Rajaram, Fossum, and Williams (2008) improved generalization in a research study by providing varied semantic contexts in which words were repeated. In comparison to the same number of repetitions in a fixed semantic context, memory-impaired people did better in a recognition task when the contexts were varied.

There are different types of generalization, including generalization across settings (probably the most important in rehabilitation), generalization across behaviors or problems, and generalization across people. The first refers to situations in which a strategy learned in one setting is used in another. Thus, if a memory-impaired person learns to use an electronic aid in a memory group but fails to use it elsewhere, generalization has not occurred. The second, generalization across behaviors or problems, refers to situations in which strategies taught to deal with one behavior or problem are applied to other behaviors or problems. For example, if someone is taught to use the PQRST procedure to improve recall of newspaper articles and then uses the same procedure to remember schoolwork, generalization has occurred. In the third type, generalization across people, when it has been established that a strategy is effective for one person, we want to know whether the same strategy is effective for others. Thus, if we demonstrate that EL learning is a good method for teaching a new computer program to John, we question whether this will also be a good strategy for Mary, Sally, and Joe. In other words, does the strategy generalize across people?

We can enhance generalization in a number of ways. For inpatients, having time at home before final discharge may lead to an increase in the application of strategies learned in the hospital. We can also educate family members and other caregivers about the nature of the memory-impaired person's difficulties and how best to handle these. Home visits, follow-up appointments, and reviews can determine whether procedures, techniques, and strategies are being maintained. Before this, however, we should address generalization as part of treatment, and, if it is not occurring spontaneously, we need to teach generalization. If someone is taught to use an electronic aid or any other memory system in the rehabilitation center, we need to observe whether or not it is used in other places, such as on the ward, at home, or at work. If it is not used, then we should encourage, prompt, or use the original teaching strategy again to ensure it is used in these other places. If a patient learns the names of therapists, friends, and neighbors through photographs in a treatment session, it is essential to make sure this learning transfers to real life. For example, we can take the patient for a walk around the center or the neighborhood to meet these people and see whether the patient can greet them by name and, if not, teach in other situations, preferably with the therapist, friend, or neighbor present. Family members and caregivers can be taught how to ensure generalization. The important thing is to consciously address generalization and not to expect it to occur spontaneously. If it does, then it is a bonus, but if not the whole rehabilitation program can be a waste of time.

## A Framework for Planning a Rehabilitation Program

I have previously described a basic framework for planning treatment (Wilson, 1992; Wilson et al., 2003) and reiterate these steps here because I have found them to be very useful for thinking about any problem I am asked to deal with in rehabilitation. Although probably first used for disruptive behaviors, the framework can be applied to memory and other cognitive deficits, motor problems, and even emotional difficulties. This framework can be used alongside the SMART goals described previously. The two are not mutually exclusive.

1. *Define the behavior to be changed.* Avoid vague and general terms like "poor memory" or "forgets easily" because it is hard to measure these, and we will not know whether our treatment has been successful. It is better to say something like "Does not use a memory aid" or "Cannot find her bed on the ward."

2. *Decide whether an operational definition is needed.* Operational definitions are useful when it is hard to pin down the problem. For example, if a patient is said to have "poor concentration" or "no self-control," one could observe the patient in situations where she or he is thought to demonstrate poor concentration or loss of self-control and, depending on the circumstances, say something like "For the purposes of this treatment, we will operationally define poor attention as an inability to work for more than 2 minutes at a task in occupational therapy" or "No self-control is operationally defined here as swearing at fellow patients, shouting at staff, and turning over chairs." Once the problems have been defined in this way, we can then measure how often they occur. In the case of memory problems, "poor memory" may be operationally defined as "does not take medication, does not remember whether he has bathed that day, and cannot find his way from the rehabilitation center to the hospital cafeteria."

3. *State the goals or aims of treatment.* As stated, it is important to specify goals clearly and unambiguously. Thus, for the memory-impaired person with the problems outlined in stage 2, we might decide, following negotiation with the patient and others, that the three goals are (1) to take medication independently three times a day for 7 consecutive days, within 1 half-hour of the specified time; (2) to use a checklist to record the date and times of baths taken and to complete this without error for 2 weeks; and (3) to learn the way to the cafeteria, taking the shortest route at lunch time each day for 2 weeks.

4. *Measure the problem(s)—that is, take baselines.* This can be carried out in a number of ways using the measures outlined previously. For the problems of our memory patient described in item 3, we would probably take a frequency count (event recording) of the number of times he takes his medication without prompting (and how close he was to the specified time) and how frequently he bathed. If the patient is a day patient, his wife might be asked to keep a record of the morning and evening medication times and the number of baths taken. We might also be interested in how many disgreements occurred over the bathing situation. With regard to finding his way to the cafeteria, if this occurred at the rehabilitation center, staff would monitor this and maybe time the patient to see how long it took him to find the cafeteria; or they might decide to count the number of prompts he needed in order to stop tak-

ing a wrong turn. The number of baseline sessions will depend on the frequency and stability of the behavior. For stable baselines such as *never* remembering to take medication without prompting, a minimum of four baselines should be carried out. For behaviors that vary considerably, one needs to ensure that the baseline is stable and one may need to do 20 or more baselines. If the behavior keeps improving during the baseline, then no further treatment may be required, because the problem is improving with time. Alternatively, one could introduce treatment and then see if the *rate* of change is faster after the introduction of an intervention. Sometimes a more detailed analysis is necessary, such as "Does time of day make a difference?" or "Is the problem worse when a particular staff member is on duty?"

5. *Consider motivators or reinforcers.* For many of the people receiving memory rehabilitation, success is sufficient motivation in and of itself. For others, the frequent use of praise, rest, and feedback may be effective. Occasionally, it might be necessary to use more tangible reinforcers such as tokens (Alderman, 2001), visits to town (Wilson, 1999), looking at magazines, or doing some other activity desired by the patient.

6. *Plan the treatment.* Several aspects need to be considered here. Not all of the following will be required in every case. The guiding principle is that anyone reading the program would know what to do. Stages to consider are:

- *What* strategy/procedure/method/technique should be used?
- *Who* should carry out the training (e.g., should everybody involved follow the procedure or just one or two people?)
- *When and where* should the training be carried out (e.g., everywhere in the center or just in one group or individual session)?
- *How* should this be carried out and *how often* (e.g., all day every day, once a week, or at some other interval)?
- *What* happens if the patient is successful? Is this sufficiently reinforcing, or should we say "well done," give her a rest, or what?
- *What* happens if the patient is unsuccessful? Do we ignore any failures, prompt the correct answer, repeat the earlier demonstration, or do something else?
- *How* will success be measured? It is important to be specific about this (e.g., "Does not repeat the question within 40 minutes" or "Takes the shortest route to the cafeteria on three consecutive occasions").
- *Who* will be responsible for keeping the records? (This might be everyone on the team, a certain staff member or family member, or some other person.)
- *Who* will be responsible for liaising between the various parties?

(This could be a case manager, a key worker, a particular therapist, or someone else.)

7. *Begin treatment.* This should be easy now that all the previous
steps have been considered and sorted.

8. *Monitor progress* as determined in step 6.

9. *Evaluate.* Is this going to be achieved through record keeping,
through a single-case experimental design, a combination of these, or
some other method? (We return to evaluation in Chapter 11).

10. *Change the treatment if necessary.* If the program has been successful, one might consider fading out the support, cues, or prompts
or applying the treatment strategy to a different problem. If the treatment has failed, one will probably abandon it. If there are some signs
of success, one might wish to modify it by, for example, trying for longer, increasing the frequency of sessions, or presenting information at
a slower rate.

11. *Plan for generalization.* The comments made in the Generalization or Transfer of Learning section apply here.

These steps can reduce the anxiety of psychologists and therapists
when they are not quite sure what to do. However experienced we are,
designing treatments for patients is often a nerve-racking task, and I
have found that when I am unsure of how to proceed, I can say to myself,
"Barbara, follow your structure." This has a calming and reassuring
effect and enables us to sink our teeth into the treatment.

CHAPTER 11

# Final Thoughts
# and a General Summary

## Principles of Good Rehabilitation

In order for rehabilitation to be ethical, effective, and personally meaningful, certain principles need to be followed. Wilson (2008) and Wilson, Gracey, et al. (in press) considered the following six core components of the rehabilitation approach followed at the Oliver Zangwill Centre to be essential to rehabilitation.

### Provide a Therapeutic Milieu

Ben-Yishay (1996) discussed the concept of the "therapeutic milieu." This refers to the organization of the physical, organizational, and social environment to ensure it provides maximum support in the process of adjustment and increased social participation. The milieu embodies a strong sense of mutual cooperation and trust, which underpins the working alliance between client and clinicians.

### Establish Goals of Rehabilitation That Are Meaningful and Functionally Relevant

Meaningful functional activity refers to all day-to-day activities that form the basis for social participation. These can be divided into vocational, educational, recreational, social, and independent living activities. It is through participation in these areas that we gain a sense of purpose and meaning in our lives. Although we may not consciously think about these activities in everyday life, they enable us to achieve certain aims or ambitions that are personally significant to us and enhance our sense of identity and well-being.

## Ensure Shared Understanding

The concept of shared understanding derives from the use of "formulation" in clinical practice (Butler, 1998). A formulation is seen as a map or guide to intervention that combines, on the one hand, a model derived from established theories and best evidence with, on the other hand, the client and family's own personal views, experiences, and stories. This concept should be applied to all individual clinical work and influence the way the entire rehabilitation program is organized. The whole team should be involved so that a shared understanding supports the philosophy and vision of the team as well as their explicit values and goals and their understanding of research and theory. Knowledge and experience should be shared with other professionals and families, and the views and contributions of past clients are also valued.

## Apply Psychological Interventions

Psychological interventions are based on certain ways of understanding feelings and behavior. Specific psychological models are used to guide work depending on the specific needs of the individual. Approaches from these models provide ways that team members can engage patients in positive change and tackle the specific problems.

## Manage Cognitive Impairments through Compensatory Strategies and Retraining Skills

Compensatory strategies are alternative ways to enable individuals to achieve a desired objective when an underlying function of the brain, such as memory, is not working effectively. Compensatory approaches to managing impairments take a number of forms, including:

1. Cognitive compensations (e.g., using a verbal strategy to compensate for a defective visual memory).
2. Using a method to enhance new learning (e.g., EL learning or spaced retrieval may lead to more efficient learning of new information or skills).
3. External aids (e.g., using a pill box to remember to take medication or an alarm to remind one to check the diary).
4. Environmental adaptations—modifying the environment to reduce cognitive demands (e.g., painting the toilet doors a dis-

tinctive color so they can be easily distinguished or working in a quiet, nondistracting room to aid concentration).

Retraining is undertaken to improve performance of a specific function of the brain or to improve performance on a particular task or activity. Although there is no evidence that we can improve memory functioning through retraining, we do know that people can improve on specific tasks through practice. Thus, by teaching people to be more independent through the use of a pager, we are not improving memory per se but rather retraining their ability to function independently. Retraining also helps to address skills lost through lack of use (e.g., lost by not being at work since an injury).

## Work Closely with Families and Caregivers

Families and caregivers sometimes say they feel like an "afterthought" in rehabilitation. They experience a significant burden after acquired brain injury and may well need support. This can be in the form of, for example, providing information and opportunities for peer support, perhaps through a relatives group; involving family and caregivers in rehabilitation; and providing individual family consultation or therapy (Yeates, 2007; Palmer, Psaila, & Yeates, in press).

## Does Rehabilitation Improve QOL?

One definition of QOL is by Ferrans (1990): "a person's sense of well-being that stems from satisfaction or dissatisfaction with the areas of life that are important to him/her" (p. 15). Stewart and King (1994) suggested there are at least two essential attributes to be considered when measuring QOL: domain and dimension. Domain refers to the content area, that is, the aspect of life that is being assessed, such as physical functioning, psychological well-being, and social relationships, whereas dimension refers to a feeling or state, such as satisfaction or importance. Bowling (2005) argued that one should measure multiple domains and more than one dimension in order to capture well-being. Petchprapai and Winkelman (2007), in a review of the literature on QOL after mild TBI, indicated that QOL is often seen as synonymous with life satisfaction. According to Meeberg (1993), however, life satisfaction is a subjective feeling referring to one's level of happiness about one's life, and QOL studies should include objective as well as subjective measures.

Subjective assessments consider feelings, perceptions, or opinions of the client, whereas objective measures look at demographic variables and socioeconomic status (May & Warren, 2001, cited by Petchprapai & Winkelman, 2007). A framework for QOL by Ferrans and Powers (1992) includes health, psychological and spiritual functioning, socio-economic, and family aspects as well as dimensions to determine the satisfaction and importance of these dimensions. One measure increasingly used to assess QOL after brain injury is the European Quality of Life Scale (EuroQol). First described by Williams (1990), it found striking similarities to relative values attached to 14 different health states in three European countries (England, the Netherlands, and Sweden). A EuroQol group was formed, and now the tool exists in a number of languages.

Some studies have looked at QOL after intervention programs. Steadman-Pare, Colantonio, Ratcliff, Chase, and Vernich (2001) interviewed 275 people between 8 and 24 years after TBI. They found that perceived mental health, self-rated health, gender (women rating QOL higher), participation in work and leisure, and availability of emotional support were significantly associated with QOL. They stressed the importance of ongoing support programs for survivors of TBI several years after injury. Corrigan, Bogner, Mysiw, Clinchot, and Fugate (2001) indicated that life satisfaction after TBI seems to be related to attaining healthy and productive lifestyles. In addition, other studies (e.g., Powell, Heslin & Greenwood, 2002) suggested that even years after brain injury, rehabilitation can yield benefits that outlive the active treatment period. Finally, Klonoff et al. (2006) found that holistic milieu-oriented rehabilitation facilitates long-term successful employment, driving, and relationship stability.

## Evaluation of Memory Rehabilitation

There is no point doing rehabilitation if it is ineffective. We have addressed the question of using goals to evaluate treatment in Chapter 9, and this often needs to be complemented with other measures. For every patient or client we see, we should ask ourselves, "Is this patient changing and, if so, is the change due to what we are doing (or have done) or would it have happened anyway?" One way that we can do this is to use single-case experimental designs, which were first used in behavioral psychology for the purpose of behavioral assessments. Single-case experimental designs allow us to evaluate an individual's response to treatment, to see whether the client is changing over time, and to determine whether any changes are due to natural recovery or to the intervention itself. In other words, we can tease out the effects of treatment from the effects of spontaneous recovery and other non-specific factors. Given that rehabilitation is planned for individuals, evaluation should take place at the individual as well as the group level, and the choice of individual or group study will again depend on the kinds of questions that need answering. For example, if we wish to find out whether a particular memory-impaired person is benefiting from EL learning, we would need to use a single-case experimental design. If we wanted to find out *how many* people appeared to be benefiting from this kind of learning, we would want to conduct a group study. Group studies average out performances, so individual differences are masked. Single-case experimental designs, on the other hand, avoid many of the problems inherent in group designs. They are often chosen specifically for their ability to evaluate an individual's progress through rehabilitation, and they are, of course, perfectly respectable as far as scientific methodology is concerned (Gianutsos & Gianutsos, 1987; Hersen & Barlow, 1982; Kazdin, 1982). The main single-case experimental designs are the ABAB or reversal designs (where A stands for baseline and B for treatment) or variations on this design and multiple baseline designs where the introduction of treatment is staggered. For an up-to-date review of these designs, see Barlow, Nock, and Hersen (2008).

As well as determining whether our treatment is effective for individuals, we sometimes need to answer questions about the efficacy of group treatment. For example, when we are running groups, we need to know whether the program or interaction has been effective. We could use a series of single-case experimental designs to do this (i.e., measure each person's change individually), or we could use a group design and compare the group receiving treatment with a control group or with a group receiving a different kind of treatment. We could use a mixture of single-case and group design (as Wilson et al., 2001, did in the NeuroPage studies where we looked both at individuals and at two groups, namely the treatment first group and the wait-list first group), or we could base our treatment on published studies and assume that because previous studies have found a certain method effective we are justified in using it. There are, of course, advantages and disadvantages to any of these methods, particularly with the latter, because we may not know whether the patients in our groups are similar to those in the published studies.

As with assessment, evaluation involves asking questions, and it is crucial that we pose the right question in such a way that it is answerable. Just as we do not ask general questions about medicine, surgery, or pharmacology, such as "Does medicine work?" or "Do drugs work?", we should not pose the question "Does rehabilitation work?" We need to make our evaluation questions more specific, such as "Do people receiving memory group treatment show less anxiety as measured by the

HADS?" (Evans & Wilson, 1992) or "Do people learn better when prevented from making mistakes during learning?" (Baddeley & Wilson, 1994). A greater, more difficult question to evaluate is "Which rehabilitation programs, strategies, or techniques work for which people under which circumstances?"

To many health service professionals, managers, and health economists, there is only one way to evaluate the effectiveness of rehabilitation, and that is through the use of randomized controlled trials, preferably under double-blind conditions. Yet psychologists and therapists cannot be blind to the treatment they are giving and in most cases neither can patients be blind to the treatment they are receiving (Mai, 1992). Single-blind trials, in which an assessor does not know which treatment has been provided, can, in some circumstances, be used. We could, for example, have an independent assessor, who does not know which treatment has been given to which person, administer the HADS to people in the memory group and to a control group. The Proceedings of the Subcommittee on TBI Rehabilitation (National Institutes of Health, 1998) suggested that evaluation studies of rehabilitation should include only those in which the researchers evaluating programs are *not* the clinicians carrying out the program.

This is not to deny the value of randomized controlled trials. There is a place for them even if we cannot make them double blind. Von Cramon, Mathes-von Cramon, and Mai (1991) examined a specific issue, namely, whether problem-solving training (PST) benefited patients with brain injury more than nonspecific training. Patients were alternately allocated to specific PST or to memory training (MT). The procedures were clearly specified, and the patients allocated to the PST benefited to a significantly greater extent than those allocated to MT as measured by posttreatment assessment. In Wilson et al.'s (2001) NeuroPage randomized controlled trial, people were randomly allocated to pager first or wait list first, so there is no doubt that we can sometimes use such designs. Despite this, we have to use a variety of research designs, including surveys and direct observation as well as single-case experimental designs and not solely randomized controlled trials in order to evaluate memory, cognitive, neuropsychological, and all other kinds of rehabilitation. In one of my favorite quotes, Andrews (1991) stated that the randomized controlled trial "is a tool to be used, not a god to be worshipped" (p. 5). He went on to say that the randomized controlled trial is an excellent tool in research where "the design is simple, where marked changes are expected, where the factors involved are relatively specific, and where the number of additional variables likely to affect the outcome is few and can be expected to be balanced out by the randomization procedure" (p. 5).

## Combining Theory and Practice

Baddeley (1993) said, "A theory of rehabilitation without a model of learning is a vehicle without an engine" (p. 235). Models of learning are important in rehabilitation, as are many others. Most survivors of brain injury will have several cognitive problems, not solely memory problems, and they will also have emotional, social, and vocational problems. Their needs are complex so we need to draw on a number of theories, models, and frameworks to reflect this multiplicity.

In 2002 I (Wilson, 2002a) published a provisional model of cognitive rehabilitation in which I argued that one model, or one group of models such as those from cognitive neuropsychology, is insufficient (1) to determine what needs to be rehabilitated, (2) to plan appropriate treatment for neuropsychological impairments, or (3) to evaluate response to rehabilitation. Rehabilitation is one of many fields that need a broad theoretical base incorporating frameworks, theories, and models from a number of different areas. If those of us in rehabilitation are constrained by one approach, this can lead to poor clinical practice because important aspects of patients' lives may be neglected. The model I proposed was a synthesis of many models used in rehabilitation and is shown in Figure 11.1.

Theoretical models can only take us so far in clinical work. We have to adapt to the individual's needs and circumstances. We know, for example, that most memory-impaired people benefit from EL learning because they are unable to remember their mistakes and, thus, cannot profit from trial-and-error learning. In practice, however, the way the principle is applied in rehabilitation will depend on the goals set, the individual's strengths and weaknesses, and the circumstances in which the learning occurs. In the Kime et al. (1996) case, in which a young woman was required to check her memory book every time her watch alarm sounded, she was initially prompted by her therapist to check the book whenever the alarm sounded and was not allowed to fail. Eventually, the young woman learned to check the book herself. Clare et al. (1999, 2000), working with patients with AD, used a number of different EL learning approaches to teach people targets they set for themselves (e.g., helping one woman to relearn the names of her grandchildren, another to relearn to tell the time, and another to check a memory board so that she did not irritate her husband by repeatedly asking him the same question). These different goals illustrate how the same EL learning principle was applied for different purposes.

For theories and models to be clinically useful, we need to use clinical experience and common sense to apply the findings. In a survey of practicing neuropsychologists working in adult brain injury reha-

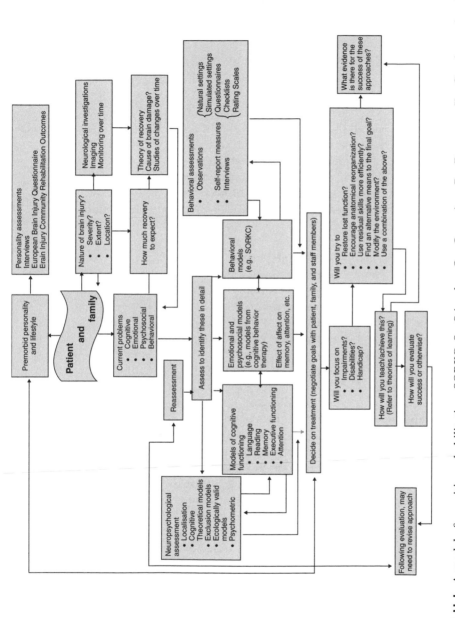

**FIGURE II.1.** A model of cognitive rehabilitation. SORKC; S = Stimulus; O = Organism; R = Response; K = Contingencies; C = Consequence. From Wilson (2002a). Copyright 2002 by Taylor & Francis Group. Reprinted by permission.

191

bilitation in the United Kingdom (Wilson, Rous, & Sopena, 2008), we found that a range of theoretical approaches was used in clinical work, with CBT being used the most and the psychoanalytical approach the least.

## Summaries of Individual Chapters

### Chapter 1

Memory is the ability to take in, store, and retrieve information. There are a number of ways in which memory can be classified. One way is to consider the length of time for which memory is stored (Baddeley & Hitch, 1974). This gives us three categories: sensory memory, which stores information for less than a quarter of a second (250 milliseconds); short-term or working memory, which holds information for a few seconds; and long-term memory, which holds information for anything from minutes to years.

Memory can also be understood in terms of the type of information that is stored. Memory for knowledge, for personal experiences, and for skills is stored differently. Tulving (1972) introduced the concept of semantic and episodic memory, with semantic memory referring to memory for general knowledge such as facts, the meanings of words, the visual appearance of objects, and the color of things. In contrast, episodic memory refers to memory for personal experiences such as where one was last weekend or when the mortgage was paid. Episodic memory allows us "to travel back in time" (Baddeley, 2002, p. 5). This requires conscious recollection and is the major handicap of most people with memory deficits.

Memory for skills or routines is known as *procedural memory*. Learning to type or to track a moving object on a screen are examples of procedural learning. The primary characteristic of this kind of learning is that it does not depend on conscious recollection; instead, the learning can be demonstrated without the need to be aware of where and how the original learning took place. Most memory-impaired people have normal or nearly normal procedural memory.

A third way we can classify memory is to consider the kind of material to be remembered. Although we may need to remember things we have seen, heard, smelled, touched, and tasted, in memory rehabilitation the main areas of concern are memory for verbal and for visual information. Some people have particular problems with just one of these types of memory, while others will have problems across the board.

A fourth way is to classify the *stages* in the process of remembering. These are the three stages required for a memory system to function.

The taking in of information is the encoding stage, retaining the information is the storage stage, and accessing the information when it is required is the retrieval stage. Although one can distinguish between these stages and patients can be found with deficits in one system only, in real life these stages interact with one another.

We can also examine memory in terms of whether one can consciously recollect specific incidents and episodes from the past (explicit memory) or whether no conscious recollection is required (implicit memory). Most memory-impaired people will have problems with explicit memory tasks, and this is likely to be the focus of memory rehabilitation, in contrast to implicit memory, which is likely to be normal or nearly normal.

Retrospective memory and prospective memory are yet other classifications. Memory for events or experiences that have already happened is retrospective and remembering to do something in the future is prospective. Episodic memory, verbal and visual memory, and explicit memory are all part of retrospective memory. Problems associated with prospective memory, leading to difficulties involved in remembering to water the plants, to pay a bill, or to take medication, are among the most common when people are asked what everyday memory problems they face (Baddeley, 2004). Memory-impaired people experience difficulties with both kinds of memory. They will have problems remembering things that happened in the past as well as things they are expected to do in the future.

The final classification for understanding memory is retrograde and anterograde amnesia. Retrograde amnesia refers to loss of memory before the onset of the memory deficit; that is, there is impaired recall of events that took place before any insult to the brain. This is very variable and may last for decades in some conditions such as encephalitis or Korsakoff's syndrome or a few minutes in some people with TBI. Anterograde amnesia refers to memory difficulties after the neurological insult and is usually the more handicapping of the two. Most memory-impaired people will have both retrograde and anterograde memory deficits.

Chapter 1 also includes a brief account of the neuroanatomical structures involved in memory functioning, including the hippocampi and surrounding areas, the limbic structures, and the frontotemporal cortex. Given the number of structures and networks involved, perhaps it is hardly surprising that memory problems are so often seen after so many kinds of brain damage. The extent to which we can expect recovery of memory functioning after an insult to the brain is discussed in Chapter 2.

## Chapter 2

Recovery can mean different things to different people; some are solely concerned with recovery of cognitive functions, others focus on survival rates, and still others only consider biological recovery such as repair of brain structures. Chapter 2 begins with some definitions of the term. My own operational definition of cognitive recovery (Wilson, 1998) is "a complete or partial resolution of cognitive deficits incurred as a result of an insult to the brain" (p. 281). Even though some partial resolution of deficits may occur in some people, this will be minimal for many of them. The adoption of a compensatory approach provides the best chance of reducing everyday problems and enhancing independent living and QOL for the majority of those with organic memory deficits.

Mechanisms of recovery include resolution from edema or swelling of the brain, diaschisis (whereby lesions caused damage to other areas of the brain through shock), plasticity or changes to the structure of the nervous system, and regeneration or regrowth of neural tissue. Changes seen in the first few minutes (e.g., after a mild head injury) probably reflect the resolution of temporary damage that has not caused structural damage. Changes seen within several days are more likely to be due to resolution of temporary structural abnormalities such as edema and vascular disruption or to the depression of enzyme metabolic activity. Recovery after several months or years is less well understood. There are several ways in which this might be achieved, including diaschisis, plasticity, and regeneration. A discussion of these mechanisms is provided.

Other issues also affect recovery. Age at insult, diagnosis, number of insults sustained by an individual, and premorbid status of the individual's brain are just a few of the probable influencing factors. These are addressed in turn. Moving on from general recovery, Chapter 2 then looks specifically at recovery from memory impairments. There is no doubt that some recovery of lost memory functioning does occur in the early weeks and months after nonprogressive brain damage; there is also no doubt that many people remain with lifelong memory problems. The picture from published studies is confusing, with some reports showing considerable improvement and others showing none. What is clear, though, is that we can improve on natural recovery through rehabilitation. Given the fact that restoration of episodic, explicit memory is unlikely in the majority of cases once the acute period is finished, compensatory approaches are the most likely to lead to change in everyday memory functioning. Treatment of semantic memory disorders is also addressed briefly in this chapter. Before beginning rehabilitation, however, a thorough assessment is required, which is the topic of Chapter 3.

## Chapter 3

A good definition of assessment for psychologists, provided as long ago as 1962 by Sundberg and Tyler, is that assessment is the systematic collection, organization, and interpretation of information about a person and his or her situation. It is also concerned with the prediction of behavior in new situations. The way this information is collected, organized, and interpreted will depend on the reason the assessment was required in the first place. Assessments are carried out to answer questions, and each question posed will determine the assessment tool to be used. Certain questions can be answered through the use of standardized tests, others need functional or behavioral assessments, and others may require specially designed procedures.

Standardized tests can help us answer questions along the following lines:

What is this person's general level of intellectual functioning?

What was the probable level of premorbid functioning?

What are this person's cognitive strengths and weaknesses?

How does this person's memory functioning compare with people of the same age in the general population?

Is the level of memory functioning consistent with what one would expect from this level of intellectual ability?

Is the memory problem global or restricted to certain kinds of material (e.g., is memory for visual material better than for verbal material)?

To what extent are the memory problems due to executive, language, perceptual, or attention difficulties?

Does this person have a high level of anxiety?

Is this person depressed?

Standardized tests are very limited when attempting to answer the following questions:

How are the memory difficulties manifested in everyday life?

What problems cause most concern to the family and the memory-impaired person?

What do we know about the cultural background and level of support available?

What coping strategies are used?

Are the problems exacerbated by depression or anxiety?

Is this person likely to be able to return to work (or school)?

Can this person live independently?

What kind of compensatory aids did this person use premorbidly?
What kind of memory compensation strategies are being used
    now?
What is the best way for this person to learn new information?

A behavioral or functional approach through observations,
self-report measures (from relatives or caregivers as well as from the
memory-impaired person), and interviews is more suited and able to
answer these treatment-related questions. The standardized and functional assessment procedures provide complementary information: The
former allows us to build up a cognitive map of a person's strengths and
weaknesses, while the latter enables us to target areas for treatment. A
number of standardized tests for assessing different aspects of memory
are suggested, together with a description of behavioral assessment procedures. In addition to tests to determine cognitive strengths and weaknesses, other aspects such mood and emotion should be assessed, and
these measures are considered in Chapter 8. Once the assessment has
been carried out, treatment needs to be designed. One of the major
ways of helping people with memory problems cope in everyday life is to
enable them to compensate through the use of external aids, the focus
of Chapter 4, written with guest contributor Narinder Kapur.

## Chapter 4

External memory aids can be classified into those that act as alerting
cues, offering a cue at a particular time and in a particular place, and
those that are representational aids, providing a stored representation
of information that is not dependent on a particular temporal or spatial
context. Alarms that help prospective memory would seem to fit neatly
into the former category, while notepads and Dictaphones are ready
examples of devices that store information for later use. The most widely
used form of representational memory aid is the written language and
electronic variants of writing. Some devices may be "multimodal," blurring this simple distinction; satellite navigation devices store representations of the outside world but also provide alerting cues at certain points
in space.

Efficient use of many external memory aids involves motivation,
patience, planning, problem solving, concentration, learning, and,
indeed, memory, so the people who need them most often have the
greatest difficulty in learning how to use them. The most commonly
used external aids are described, and consideration is given regarding
how to teach their use. Nonelectronic aids are more widely used than

electronic ones, and certain characteristics are predictive of the use of external aids. These include age (younger patients are better in their use than older people) and severity of deficit (very severely memory-impaired people compensate less well). Those who used aids premorbidly are more likely to compensate. Those without widespread cognitive deficits are also more likely to use aids than those with such deficits. Scherer (2005) pointed out that successful use of external aids depends on a good match between a number of variables, including insight and motivation; past use of memory aids; cognitive, emotional, and motivational characteristics; everyday demands on memory; family/work support; the various cognitive and behavioral strategies; and types of memory aids available to the clinician.

This chapter also provides a description of how to set up a memory aids clinic or resource center, including funding, staffing, the range of aids and resources needed, finding and cataloging these aids, and research and development.

Because environmental aids were only touched on in Chapter 4, a little more is added here. Kapur et al. (2004) classified nonelectronic aids into environmental and portable external aids. The environmental aids are further subdivided into proximal and distal aids. The proximal environment covers the design and contents of a room or vehicle and the equipment an individual uses in everyday settings. Items that are not specific to a particular environment, such as notebooks, clocks, and computers, are considered under different sections. In his excellent book *The Psychology of Everyday Things*, Norman (1988) argued that knowledge should be in the world rather than in the head. By this, he means that if we approach a door it should be obvious whether or not we should push or pull it. If we are using a stove, it should be obvious which knob works which burner. We should not have to remember these things, because the design should make it obvious. This is the same principle behind the concept of environmental memory aids.

Just as people with severe physical disabilities can use environmental control systems to enable them to open and close doors, turn the pages of a book, answer the telephone, and so forth, so can people with cognitive deficits avoid the need to use memory provided the environment is structured in a certain way. Thus, someone with severe executive deficits may be able to function in a structured environment, with no distractions and where there is no need to problem solve because the task at hand is clear and unambiguous. Similarly, people with severe memory problems may not be handicapped in environments where there are no demands made on memory. Thus, if doors, cupboards, drawers, and storage jars are clearly labeled, if rooms are cleared of dangerous equipment, if someone reminds or accompanies the memory-impaired person when it is time to go to the dentist or to eat dinner, the person may cope reasonably well.

Kapur et al. (2004) gave other examples. Items can be left by the front door for people who forget to take belongings with them when they leave the house; a message can be left on the mirror in the hallway; and a simple flowchart can be used to help people search in likely places when they cannot find a lost belonging (Moffat, 1989). Cars, mobile phones, and other items may have intrinsic alarms to remind people to do things. These can be paired with voice messages to remind people why the alarm is ringing. Modifications can also be made to verbal environments to avoid irritating behavior such as the repetition of a question, story, or joke. It might be possible to identify a trigger or an antecedent that elicits this behavior. Thus, by eliminating the trigger, one can avoid the repetitious behavior. For example, in response to the question "How are you today?", one young head-injured man would always say, "Just getting over my hangover." If staff simply said "Good morning," however, he replied, "Good morning," so the repetitious comments about his supposed hangover were avoided.

Proximal environmental aids, therefore, involve structuring the immediate environment and organizing the equipment or material in the environment to reduce the load on memory. Distal environmental aids, on the other hand, involve the wider environment and include the layout of buildings, shopping centers, streets, and towns. Smart houses are already in existence to help "disable the disabling environment" (Slaven, personal communication, 1999) described by Wilson and Evans (2000) and Gibbs (2000). Layouts of shopping centers, office buildings, hospitals, and residential homes differ in ease of negotiating. In some the sign postings, color coding, alarm systems, and warning signs greatly reduce the chances of getting lost or falling downstairs. Improvement in the organization of these wider environments can, like the proximal environmmental aids, reduce the memory load.

## Chapter 5

This chapter considers mnemonics and rehearsal strategies. Mnemonics are systems that enable us to remember things more easily. Sometimes the term is used to describe anything that improves memory, including external memory aids, but more often it refers to internal strategies that are consciously learned and require considerable effort to put into practice (Harris, 1984). Verbal and visual mnemonic systems as well as motor movements for improving recall are elucidiated, and research into their use with memory-impaired people is presented.

Despite the fact that some individuals can benefit from mnemonics, not everybody with memory impairments will be able to use these spontaneously. Their efficacy can be enhanced if therapists and others recognize that mnemonics can be used to achieve faster learning for particular pieces of information, such as names of a few people or a new address. It may help to use two or three strategies, such as visual imagery, vanishing cues, and spaced retrieval/expanding rehearsal, to improve learning of one piece of information.

New information should be taught one step at a time. We need to take on broad individual preferences and styles; we should focus on things that the person with memory impairments wants and needs to learn and will be useful in everyday life. Generalization or the transfer to real life must always be built in to the training program.

Rehearsal simply means to practice, repeat, or go over something until it is remembered. Rote rehearsal, or simply repeating material, is widely used by the general population, but it is not a particularly good learning strategy for people with memory deficits. We can hear or read something many times over and still not remember it. In this situation, it is a case of "going in one ear and out the other." In addition to expanded rehearsal/spaced retrieval, which is addressed at some length in Chapter 6, other rehearsal strategies exist, including PQRST, first described by Robinson (1970), and the similar method of SQR3 (Rowntree, 1982). PQRST stands for **P**review, **Q**uestion, **R**ead, **S**tate, and **T**est, and SQR3 stands for **S**urvey, **Q**uestion, **R**ead, **R**ecall, and **R**eview. In practice, the stages followed are virtually identical. The PQRST procedure is described, and research of its effectiveness with memory-impaired people is considered together with reasons why it works. Using the procedure in clinical practice is also addressed.

## Chapter 6

How to improve new learning is the topic of this chapter. Three methods are considered in detail, namely errorless (EL) learning, spaced retrieval (otherwise known as expanded rehearsal), and the method of vanishing cues (VC). EL learning is a teaching technique whereby people are prevented, as far as possible, from making mistakes while they are learning a new skill or acquiring new information. This can be carried out in a number of ways such as providing spoken or written instructions or guiding the person through a task. The principle is to avoid, as far as possible, mistakes being made during learning and to minimize the possibility of erroneous responses: In order to benefit from our mistakes (trial-and-error learning), we need to be able to remember our mistakes. People with very poor memory functioning cannot do this, so the very fact of making an erroneous response can strengthen that response. Explicit memory is the system that allows us to correct errors; implicit memory is not equipped to do this and people with amnesia are dependent on implicit memory. The theoretical underpinnings of EL learning are discussed, as is the efficacy of EL learning with survivors of brain injury.

There is now considerable evidence that EL learning is superior to errorful learning for people with severe memory deficits. In a meta-analysis of EL learning, Kessels and de Haan (2003) found a large and statistically significant effect size of EL learning treatment. However, there are conflicting views about the benefits of EL learning for people with less severe memory impairments. There is also some debate about the benefits of EL learning for problems other than episodic memory deficits.

It should be remembered that EL learning is not a program of treatment. Instead, it is a description, or an approach, whereby the task is manipulated to eliminate or reduce errors (Fillingham et al., 2003). There are many different ways to reduce the likelihood of errors, such as providing written instructions, guiding someone through a particular task, and modeling the steps of a procedure little by little. Spaced retrieval, also known as expanded or expanding rehearsal, involves the presentation of material to be remembered followed by immediate testing. People with a normal immediate memory span (and this includes most memory-impaired people) will be able to do this. The tester then waits for a second or two and requests the information again. The test interval is very gradually increased until the information is learned. Spaced retrieval may work because it is a form of distributed practice (i.e., distributing the learning trials over a period of time rather than amassing them together in one block). Distributed practice increases the likelihood of learning. Massed practice is a less efficient learning strategy than distributed practice (Baddeley, 1999), a phenomenon described in the 1930s (Baddeley & Longman, 1978; Lorge, 1930). The method has been used to help people with TBI, stroke, encephalitis, and dementia. We look at studies in which spaced retrieval has been combined with EL learning and used alone. A combination of the two is preferred. It appears to be a powerful learning strategy for people with progressive as well as nonprogressive conditions.

VC is a method whereby prompts are provided and then gradually faded out. For example, someone learning a new name might be expected first to copy the whole name, then the last letter would be deleted; the name would be copied again and the last letter inserted by the person copying the name; then the last two letters would be deleted and the process repeated until all letters were completed by the person learning the name. This is similar to the method of backward chaining used to teach new skills to people with learning disabilities.

Glisky et al. (1986) were the first to report VC with memory-impaired people, and since then several studies have been carried out not only with nonprogressive patients but also with people with dementia. There are mixed results in published research articles. The main problem with VC is that it may work only when there is at least one letter left. Even though the original Glisky et al. (1986) study found that all their patients eventually learned computer terminology without the initial letter, the learning was slow and took many trials (unlike implicit memory, which occurs unconsciously and without such effort). If VC is the method selected to teach new information, then it is suggested that it be combined with EL learning principles.

A study by Ehlhardt et al. (2008) provides the following guidelines for teaching new information to memory-impaired people:

1. The intervention targets should be clearly delineated and/or task analyses used when training multistep procedures.
2. Errors should be constrained, and the output of clients should be controlled when they are acquiring new or relearning information and procedures.
3. Sufficient practice should be provided.
4. Practice should be distributed.
5. Variation in the form of multiple examples should be provided to avoid hyperspecificity of learning and enhance generalization.
6. Strategies to promote more effortful processing (e.g., verbal elaboration, imagery) should be used.
7. New learning should focus on ecologically valid targets.

## Chapter 7

The provision of rehabilitation through memory groups is examined. Group therapy is desirable for several reasons. Memory-impaired people may benefit from interaction with others having similar problems. Sometimes those with memory impairment fear they are losing their sanity, and this fear may be alleviated by observing others with similar problems. Groups can reduce anxiety and distress. They can instill hope and show patients that they are not alone. In addition, it may be easier to accept advice from peers than from therapists and to use strategies that peers are using rather than strategies recommended by professional staff.

Groups can be open or closed, homogeneous or heterogeneous, and for people from a single diagnostic category or a mixture of categories. All have advantages and disadvantages. Different types of groups are described in detail, including inpatient group, outpatient group, day patient group, groups for people with dementia, and a group for families and caregivers.

Self-help and support groups are also valuable, and some charities that help support people with memory problems are described: Headway (the Brain Injuries Association), the Encephalitis Society, and the Alzheimer's Society. Wearing (1992) pointed out that all self-help groups have the same broad aims. First, they provide support for patients and families in a social network of people who understand the problem. Second, they inform patients and families about the particular problem they were set up to help and how to deal with this problem. Third, they access services in the community. Fourth, they lobby for better care and support services. Fifth, they increase public awareness of the problem. Sixth, they are able to educate themselves about the condition through long-term liaison with professionals and families. Seventh, they promote research to advance knowledge.

## Chapter 8

The area of interest in this chapter is disorders of emotion and mood that accompany memory impairment. In addition to poor memory, those requiring rehabilitation are likely to be anxious or depressed. They may have mood swings, feel fearful, and possibly suffer from PTSD. These problems need to be addressed alongside the memory and other cognitive deficits. It is not always easy to separate cognitive, emotional, and psychosocial problems from one another. Not only does emotion affect how we think and behave, but also cognitive deficits can be exacerbated by emotional distress (Dalgleish & Cox, 2002) and can cause apparent behavior problems (Wilson, 1999).

Psychosocial difficulties can result in increased emotional and behavioral problems, and anxiety can reduce the effectiveness of intervention programs. There is clearly an interaction between all these aspects of human functioning and, indeed, this is the core assumption of the holistic approach to brain injury rehabilitation pioneered by Diller (1976), Ben-Yishay (1978), and Prigatano (1986). Prigatano (1994) suggested that holistic programs result in less emotional distress, increased self-esteem, and greater productivity. It is clear from a number of studies that mood and emotional disorders are common after brain injury. In their population-based study in South Carolina, Horner et al. (2008) interviewed by telephone 1,560 adults who had sustained a TBI approximately 1 year earlier. Of these, 40% had clinically significant mood and anxiety disorders, a further 12.6% had probable disorders, and 27.5% had possible disorders. Thus, the vast majority of the sample were reporting some mood and anxiety problems. Some assessment tools for disorder of mood and emotion are outlined along with strengths and weaknesses.

Also included in this chapter are measures to assess the recognition of emotional expressions. With regard to treatment of emotional difficulties, we again examine group treatments as well as individual psychological support. A structure is provided for a mood management group and for a psychological support group. Individual psychological support is mostly derived from CBT, which is now very much part of brain injury rehabilitation. Tyerman and King (2004) discussed psychotherapy with people with different cognitive deficits and suggested ways to circumvent problems. For those with memory problems, for example, they suggested notes, audio- and videotapes of sessions, frequent repetitions, mini-reviews, telephone reminders to complete homework tasks, and use of family members as cotherapists. The chapter also includes a brief account of treatment for disorders of emotional perception after brain injury.

## Chapter 9

One of the main changes in rehabilitation over the past decade has been the adoption of goal setting to plan and evaluate rehabilitation. In the Wilson, Rous, and Sopena (2008) survey, all 54 respondents said they used a goal-planning approach to rehabilitation. A goal is defined as something the person receiving rehabilitation wants to do, something that is relevant and meaningful to him or to her, and something reflecting his or her longer term aims. Because rehabilitation is ultimately concerned with enabling people to participate effectively in valued activities (Hart & Evans, 2006), memory rehabilitation should set appropriate goals that should be the main focus of intervention, and whether or not they are achieved is, or should be, one of the main ways of evaluating the success of memory rehabilitation.

There are several advantages to a goal-setting approach. First, it makes certain that the aims of the admission are clearly documented. Second, in addition to the rehabilitation team, patients, relatives, and caregivers become involved. Third, it promotes team work. Fourth, it incorporates a measure of outcome. Fifth, it removes the artificial distinction between outcome and client-centered activity. Goal attainment scaling (Kiresuk & Sherman, 1968) can be used to weight the goals and thus make them more comparable.

Goals are usually negotiated among patients, families, and professional staff and should follow SMART principles: **S**pecific, **M**easurable,
**A**chievable, **R**ealistic, and **T**ime based. It is important to review goals
regularly, and if they are not achieved, the reasons for this should be
recorded. Although goals will differ for people at different stages of the
recovery or rehabilitation process and for people with different degrees
of severity, some aspects will be common to all. Collicutt-McGrath
(2008) discussed life goals that are likely to affect all rehabilitation
patients. Like all goals, memory goals are broken down into short-term
and action plans. Typically, long-term goals are those expected to be
achieved by the time of discharge from the program. Short-term goals
are steps toward the long-term goal and are usually expected to be
achieved in 1 or 2 weeks. Action plans are steps taken by someone other
than the client to help achieve a short-term goal. Examples are provided
of goals for inpatients, day patients, and outpatients. Using goals to measure the success of rehabilitation is also addressed in this chapter.

## Chapter 10

Guidelines on planning a memory rehabilitation program are considered. First, we present some general tips from Kapur (2008) on taking
it easy, being organized, concentrating better, and using memory aids.
Each patient or client then needs to have his or her cognitive and emotional strengths and weaknesses assessed. Standardized tests should be
complemented with observations, interviews, and self-report measures.
Goals should be set following the principles presented in Chapter 9.
Suggestions are provided on selecting the best strategy or strategies for
attaining the goals. Examples are provided from Kime (2006), and a single-case study showing the natural history of the development of a compensatory system is reproduced from Wilson, J. C., and Hughes (1997).

Finally, a framework is presented to help readers plan a rehabilitation program. This framework can be applied to most of the problems one is likely to face when working with survivors of brain injury,
although the examples here are specifically for memory rehabilitation.

## Chapter 11

The present chapter has examined good principles for rehabilitation,
QOL issues, evaluation of treatment, and integrating theory and prac-
tice. I would like to end with some comments from my colleague, Jim
Malec. In his paper "Mayo Brain Injury Rehabilitation: What We've
Learned in the Past 20 years," presented at the Fifteenth Annual Brain

Injury Conference at the Mayo Clinic, Rochester, Minnesota, in June 2008, Malec pointed out that "life can be and often is good even after brain injury" and offered the following advice: Get in with the patients right away and stick with them and their families; bring hope early and often; trying to make the patient "confront reality" is for amateurs; brain injury rehabilitation takes special people. Malec then went on to say, in commonsense terminology, that rehabilitation "is about teamwork, it's about family, it's about networking, evaluating what you're doing makes it better, in rehab one size does not fit all, with ongoing research brain injury rehab is constantly improving."

In conclusion to the book as a whole, I would like to say that the audience I have had in mind throughout consists of those professionals whose aim is to improve the lives of people with memory difficulties caused by neurological damage to the brain. These include clinical psychologists, neuropsychologists, occupational therapists, and speech therapists involved in rehabilitating adults with nonprogressive memory impairment. It should also provide guidance and understanding for those working in the field of dementia. The book may also appeal to psychiatrists, neurologists, nurses, physiotherapists, and social workers familiar with, or wishing to increase their knowledge of, rehabilitation of memory. Finally, the book's extensive and, I hope, thorough coverage of all areas in its chosen field may appeal to teachers and students needing to extend and update their understanding of all issues involved in memory rehabilitation.

I hope that the individual reader will gain an understanding of the principles involved in memory rehabilitation and, if in a position to do so, be able to plan and implement practical programs to reduce problems in everyday life. By reading this book, the reader should be able to understand the current principles of memory rehabilitation and appreciate how these have derived from theoretical studies. The professional therapist should be able to carry out appropriate assessments, set goals, implement strategies, understand how to teach these strategies, recognize the importance of dealing with the emotional consequences of memory impairment, and evaluate their treatment programs. Above all they will know how to reduce the everyday memory problems of survivors of brain injury.

And the future? There is no doubt that we will see new developments in technology and external aids, and it is hoped that these will benefit memory-impaired people. This will require understanding, patience, and ingenuity from those working in the field. The increasing use of sophisticated brain imaging technology such as positron emission tomography is enhancing our conception of brain damage (see, e.g., Frith, 2007), but whether this will help us with our rehabilitation programs remains to be seen.

New assessment procedures are likely to appear to help us grasp the strengths and weaknesses of our patients. New treatments, perhaps pharmacological ones, which can be combined with our current rehabilitation techniques, may well be just around the corner, and better evaluation of our interventions would be welcome. Perhaps the best future development would be that all memory-impaired people and their families can access appropriate rehabilitation for their cognitive, emotional, and psychosocial needs.

# Resources

## Websites That Provide Memory Aids

*alzstore.com*

A range of materials, including books, alarm systems, etc., that may be suitable for patients with Alzheimer's disease or their caregivers.

*bindependent.com*

Alarm watches and other electronic reminders.

*cobolt.co.uk* and *onlineshop.rnib.org.uk*

A range of devices, including memory aids, for the visually impaired.

*connevans.co.uk*

Photophone, alerting devices, vibrating watches, alarms for the hearing impaired.

*dayclocks.co.uk*

Clocks that indicate the date or the date and time.

*enablingdevices.com*

Various types of aids, including vibrating cuing devices.

*epill.com*

Various types of pillboxes and electronic reminders.

*euroffice.co.uk*

Range of Post-it Note items, White boards, filofaxes, etc.

*hagger.co.uk* and *independentliving.com*

Aids for a range of disabilities, including visual, auditory, motor, and some memory aids.

*medicalarm.co.uk*

Pillboxes, watch alarms.

*onlineorganizing.com*

Various organization aids, including MotivAider (vibrating alarm device).

*qstartreminders.com*

In-car/automobile voice reminders.

*Relax-uk.com*

Message-alarm watch, sleep-tracking watch with alarm.

*silverphone.co.uk*

Phones designed for the elderly, which may be suitable for the visually/ cognitively impaired.

*talkingproducts.co.uk*

Voice messaging systems, including mini-voice recorder.

*thart@einstein.edu*

A useful catalog of portable electronic devices to improve memory and organization (can be obtained from Dr. Tessa Hart in Philadelphia).

# Societies Offering Advice/Information

## *United Kingdom*

**Alzheimer's Society**
Devon House, 58 St. Katharine's Way, London E1W 1JX
Tel: 020 7423 3500
Fax: 020 7423 3501
Website: *www.alzheimers.org.uk*
E-mail: *enquiries@alzheimers.org.uk*

**British Epilepsy Association**
New Anstey House, Gate Way Drive, Yeadon, Leeds LS19 7XY
Tel: 0113 210 8800
Website: *www.epilepsy.org.uk*

**Carers UK**
20 Great Dover Street, London SE1 4LX
Tel: 020 7378 4999
Fax: 020 7378 9781
Website: *www.carersuk.org*
E-mail: *info@carersuk.org*

**Disabled Living Foundation**
380-384 Harrow Road, London W9 2HU
Tel: 020 7289 6111/Help line: 0845 130 9177
Website: *www.dlf.org.uk*
E-mail: *info@dlf.org.uk*

**Encephalitis Society**
7b Saville Street, Malton, North Yorkshire YO17 7LL
Tel: 01653 692 583/Support line 01653 699 599
Website: *www.encephalitis.info*
E-mail: *mail@encephalitis.info*

**Headway—the Brain Injuries Association**
7 King Edward Court, King Edward Street, Nottingham NG1 1EW
Tel: 0115 9240800/Help line: 0808 800 2244
Fax: 0115 958 4446
Website: *www.headway.org.uk*
E-mail: *info@headway.org.uk*

**Help the Aged**
207-221 Pentonville Road, London N1 9UZ
Tel: 020 7278 1114
Fax: 020 7278 1116
Website: *www.helptheaged.org.uk*
E-mail: *info@helptheaged.org.uk*

**Huntington's Disease Association**
Neurosupport Centre, Liverpool L3 8LR
Tel: 0151 298 3298
Fax: 0151 298 9440
Website: *www.hda.org.uk*
E-mail: *info@hda.org.uk*

**Mental Health Foundation**
Sea Containers House, 9th Floor, 20 Upper Ground, London SE1 9QB
Tel: 020 7803 1101
Fax: 020 7803 1111
Website: *www.mentalhealth.org.uk*
E-mail: *mhf@mhf.org.uk*

**MIND—National Association for Mental Health**
15-19 Broadway, London E15 4BQ
Tel: 0845 766 0163
Website: *www.mind.org.uk*
E-mail: *contact@mind.org.uk*

**Multiple Sclerosis Society**
MS National Centre, 372 Edgware Road, London NW2 6ND
Tel: 020 8438 0700
Fax: 020 8438 0701
Website: *www.mssociety.org.uk*

**National Society for Epilepsy**
Chesham Lane, Chalfont St. Peter, Bucks SL9 0RJ
Tel: 01494 601 300
Fax: 01494 871 927
Website: *www.epilepsynse.org.uk*

**Oliver Zangwill Centre for Neuropsychological Rehabilitation**
The Princess of Wales Hospital, Lynn Road, Ely, Cambridgeshire CB6 1DN
Tel: 01353 652165
Fax: 01353 652164
Website: *www.ozc.nhs.uk*
E-mail: *andrew.bateman@ozc.nhs.uk*

**Parkinson's Disease Society**
215 Vauxhall Bridge Road, London SW1V IEJ
Tel: 0808 800 0303
Website: *www.parkinsons.org.uk*
E-mail: *enquiries@parkinsons.org.uk*

**RADAR (Royal Association for Disability and Rehabilitation)**
12 City Forum, 250 City Road, London EC1V 8AF
Tel: 020 7250 3222
Fax: 020 7250 0212
Website: *www.radar.org.uk*
E-mail: *radar@radar.org.uk*

**Stroke Association**
Stroke House, 240 City Road, London EC1V 2PR
Tel: 020 7566 0300
Fax: 020 7490 2686
Website: *www.stroke.org.uk*

## United States

*General*

**Acoustic Neuroma Association**
600 Peachtree Parkway, Suite 108, Cumming, GA 30041
Tel: 770-205-8211, 877-200-8211
Fax: 770-205-0239, 877-202-0239
Website: *www.anausa.org*
E-mail: *info@anausa.org*

**Brain Injury Association of America\***
1608 Spring Hill Road, Suite 110, Vienna, VA 22182
Tel: 703-761-0750
Fax: 703-761-0755
Website: *www.biausa.org*

---

\*Most states also have a brain injury association.

**Brain Trauma Foundation**
708 Third Avenue, New York, NY 10017
Tel: 212-772-0608
Fax: 212-772-0357
Website: *www.braintrauma.org*

**Epilepsy Foundation of America**
8301 Professional Place, Landover, MD 20785
Tel: 800-332-1000
Website: *www.epilepsyfoundation.org*

**Family Caregiver Alliance/ National Center on Caregiving**
180 Montgomery Street, Suite 1100, San Francisco, CA 94104
Tel: 415-434-3388, 800-445-8106
Fax: 415-434-3508
Website: *www.caregiver.org*
E-mail: *info@caregiver.org*

**North American Brain Injury Society**
PO Box 1804, Alexandria, VA 22313
Tel: 703-960-6500
Fax: 703-960-6603
Website: *www.nabis.org*

**National Institute of Mental Health (NIMH)**
6001 Executive Boulevard, Room 8184, MSC 9663, Bethesda, MD
20892-9663
Tel: 301-443-4513, 866-615-NIMH (6464), 301-443-8431 (TTY)
Fax: 646-638-1546
Website: *www.nimh.nih.gov*
E-mail: *nimhinfo@nih.gov*

**National Institute on Disability and Rehabilitation Research (NIDRR)**
U.S. Department of Education Office of Special Education and Rehabilita-
tive Services, 400 Maryland Avenue, SW, Washington, DC 20202-7100
Tel: 202-245-7460, 202-245-7316 (TTY)
Website: *www.ed.gov/about/offices/list/osers/nidrr*

**National Organization for Rare Disorders (NORD)**
55 Kenosia Avenue, PO Box 1968, Danbury, CT 06813-1968
Tel: 203-744-0100, Voice mail 800-999-NORD (6673)
Fax: 203-798-2291
Website: *www.rarediseases.org*
E-mail: *orphan@rarediseases.org*

**National Rehabilitation Information Center (NARIC)**
4200 Forbes Boulevard, Suite 202, Lanham, MD 20706-4829
Tel: 301-459-5900, 301-459-5984 (TTY), 800-346-2742
Fax: 301-562-2401
Website: *www.naric.com*
E-mail: *naricinfo@heitechservices.com*

## Alzheimer's Disease

**Alzheimer's Association**
225 North Michigan Avenue, 17th Floor, Chicago, IL 60601-7633
Tel: 312-335-8700
Fax: 866-699-1246
Website: *www.alz.org*
E-mail: *info@alz.org*

**Alzheimer's Disease Education and Referral Center (ADEAR)**
PO Box 8250, Silver Spring, MD 20907-8250
Tel: 301-495-3311, 800-438-4380
Fax: 301-495-3334
Website: *www.nia.nih.gov/alzheimers*
E-mail: *adear@nia.nih.gov*

**Alzheimer's Drug Discovery Foundation** (formerly Institute for the Study
of Aging)
1414 Avenue of the Americas, Suite 1502, New York, NY 10019
Tel: 212-935-2402
Fax: 212-935-2408
Website: *www.alzdiscovery.org*
E-mail: *hfillit@alzdiscovery.org*

**Alzheimer's Foundation of America**
322 Eighth Avenue, 7th Floor, New York, NY 10001
Tel: 866-AFA-8484 (232-8484)
Fax: 646-638-1546
Website: *www.alzfdn.org*
E-mail: *info@alzfdn.org*

**American Health Assistance Foundation**
22512 Gateway Center Drive, Clarksburg, MD 20871
Tel: 301-948-3244, 800-437-AHAF (2423)
Fax: 301-948-4403
Website: *www.ahaf.org*
E-mail: *info@ahaf.org*

**Association for Frontotemporal Dementias (AFTD)**
1616 Walnut Street, Suite 1100, Philadelphia, PA 19103
Tel: 267-514-7221, 866-507-7222
Website: *www.ftd-picks.org*
E-mail: *info@ftd-picks.org*

**C-Mac Informational Services/Caregiver News** (for Alzheimer's-type
dementia caregivers)
120 Clinton Lane, Cookeville, TN 38501-8946
Website: *www.caregivernews.org*
E-mail: *caregiver_cmi@hotmail.com*

**John Douglas French Alzheimer's Foundation**
11620 Wilshire Boulevard, Suite 270, Los Angeles, CA 90025
Tel: 310-445-4650, 800-477-2243
Fax: 310-479-0516
Website: *www.jdfaf.org*
E-mail: *jdfaf@earthlink.net*

**Lewy Body Dementia Association**
PO Box 451429, Atlanta, GA 31145-9429
Tel: 404-935-6444, 800-LEWYSOS (539-9767)
Fax: 480-422-5434
Website: *www.lbda.org*
E-mail: *lbda@lbda.org*

**National Family Caregivers Association**
10400 Connecticut Avenue, Suite 500, Kensington, MD 20895-3944
Tel: 301-942-6430, 800-896-3650
Fax: 301-942-2302
Website: *www.thefamilycaregiver.org*
E-mail: *info@thefamilycaregiver.org*

**National Hospice and Palliative Care Organization/
National Hospice Foundation**
1731 King Street, Suite 100, Alexandria, VA 22314
Tel: 703-837-1500, Help line: 800-658-8898
Fax: 703-837-1233
Website: *www.nhpco.org*
E-mail: *nhpco_info@nhpco.org*

**National Respite Network and Resource Center**
800 Eastowne Drive, Suite 105, Chapel Hill, NC 27514
Tel: 919-490-5577, x222
Fax: 919-490-4905
Website: *www.archrespite.org*

**Well Spouse Association**
63 West Main Street, Suite H, Freehold, NJ 07728
Tel: 800-838-0879, 732-577-8899
Fax: 732-577-8644
Website: *www.wellspouse.org*
E-mail: *info@wellspouse.org*

## Huntington's Disease

**Hereditary Disease Foundation**
3960 Broadway, 6th Floor, New York, NY 10032
Tel: 212-928-2121
Fax: 212-928-2172
Website: *www.hdfoundation.org*
E-mail: *curehd@hdfoundation.org*

**Huntington's Disease Society of America**
505 Eighth Avenue, Suite 902, New York, NY 10018
Tel: 212-242-1968, 800-345-HDSA (4372)
Fax: 212-239-3430
Website: *www.hdsa.org*
E-mail: *hdsainfo@hdsa.org*

*Multiple Sclerosis*

**Accelerated Cure Project for Multiple Sclerosis**
300 Fifth Avenue, Waltham, MA 02451
Tel: 781-487-0008
Fax: 781-487-0009
Website: *www.acceleratedcure.org*
E-mail: *info-web05@acceleratedcure.com*

**American Autoimmune Related Diseases Association**
22100 Gratiot Avenue, East Detroit, MI 48201-2227
Tel: 586-776-3900, 800-598-4668
Fax: 586-776-3903
Website: *www.aarda.org*
E-mail: *aarda@aarda.org*

**Clearinghouse on Disability Information**
Office of Special Education and Rehabilitative Services
Communications and Customer Service Team
550 12th Street, SW, Room 5133, Washington, DC 20202-2550
Tel: 202-245-7307, 202-205-5637 (TTD)
Fax: 202-450-7636
Website: *www.ed.gov/about/offices/list/osers/codi.html*

**Multiple Sclerosis Association of America**
706 Haddonfield Road, Cherry Hill, NJ 08002
Tel: 856-488-4500, 800-532-7667
Fax: 856-661-9797
Website: *www.msassociation.org*
E-mail: *msaa@msassociation.org*

**Multiple Sclerosis Foundation**
6350 North Andrews Avenue, Fort Lauderdale, FL 33309-2130
Tel: 954-776-6805, 888-MSFOCUS (673-6287)
Fax: 954-351-0630
Website: *www.msfocus.org*
E-mail: *support@msfocus.org*

**National Ataxia Foundation (NAF)**
2600 Fernbrook Lane North, Suite 119, Minneapolis, MN 55447-4752
Tel: 763-553-0020
Fax: 763-553-0167
Website: *www.ataxia.org*
E-mail: *naf@ataxia.org*

**National Multiple Sclerosis Society**
733 Third Avenue, 6th Floor, New York, NY 10017-3288
Tel: 212-986-3240, 800-344-4867 (FIGHTMS)
Fax: 212-986-7981
Website: *www.nationalmssociety.org*
E-mail: *nat@nmss.org*

**Paralyzed Veterans of America (PVA)**
801 18th Street, NW, Washington, DC 20006-3517
Tel: 202-USA-1300 (872-1300), 800-555-9140
Fax: 202-785-4452
Website: *www.pva.org*
E-mail: *info@pva.org*

## Parkinson's Disease

**American Parkinson Disease Association**
135 Parkinson Avenue, Staten Island, NY 10305-1425
Tel: 718-981-8001, 800-223-2732, California: 800-908-2732
Fax: 718-981-4399
Website: *www.apdaparkinson.org*
E-mail: *apda@apdaparkinson.org*

**Bachmann–Strauss Dystonia and Parkinson Foundation**
551 Fifth Avenue, Suite 520, New York, NY 10176
Tel: 212-682-9900
Fax: 212-987-0662
Website: *www.dystonia-parkinsons.org*
E-mail: *Bachmann.Strauss@mssm.edu*

**Michael J. Fox Foundation for Parkinson's Research**
Church Street Station, PO Box 780, New York, NY 10008-0780
Tel: 212-509-0995
Website: *www.michaeljfox.org*

**National Parkinson Foundation**
1501 NW 9th Avenue, Bob Hope Road, Miami, FL 33136-1494
Tel: 305-243-6666, 800-327-4545
Fax: 305-243-5595
Website: *www.parkinson.org*
E-mail: *contact@parkinson.org*

**Parkinson Alliance**
PO Box 308, Kingston, NJ 08528-0308
Tel: 609-688-0870, 800-579-8440
Fax: 609-688-0875
Website: *www.parkinsonalliance.org*
E-mail: *admin@parkinsonalliance.org*

**Parkinson's Action Network**
1025 Vermont Avenue, NW, Suite 1120, Washington, DC 20005
Tel: 800-850-4726, 202-638-4101
Fax: 202-638-7257
Website: *www.parkinsonsaction.org*
E-mail: *info@parkinsonsaction.org*

**Parkinson's Disease Foundation (PDF)**
1359 Broadway, Suite 1509, New York, NY 10018
Tel: 212-923-4700, 800-457-6676
Fax: 212-923-4778
Website: *www.pdf.org*
E-mail: *info@pdf.org*

**Parkinson's Institute and Clinical Center**
675 Almanor Avenue, Sunnyvale, CA 94085
Tel: 408-734-2800, 800-786-2958
Fax: 408-734-8522
Website: *www.thepi.org*
E-mail: *info@thepi.org*

**Parkinson's Resource Organization**
74090 El Paseo Drive, Suite 102, Palm Desert, CA 92260-4135
Tel: 760-773-5628, 310-476-7030, 877-775-4111
Fax: 760-773-9803
Website: *www.parkinsonsresource.org*
E-mail: *info@parkinsonsresource.org*

**WE MOVE (Worldwide Education and Awareness for Movement Disorders)**
204 West 84th Street, New York, NY 10024
Tel: 212-875-8312
Fax: 212-875-8389
Website: *www.wemove.org*
E-mail: *wemove@wemove.org*

## Stroke

**American Health Assistance Foundation**
22512 Gateway Center Drive, Clarksburg, MD 20871
Tel: 301-948-3244, 800-437-AHAF (2423)
Fax: 301-948-4403
Website: *www.ahaf.org*
E-mail: *info@ahaf.org*

**American Stroke Association: A Division of American Heart Association**
7272 Greenville Avenue, Dallas, TX 75231-4596
Tel: 1-888-4STROKE (478-7653)
Fax: 214-706-5231
Website: *www.strokeassociation.org*
E-mail: *strokeassociation@heart.org*

**Brain Aneurysm Foundation**
269 Hanover Street, Building 3, Hanover, MA 02339
Tel: 781-826-5556, 888-BRAIN02 (272-4602)
Website: *www.bafound.org*
E-mail: *office@bafound.org*

**Brain Attack Coalition**
31 Center Drive, Room 8A07, Bethesda, MD 20892-2540
Tel: 301-496-5751
Fax: 301-402-2186
Website: *www.stroke-site.org*

**Children's Hemiplegia and Stroke Association (CHASA)**
4101 West Green Oaks, Suite 305, PMB 149, Arlington, TX 76016
Tel: 817-492-4325
Website: *www.hemikids.org*
E-mail: *info437@chasa.org*

**Hazel K. Goddess Fund for Stroke Research in Women**
785 Park Avenue, New York, NY 10021-3552
Tel: 212-713-6789
Fax: 212-288-2160
Website: *www.thegoddessfund.org*
E-mail: *info@thegoddessfund.org*

**Heart Rhythm Foundation**
1400 K Street, NW, Suite 500, Washington, DC 20005
Tel: 202-464-3404
Fax: 202-464-3405
Website: *www.heartrhythmfoundation.org*
E-mail: *support@heartrhythmfoundation.org*

**National Aphasia Association**
350 Seventh Avenue, Suite 902, New York, NY 10001
Tel: 212-267-2814, 800-922-4NAA (4622)
Fax: 212-267-2812
Website: *www.aphasia.org*
E-mail: *naa@aphasia.org*

**National Stroke Association**
9707 East Easter Lane, Suite B, Centennial, CO 80112-3747
Tel: 303-649-9299, 800-STROKES (787-6537)
Fax: 303-649-1328
Website: *www.stroke.org*
E-mail: *info@stroke.org*

**Stroke Clubs International**
805 12th Street, Galveston, TX 77550
Tel: 409-762-1022
E-mail: *strokeclubs@earthlink.net*

## Australia

**Alzheimer's Australia**
PO Box 4019, Hawker, ACT 2614
Tel: 61 (2) 6254 4233
Website: *www.alzheimers.org.au*

**Australian Huntington's Disease Association**
PO Box 580, North Adelaide, SA 5006
Website: *www.huntingtonsaustralia.asn.au*
E-mail: *national@huntingtonsaustralia.asn.au*

**Brain Injury Australia**
PO Box 874, Auburn NSW 1835
Tel: (02) 8507 6555
Fax: (02) 8507 6556
Website: *www.braininjuryaustralia.org.au*
E-mail: *admin@braininjuryaustralia.org.au*

**MS Australia**
117 Division Street, Deakin, ACT 2600
Tel: 612 6285 2999
Fax: 612 6281 0817
Website: *www.msaustralia.org.au*
E-mail: *admin@ms.org.au*

**National Stroke Foundation**
Level 7, 461 Bourke Street, Melbourne, VIC 3000
Tel: 61 3 9670 1000
Fax: 61 3 9670 9300
Website: *www.strokefoundation.com.au*
E-mail: admin@strokefoundation.com.au

**Parkinson's Australia**
Frewin Centre, Frewin Place, Scullin, ACT 2614
Tel: (02) 6278 8916
Website: *www.parkinsons.org.au*
E-mail: *norman.marshall@parkinsonsaustralia.org.au*

## Canada

**Alzheimer Society of Canada**
20 Eglinton Avenue W, Suite 1600, Toronto, ON M4R 1K8
Tel: 416-488-8772, Toll-free: 800-616-8816 (valid only in Canada)
Fax: 416-488-3778
Website: *www.alzheimer.ca*
E-mail: *info@alzheimer.ca*

**Heart and Stroke Foundation**
222 Queen Street, Suite 1402, Ottawa, ON K1P 5V9
Tel: 613-569-4361
Fax: 613-569-3278
Website: *www.heartandstroke.ca*

**Huntington Society of Canada**
151 Frederick Street, Suite 400, Kitchener, ON N2H 2M2
Tel: 519-749-7063
Fax: 519-749-8965
Website: *www.huntingtonsociety.ca*
E-mail: *info@huntingtonsociety.ca*

**Multiple Sclerosis Society of Canada**
174 Bloor E. Toronto, ON M4W3R8
Tel: 416-922-6065
Fax: 416-922-7538
Website: *www.mssociety.ca*
E-mail: *info@mssociety.ca*

**Parkinson Society Canada**
4211 Yonge Street, 316 Toronto, ON M2P 2A9
Tel: 416-227-9700, Toll-free: 800-565-3000
Fax: 416-227-9600
Website: *www.parkinson.ca*
E-mail: *general.info@parkinson.ca*

**Brain Injury Association of Canada**
28 Caron, Gatineau, Québec J8Y 1Y7
Tel: 819-777-2492, Toll-free: 866-977-2492
Fax: 819-595-2458
Website: *www.biac-aclc.ca*
E-mail: *info@biac-aclc.ca*

## Czech Republic

**Aging**
*www.zivot90.cz*
*www.tretivek.cz*
*www.treninkpameti.webnode.com*
*www.ddfrantiskov.cz*

**Alzheimer's Disease**

*www.alzheimer.cz*

**Brain Injury**

*www.cerebrum2007.cz*

**Huntington's Disease**

*www.huntington.cz*

**Multiple Sclerosis**

*www.roska.eu*

**Parkinson's Disease**

*www.parkinsonovachoroba.cz*

**Stroke**

*www.sdruzenicmp.cz*

## Finland

**Alzheimer-Keskusliitto Ry (Alzheimer's disease)**
Luotsikatu 4 E, 00160 Helsinki
Tel: 358-9-6226 200
Fax: 358-9-6226 2020
Website: *www.alzheimer.fi*
E-mail: *toimisto@alzheimer.fi*

**Aivovammaliitto Ry (Brain Injury)**
Nordenskiöldinkatu 18 A, 00250 Helsinki
Tel: 358-9-836 6580
Website: *www.aivovammaliitto.fi*
E-mail: *aivovammaliitto@aivovammaliitto.fi*

**Suomen MS-liitto Ry (Multiple Sclerosis)**
PL 15 (Seppäläntie 90), Masku 21251
Tel: 358-2-439 2111
Fax: 358-2-439 2133
Website: *www.ms-liitto.fi*
E-mail: *tiedotus@ms-liitto.fi*

**Suomen Parkinson-liitto Ry (Parkinson's Disease)**
Erityisosaamiskeskus Suvituuli, Suvilinnantie 2, PL 905, 20101 Turku
Tel: 358-2-2740 400
Fax: 358-2-2740 444
Website: *www.parkinson.fi*
E-mail: *parkinson-liitto@parkinson.fi*

**Aivohalvaus- ja afasialiitto (Stroke)**
Suvilinnantie 2, 20900 Turku
Tel: 358-2-2138 200
Fax: 358-2-2138 210
Website: *www.stroke.fi*
E-mail: *aivohalvaus.dysfasia@stroke.fi*

## Greece

**Athens Association of Alzheimer's Disease and Related Disorders**
Markou Mousourou 89, 11636 Athens
Tel: 30 210 70 13 271
Website: *www.alzheimerathens.gr*
E-mail: *info@alzheimerathens.gr*

## Hong Kong

**Hong Kong Alzheimer's Disease Association**
G/F, Wang Yip House, Wang Tau Hom Estate, Kowloon, Hong Kong Special Administrative Region, China
Tel: 852 23381120
Fax: 852 23380772
Website: *www.hkada.org.hk*

**Hong Kong Parkinson's Disease Foundation**
Hong Kong Parkinson's Disease Foundation, Department of Medicine, Queen Mary Hospital, University of Hong Kong, 102 Pokfulam Road, Hong Kong Special Administrative Region, China
Tel: 852 81005223
Fax: 852 29741171
Website: *www.hkpdf.org.hk*
E-mail: *info@hkpdf.org.hk*

**Hong Kong Stroke Society**
Room 346, L-Block, Queen Mary Hospital, Department of Neurology
Tel: 852 28553315
Fax: 852 28551171
Website: *www.stroke.org.hk*
E-mail: *secretary@stroke.org.hk*

**Hong Kong Society for Rehabilitation**
6/F, 7 Sha Wan Drive, Pokfulam, Hong Kong Special Administrative
Region, China
Tel: 852 28176277
Fax: 852 28551947
Website: *www.rehabsociety.org.hk*
E-mail: *enquiry@rehabsociety.org.hk*

## The Netherlands

**Alzheimer Nederland**
Postbus 183, 3980 CD Bunnik
Tel: 030-659 69 00
Fax: 030-659 69 01
Website: *www.alzheimer-nederland.nl*
E-mail: *info@alzheimer-nederland.nl*

**Hartstichting (Heart and Stroke)**
Bordewijklaan 3, 2591 XR Den Haag
Tel: 070-315 55 55
Fax: 070-335 28 26
Website: *www.hartstichting.nl*
E-mail: *info@hartstichting.nl*

**Hersenstichting Nederland (Brain Injury Association)**
Koediefstraat 5, 2511 CG Den Haag
Tel: 070-360 48 16
Fax: 070-360 99 46
Website: *www.hersenstichting.nl*
E-mail: *info@hersenstichting.nl*

**MS Vereniging Nederland**
Laan van Meerdervourt 51, Postbus 30 470, 2500 GL Den Haag
Tel: 070-374 77 77
Fax: 070-374 77 70
Website: *www.msvereniging.nl*
E-mail: *info@msvn.nl*

**Parkinson Patiënten Vereniging**
Kosterijland 12, 3981 AJ Bunnik
Tel: 030-656 13 69
Website: *www.parkinson-vereniging.nl*
E-mail: *info@parkinson-vereniging.nl*

**Vereniging Cerebraal (Cerebral Association)**
Palestrinastraat 1b, 3533 EH Utrecht
Tel: 030-296 65 75
Website: *www.cerebraal.nl*
E-mail: *secr@cerebraal.nl*

**Vereniging van Huntington (Association of Huntington)**
Laan van Meerdervoort 51, 2517 AE Den Haag
Tel: 070-314 88 88
Fax: 070-314 88 80
Website: *www.huntington.nl*

## New Zealand

**Alzheimers New Zealand**
Level 3 Adelphi Finance House, 15 Courtney Place, Wellington
Website: *www.alzheimers.org.nz*
E-mail: *nationaloffice@alzheimers.org.nz*

**Brain Injury Association of New Zealand**
PO Box 83, Albany Village 0755, Auckland
Tel: (09) 414 5693
Fax: (09) 415 5643
Website: *www.brain-injury.org.nz*
E-mail: *national@brain-injury.org.nz*

**Head Injury Society of New Zealand**
PO Box 1168, Hamilton
Tel: Toll free: 0508 444 357/Phone: (07) 839 1182
Website: *www.head-injury.org.nz*
E-mail: *headinjury@xtra.co.nz*

**Huntington's Disease Association of New Zealand**
PO Box 78, Cust, North Canterbury, NZ
Tel: (64) 3-3125 612
Fax: (64) 4-232 5365
Website: *www.huntingtons.org.nz*

**Multiple Sclerosis Society of New Zealand**
Level 2, 85 The Terrace, PO Box 2627, Wellington 6140
Tel: (64) 4 499 4677
Fax: (64) 4 499 4675
Website: *www.msnz.org.nz*

**Parkinson's New Zealand**
PO Box 11 067, Wellington 6142
Tel: (04) 472 2796
Fax: (04) 472 2162
Website: *www.parkinsons.org.nz*
E-mail: *info@parkinsons.org.nz*

**Stroke Foundation of New Zealand**
PO Box 12482, L1, Federation House, 95-99 Molesworth Street,
Wellington
Tel: (04) 472 8099/Toll free: 0800 STROKE (0800 78 76 53)
Website: *www.stroke.org.nz*
E-mail: *strokenz@stroke.org.nz*

## Singapore

**Alzheimer's Disease Association**
Blk 157 Lorong 1 Toa Payoh, #01-1195 Singapore 310157
Tel: 65 6353-8734
Fax: 65 6353-8518
Website: *www.alzheimers.org.sg*
E-mail: *alzheimers.tp@pacific.net.sg*

**Parkinson's Disease Society of Sinapore**
c/o SNSA, 26 Dunearn Road, Singapore 309423
Tel: 65 6353-5338
Fax: 65 6358-4139
Website: *www.parkinsonsingapore.com*
E-mail: *pdsspore@gmail.com*

**Singapore Brain and Spine Injury Foundation**
c/o Department of Neurosurgery, National Neuroscience Institute
11 Jalan Tan Tock Seng, Singapore 308433
Website: *www.sbsif.org.sg*
E-mail: *info@sbsif.com.sg*

**Singapore National Stroke Association**
26 Dunearn Road, Singapore 309423
Tel: 65 6358-4138
Fax: 65 6358-4139
Website: *www.snsa.org.sg*
E-Mail: *sporensa@singnet.com.sg*

## *South Africa*

**Alzheimer's South Africa**
Tel: 011 478 2234
Website: *www.alzheimers.org.za*
E-mail: *info@alzheimers.org.za*

**Heart and Stroke Foundation**
PO Box 15139, Vlaeberg 8018
Tel: (021) 447 4222
Fax: (021) 447 0322
Website: *www.heartfoundation.co.za*
E-mail: *heart@heartfoundation.co*

**Huntington's Society of South Africa**
PO Box 44501, Claremonte, Cape Town, 7735 Südafrika
Tel: (27) 21 - 938 4911
Fax: (27) 21 - 761 4438
E-mail: *jschron@iafrica.com*

**Multiple Sclerosis South Africa**
Tel: MSSA Help Line 0860 456772
Website: *www.multiplesclerosis.co.za*
E-mail: *msu@multiplesclerosis.co.za*

**Parkinson Association of South Africa**
304 Oak Avenue, Standard Bank Building, 3rd floor, Ferndale,
Randburg 2194
Tel: (27) 011-787-8792
Fax: (27) 011-787-2047
Website: *www.parkinsons.co.za*
E-mail: *office@parkinsons.co.za*

# References

Abel, S., Schultz, A., Radermacher, I., Willmes, K., & Huber, W. (2005). Decreasing and increasing cues in naming therapy for aphasia. *Aphasiology, 19*(9), 831–848.

Achté, K. A., Hillbom, E., & Aalberg, V. (1969). Psychoses following war brain injuries. *Acta Psychiatrica Scandinavica, 45*(1), 1–18.

Achté, K. A., Lönnqvist, J., & Hillbom, E. (1970). Suicides of war brain injured veterans. *Psychiatrica Fennica, 1,* 231–239.

Alderman, N. (2001). Management of challenging behaviour. In R. L. Wood & T. M. McMillan (Eds.), *Neurobehavioural disability and social handicap following traumatic brain injury.* Hove, UK: Psychology Press.

Alderman, N., Fry, R. K., & Youngson, H. A. (1995). Improvement of self-monitoring skills, reduction of behaviour disturbance and the dysexecutive syndrome: Comparison of response cost and a new programme of self-monitoring training. *Neuropsychological Rehabilitation, 5*(3), 193–221.

Almli, C., & Finger, S. (1988). Toward a definition of recovery of function. In S. Finger, T. E. LeVere, C. Almli, & D. G. Stein (Eds.), *Brain injury and recovery: Theoretical and controversial issues.* New York: Plenum Press.

Almli, C., & Finger, S. (1992). Brain injury and recovery of function: Theories and mechanisms of functional reorganization. *Journal of Head Trauma Rehabilitation, 7*(2), 70–77.

Anderson, S. W. (1996). Cognitive rehabilitation in closed head injury. In M. Rizzo & D. Tranel (Eds.), *Head injury and post-concussion syndrome.* New York: Churchill Livingstone.

Andrews, K. (1991). The limitations of randomized controlled trials in rehabilitation research. *Clinical Rehabilitation, 5*(1), 5–8.

Arco, L. (2008). Neurobehavioural treatment for obsessive–compulsive disorder in an adult with traumatic brain injury. *Neuropsychological Rehabilitation, 18*(1), 109–124.

Arkin, S. M. (2000). Alzheimer memory training: Students replicate learning successes. *American Journal of Alzheimer's Disease and Other Dementias, 15*(3), 152–162.

Arkin, S. M. (2001). Alzheimer rehabilitation by students: Interventions and outcomes. *Neuropsychological Rehabilitation, 11*(3), 273–317.

Arnott, S. R., Grady, C. L., Hevenor, S. J., Graham, S., & Alain, C. (2005). The functional organization of auditory working memory as revealed by fMRI. *Journal of Cognitive Neuroscience, 17*(5), 819–831.

Atkinson, R. C., & Shiffrin, R. M. (1971). The control of short-term memory. *Scientific American, 225*(2), 82–90.

Attella, M. J., Nattinville, A., & Stein, D. G. (1987). Hormonal state affects recovery from frontal cortex lesions in adult female rats. *Behavioral and Neural Biology, 48*(3), 352–367.

Azmitia, E. C. (2007). Cajal and brain plasticity: Insights relevant to emerging concepts of mind. *Brain Research Reviews, 55*(2), 395–405.

Bäckman, L., & Dixon, R. A. (1992). Psychological compensation: A theoretical framework. *Psychological Bulletin, 112*(2), 259–283.

Baddeley, A. D., & Hitch, G. J. (1974). Working memory. In G. H. Bower (Ed.), *The psychology of learning and motivation.* New York: Academic Press.

Baddeley, A. D. (1986). *Working memory.* Gloucester, UK: Clarendon Press.

Baddeley, A. D. (1992). Memory theory and memory therapy. In B. A. Wilson & N. Moffat (Eds.), *Clinical management of memory problems* (2nd ed.). London: Chapman & Hall.

Baddeley, A. D. (1993). A theory of rehabilitation without a model of learning is a vehicle without an engine: A comment on Caramazza and Hillis. *Neuropsychological Rehabilitation, 3*(3), 235–244.

Baddeley, A. D. (1997). *Human memory: Theory and practice* (2nd ed.). Hove, UK: Psychology Press.

Baddeley, A. D. (1999). *Essentials of human memory.* Hove, UK: Psychology Press.

Baddeley, A. D. (2000). The episodic buffer: A new component of working memory? *Trends in Cognitive Sciences, 4*(11), 417–423.

Baddeley, A. D. (2002). *The handbook of memory disorders* (2nd ed.). Chichester, UK: Wiley.

Baddeley, A. D. (2004). The psychology of memory. In A. D. Baddeley, M. D. Kopelman, & B. A. Wilson (Eds.), *The essential handbook of memory disorders for clinicians.* Chichester, UK: Wiley.

Baddeley, A. D., Emslie, H., & Nimmo-Smith, I. (1992). *The speed and capacity of language-processing test.* Bury St. Edmunds, UK: Thames Valley Test Company.

Baddeley, A. D., & Hitch, G. J. (1974). Working memory. In G. H. Bower

(Ed.), *The psychology of learning and motivation: Advances in research and theory.* New York: Academic Press.

Baddeley, A. D., & Longman, D. J. A. (1978). The influence of length and frequency of training session on the rate of learning to type. *Ergonomics, 21*(8), 627–635.

Baddeley, A. D., Nimmo-Smith, I., & Emslie, H. (1994). *Doors and people.* Bury St. Edmunds, UK: Thames Valley Test Company.

Baddeley, A. D., & Wilson, B. A. (1986). Amnesia, autobiographical memory, and confabulation. In D. C. Rubin (Ed.), *Autobiographical memory.* Cambridge, UK: Cambridge University Press.

Baddeley, A. D., & Wilson, B. A. (1988a). Comprehension and working memory: A single case neuropsychological study. *Journal of Memory and Language, 27*(5), 479–498.

Baddeley, A. D., & Wilson, B. A. (1988b). Frontal amnesia and the dysexecutive syndrome. *Brain and Cognition, 7*(2), 212–230.

Baddeley, A. D., & Wilson, B. A. (1994). When implicit learning fails: Amnesia and the problem of error elimination. *Neuropsychologia, 32*(1), 53–68.

Baddeley, A. D., & Wilson, B. A. (2002). Prose recall and amnesia: Implications for the structure of working memory. *Neuropsychologia, 40*(10), 1737–1743.

Baer, D. M., Wolf, M. M., & Risley, T. R. (1968). Some current dimensions of applied behavior analysis. *Journal of Applied Behavior Analysis, 1*(1), 91–97.

Bak, T. H., Antoun, N., Balan, K. K., & Hodges, J. R. (2001). Memory lost, memory regained: Neuropsychological findings and neuroimaging in two cases of paraneoplastic limbic encephalitis with radically different outcomes. *Journal of Neurology, Neurosurgery, and Psychiatry, 71*(1), 40–47.

Barlow, D. H., Nock, M. K., & Hersen, M. (2008). *Single case experimental designs: Strategies for studying behavior change* (3rd ed.). New York: Allyn & Bacon.

Bateman, A., Brentnall, S., Evans, J., Gartland, D., Gracey, F., Keohane, C., et al. (2005). Outcomes of intensive neuropsychological rehabilitation: The relationship between the Dysexecutive Questionnaire (DEX), European Brain Injury Questionnaire (EBIQ) and SMART goal attainment. *Brain Impairment, 6*, 132.

Baxter, L., Spencer, B., & Kerrigan, J. F. (2007). Clinical application of functional MRI for memory using emotional enhancement: Deficit and recovery with limbic encephalitis. *Epilepsy and Behavior, 11*(3), 454–459.

Beardsall, L., & Huppert, F. A. (1991). A comparison of clinical, psychometric and behavioural memory tests: Findings from a community study of the early detection of dementia. *International Journal of Geriatric Psychiatry, 6*(5), 295–306.

Beck, A. T. (1970). Cognitive therapy: Nature and relation to behavior therapy. *Behavior Therapy, 1,* 184–200.

Beck, A. (1987). *The Beck Depression Inventory.* San Antonio, TX: Psychological Corporation.

Becker, J. T., & Overman, A. A. (2004). The memory deficit in Alzheimer's disease. In A. D. Baddeley, M. D. Kopelman, & B. A. Wilson (Eds.), *The essential handbook of memory disorders for clinicians.* Chichester, UK: Wiley.

Behrmann, M., Marotta, J., Gauthier, I., Tarr, M. J., & McKeeff, T. J. (2005). Behavioral change and its neural correlates in visual agnosia after expertise training. *Journal of Cognitive Neuroscience, 17*(4), 554–568.

Benke, T., Hohenstein, C., Poewe, W., & Butterworth, B. (2000). Repetitive speech phenomena in Parkinson's disease. *Journal of Neurology, Neurosurgery, and Psychiatry, 69*(3), 319–324.

Bennett-Levy, J., & Powell, G. E. (1980). The Subjective Memory Questionnaire (SMQ). An investigation into the self-reporting of "real-life" memory skills. *British Journal of Social and Clinical Psychology, 19,* 177–188.

Benton, A. L. (1974). *Revised Visual Retention Test* (4th ed.). New York: Psychological Corporation.

Ben-Yishay, Y. (1978). *Working approaches to remediation of cognitive deficits in brain damaged persons* (Rehabilitation Monograph No. 59). New York: New York University Medical Center.

Ben-Yishay, Y. (1996). Reflections on the evolution of the therapeutic milieu concept. Historical aspects of neuropsychological rehabilitation. *Neuropsychological Rehabilitation, 6*(4), 327–343.

Ben-Yishay, Y. (2000). Post-acute neuropsychological rehabilitation: A holistic perspective. In A. L. Christensen & B. P. Uzzell (Eds.), *International handbook of neuropsychological rehabilitation* (Critical issues in neuropsychology series). Amsterdam, The Netherlands: Kluwer Academic.

Berg, I. J., Koning-Haanstra, M., & Deelman, B. G. (1991). Long-term effects of memory rehabilitation: A controlled study. *Neuropsychological Rehabilitation, 1,* 97–111.

Berger, G., Bernhardt, T., Schramm, U., Muller, R., Landsiedel-Anders, S., Kratzsch, T., et al. (2004). No effects of a combination of caregivers support group and memory training/music therapy in dementia patients from a memory clinic population. *International Journal of Geriatric Psychiatry, 19*(3), 223–231.

Bernhardt, E., Maurer, K., & Frolich, L. (2002). Der Einfluss eines alltagsbezogenenkognitivenTrainings auf die Aufmerksamkeits und Gedaechtnisleisung vonPersonen mir Demenz [Influence of a memory training program on attention and memory performance of patients with dementia]. *Zeitschrift fuer Gerontolgie and Geriatrie, 35,* 32–38.

Berry, E., Kapur, N., Williams, L., Hodges, S., Watson, P., Smyth, G., et al. (2007). The use of a wearable camera, SenseCam, as a pictorial diary to improve autobiographical memory in a patient with limbic encephalitis: A preliminary report. *Neuropsychological Rehabilitation, 17*(4–5), 582–601.

Berthier, M. L., Kulisevsky, J. J., Gironell, A., & López, O. L. (2001). Obsessive–compulsive disorder and traumatic brain injury: Behavioral, cognitive, and neuroimaging findings. *Neuropsychiatry, Neuropsychology, and Behavioral Neurology, 14*(1), 23–31.

Bion, W. (1968). *Experiences in groups.* London: Tavistock.

Bird, M. (2001). Behavioural difficulties and cued recall of adaptive behaviour in dementia: Experimental and clinical evidence. *Neuropsychological Rehabilitation, 11*(3), 357–375.

Bjork, R. A. (1988). Retrieval practice and the maintenance of knowledge. In M. M. Gruneberg, P. E. Morris, & R. N. Sykes (Eds.), *Practical aspects of memory: Current research and issues: Vol. 2. Clinical and educational implications.* Chichester, UK: Wiley.

Blake, D. D., Weathers, F. W., Nagy, L. M., Kaloupek, D. G., Gusman, F. D., Charney, D. S., et al. (1995). The development of a clinician-administered PTSD scale. *Journal of Traumatic Stress, 8*(1), 75–90.

Boman, I. L. (2007). Using electronic aids to daily living after acquired brain injury: A study of the learning process and the usability. *Disability and Rehabilitation: Assistive Technology, 2*(1), 23–33.

Bornhofen, C., & McDonald, S. (2008). Emotion perception deficits following traumatic brain injury: A review of the evidence and rationale for intervention. *Journal of the International Neuropsychological Society, 14*(4), 511–525.

Bourgeois, M. S. (2007). *Memory books and other graphic cuing systems: Practical communication and memory aids for adults with dementia.* Baltimore, MD: Health Professions Press.

Bowen, A., Neumann, V., Conner, M., Tennant, A., & Chamberlain, M. A. (1998). Mood disorders following traumatic brain injury: Identifying the extent of the problem and the people at risk. *Brain Injury, 12*(3), 177–190.

Bowling, A. (2005). *Measuring health: A review of quality of life measurement scales* (3rd ed.). Maidenhead, UK: Open University Press.

Brasted, P. J., Bussey, T. J., Murray, E. A., & Wise, S. P. (2005). Conditional motor learning in the nonspatial domain: Effects of errorless learning and the contribution of the fornix to one-trial learning. *Behavioral Neuroscience, 119*(3), 662–676.

Braun, J. J. (1978). Time and recovery from brain damage. In S. Finger (Ed.), *Recovery from brain damage: Research and theory.* New York: Plenum Press.

Breuning, E., Van Loon-Vervoorn, W. A., & Van Dieren, M. P. (1989). [Memory training with Korsakov patients.] *Tijdschrift voor Alcohol, Drugs en Andere Psychotrope Stoffen, 15*(6), 213–221.

Brewin, C. R., Dalgleish, T., & Joseph, S. (1996). A dual representation theory of posttraumatic stress disorder. *Psychological Review, 103,* 670–686.

Broadbent, D. E., Cooper, P. F., Fitzgerald, P., & Parkes, K. R. (1982). The Cognitive Failures Questionnaire (CFQ) and its correlates. *The British Journal of Clinical Psychology, 21*(1), 1–16.

Brodtmann, A., Puce, A., Darby, D., & Donnan, G. (2007). fMRI demonstrates diaschisis in the extrastriate visual cortex. *Stroke, 38*(8), 2360–2363.

Broman, M., Rose, A. L., Hotson, G., & Casey, C. M. (1997). Severe anterograde amnesia with onset in childhood as a result of anoxic encephalopathy. *Brain, 120*(3), 417–433.

Brooks, D. N., & Baddeley, A. D. (1976). What can amnesic patients learn? *Neuropsychologia, 14*(1), 111–122.

Brooks, N., Campsie, L., Symington, C., Beattie, A., & McKinlay, W. (1987). The effects of severe head injury on patient and relative within several years of injury. *Journal of Head Trauma Rehabilitation, 2,* 1–13.

Brown, R. (2004). Psychological and psychiatric aspects of brain disorder: Nature, assessment and implications for clinical neuropsychology. In L. H. Goldstein & J. E. McNeil (Eds.), *Clinical neuropsychology: A practical guide to assessment and management for clinicians.* Chichester, UK: Wiley.

Brunberg, J. A., Frey, K. A., Horton, J. A., & Kuhl, D. E. (1992). Crossed cerebellar diaschisis: Occurrence and resolution demonstrated with PET during carotid temporary balloon occlusion. *American Journal of Neuroradiology, 13*(1), 58–61.

Brush, J. A., & Camp, C. J. (1998). *A therapy technique for improving memory: Spaced retrieval.* Beachwood, OH: Menora Park Centre for Senior Living.

Bryant, R. A. (2001a). Posttraumatic stress disorder and mild brain injury: Controversies, causes and consequences. *Journal of Clinical and Experimental Neuropsychology, 23*(6), 718–728.

Bryant, R. A. (2001b). Posttraumatic stress disorder and traumatic brain injury: Can they co-exist? *Clinical Psychology Review, 21*(6), 931–948.

Bryant, R. A., Marosszeky, J. E., Crooks, J., & Gurka, J. A. (2000). Posttraumatic stress disorder after severe traumatic brain injury. *American Journal of Psychiatry, 157,* 629–631.

Burgess, P. W., Alderman, N., Evans, J., Emslie, H., & Wilson, B. A. (1998). The ecological validity of tests of executive function. *Journal of the International Neuropsychological Society, 4*(6), 547–558.

Burgess, P. W., Veitch, E., de Lacy Costello, A., & Shallice, T. (2000). The cognitive and neuroanatomical correlates of multitasking. *Neuropsychologia, 38*(6), 848–863.

Bush, S. S., Ruff, R. M., Tröster, A. I., Barth, J. T., Koffler, S. P., Pliskin, N. H., et al. (2005). Symptom validity assessment: Practice issues and medical necessity NAN Policy & Planning Committee. *Archives of Clinical Neuropsychology, 20*(4), 419–426.

Bussman-Mork, B. A., Hildberandt, H., Giesselmann, H., & Sachsenheimer, W. (2000). Behandlung mittelschwerer sprachlicher gedachtnisstorungen: Ein vergleich mehrerer methoden [Treatment of verbal memory disorders: A comparison of several methods]. *Neurologie und Rehabilitation, 6*(4), 195–204.

Butler, G. (1998). Clinical formulation. In A. Bellack & M. Hersen (Eds.), *Comprehensive clinical psychology.* Oxford, UK: Pergamon Press.

Butters, N., & Albert, M. S. (1982). Processes underlying failures to recall remote events. In L. S. Cermak (Ed.), *Human memory and amnesia.* Hillsdale, NJ: Erlbaum.

Cajal, S. R. (1888). Estructura de los centros nerviosos de las aves [Structure of the nerve centers of birds]. *Revista Trimestral de Histología Normal y Patológica, 1,* 1–10.

Camp, C. J. (1989). Facilitation of new learning in Alzheimer's disease. In G. Gilmore, P. Whitehouse, & M. Wykle (Eds.), *Memory and aging: Theory, research and practice.* New York: Springer.

Camp, C. J., Bird, M., & Cherry, K. (2000). Retrieval strategies as a rehabilitation aid for cognitive loss in pathological aging. In R. D. Hill, L. Bäckman, & A. Stigsdotter-Neely (Eds.), *Cognitive rehabilitation in old age.* New York: Oxford University Press.

Camp, C. J.. & Foss, J. W. (1997). Designing ecologically valid memory interventions for persons with dementia. In D. G. Payne & F. G. Conrad (Eds.), *Intersections in basic and applied memory research* (pp. 311–325). Mahwah, NJ: Erlbaum.

Camp, C. J., Foss, J. W., Stevens, A. B., & O'Hanlon, A. M. (1996). Improving prospective memory performance in persons with Alzheimer's disease. In M. A. Brandimonte, G. O. Einstein, & M. A. McDaniel (Eds.), *Prospective memory: Theory and application.* Mahwah, NJ: Erlbaum.

Caplan, B. (1987). *Rehabilitation psychology desk reference.* Rockville, MD: Aspen.

Carlomagno, S., Van Eeckhout, P., Blasi, V., Belin, P., Samson, Y., & Deloche, G. (1997). The impact of functional neuroimaging methods on the development of a theory for cognitive remediation. *Neuropsychological Rehabilitation, 7*(4), 311.

Carney, N., Chesnut, R. M., Maynard, H., Mann, N. C., Patterson, P., & Helfand, M. (1999). Effect of cognitive rehabilitation on outcomes for persons with traumatic brain injury: A systematic review. *Journal of Head Trauma Rehabilitation, 14*(3), 277–302.

Carver, C. S., & Scheier, M. F. (1990). Origins and functions of positive and negative affect: A control-process view. *Psychological Review, 97*(1), 19–35.

Cavaco, S., Anderson, S. W., Allen, J. S., Castro-Caldas, A., & Damasio, H. (2004). The scope of preserved procedural memory in amnesia. *Brain, 127*(8), 1853–1867.

Cermak, L. S. (1975). Imagery as an aid to retrieval for Korsakoff patients. *Cortex, 11*(2), 163–169.

238 References

Cermak, L. S., & O'Connor, M. (1983). The anterograde and retrograde retrieval ability of a patient with amnesia due to encephalitis. *Neuropsychologia, 21*(3), 213–234.

Chan, D., Fox, N. C., Scahill, R. I., Crum, W. R., Whitwell, J. L., Leschziner, G., et al. (2001). Patterns of temporal lobe atrophy in semantic dementia and Alzheimer's disease. *Annals of Neurology, 49*(4), 433–442.

Chan, M., Estève, D., Escriba, C., & Campo, E. (2008). A review of smart homes: Present state and future challenges. *Computer Methods and Programs in Biomedicine, 91*(1), 55–81.

Cheek, P., Nikpour, L., & Nowlin, H. D. (2005). Aging well with smart technology. *Nursing Administration Quarterly, 29*(4), 329–338.

Chemerinski, E., & Levine, S. R. (2006). Neuropsychiatric disorders following vascular brain injury. *Mount Sinai Journal of Medicine, New York, 73*(7), 1006–1014.

Clare, L. (2008). *Neuropsychological rehabilitation and people with dementia* (1st ed.). Hove, UK: Psychology Press.

Clare, L., & Wilson, B. A. (1997). *Coping with memory problems: A practical guide for people with memory impairments, their relatives, friends and carers.* Bury St. Edmunds, UK: Thames Valley Test Company.

Clare, L., Wilson, B. A., Breen, K., & Hodges, J. R. (1999). Errorless learning of face-name associations in early Alzheimer's disease. *Neurocase, 5*, 37–46.

Clare, L., Wilson, B. A., Carter, G., Breen, K., Gosses, A., & Hodges, J. R. (2000). Intervening with everyday memory problems in dementia of Alzheimer type: An errorless learning approach. *Journal of Clinical and Experimental Neuropsychology, 22*(1), 132–146.

Clare, L., Wilson, B. A., Carter, G., & Hodges, J. R. (2003). Cognitive rehabilitation as a component of early intervention in Alzheimer's disease: A single case study. *Aging & Mental Health, 7*(1), 15–21.

Clare, L., Wilson, B. A., Carter, G., Hodges, J. R., & Adams, M. (2001). Long-term maintenance of treatment gains following a cognitive rehabilitation intervention in early dementia of Alzheimer type: A single case study. *Neuropsychological Rehabilitation, 11*(3), 477–494.

Clare, L., Wilson, B. A., Carter, G., Roth, I., & Hodges, J. R. (2002). Relearning face-name associations in early Alzheimer's disease. *Neuropsychology, 16*(4), 538–547.

Clare, L., & Woods, R. T. (Eds.). (2001). *Cognitive rehabilitation in dementia* [Special issue]. *Neuropsychological Rehabilitation, 11*(3/4).

Clare, L., & Woods, R. T. (2004). Cognitive training and cognitive rehabilitation for people with early-stage Alzheimer's disease: A review. *Neuropsychological Rehabilitation, 14*, 385–401.

Cockburn, J., & Smith, P. T. (1989). *The Rivermead Behavioural Memory Test supplement three: Elderly people.* Bury St. Edmunds, UK: Thames Valley Test Company.

Code, C., & Herrmann, M. (2003). The relevance of emotional and psychosocial factors in aphasia to rehabilitation. *Neuropsychological Rehabilitation, 13*(1–2), 109–132.

Cohen, N. J., & Corkin, S. (1981). *The amnesic patient H. M.: Learning and retention of a cognitive skill.* Paper presented at the Society for Neuroscience, Los Angeles.

Cole, E. (1999). Cognitive prosthetics: An overview to a method of treatment. *NeuroRehabilitation, 12*(1), 39–51.

Cole, E., & Dehdashti, P. (1990). Interface design as a prosthesis for an individual with a brain injury. *ACM SIGCHI Bulletin, 22*(1), 28–32.

Collicut-McGrath, J. (2008). Post-acute in-patient rehabilitation. In A. Tyerman & N. S. King (Eds.), *Psychological approaches to brain injury rehabilitation.* Oxford, UK: BPS Blackwell.

*Concise Oxford English Dictionary* (10th ed.). (1999). Oxford, UK: Oxford University Press.

Conover, J. C., & Notti, R. Q. (2008). The neural stem cell niche. *Cell and Tissue Research, 331*(1), 211–224.

Corkin, S. (1996). Acquisition of motor skill after bilateral medial temporal-lobe excision. *Neurocase, 2*(4), 259–298.

Corrigan, J. D., Bogner, J. A., Mysiw, W. J., Clinchot, D., & Fugate, L. (2001). Life satisfaction after traumatic brain injury. *The Journal of Head Trauma Rehabilitation, 16*(6), 543–555.

Corwin, J., & Bylsma, F. W. (1993). Translation of excerpts from Andre Rey's *Psychological examination of traumatic encephalopathy* and P. A. Osterreith's *The Complex Figure Copy Test. The Clinical Neuropsychologist, 7,* 3–15.

Coughlan, A. K., & Hollows, S. (1985). *The Adult Information Processing Battery.* Leeds, UK: A.K. Coughlan.

Coughlan, A. K., & Storey, P. (1988). The Wimbledon Self-Report Scale: Emotional and mood appraisal. *Clinical Rehabilitation, 2*(3), 207–213.

Craik, F. I. M., & Lockhart, R. S. (1972). Levels of processing: A framework for memory research. *Journal of Verbal Learning and Verbal Behavior, 11*(6), 671–684.

Craik, F. I. M., & Watkins, M. J. (1973). The role of rehearsal in short-term memory. *Journal of Verbal Learning and Verbal Behavior, 12,* 599–607.

Craik, F. I. M., Winocur, G., Palmer, H., Binns, M. A., Edwards, M., Bridges, K., et al. (2007). Cognitive rehabilitation in the elderly: Effects on memory. *Journal of the International Neuropsychological Society, 13*(1), 132–142.

Crawford, J., Smith, G., Maylor, E., Della Sala, S., & Logie, R. (2003). The Prospective and Retrospective Memory Questionnaire (PRMQ): Normative data and latent structure in a large non-clinical sample. *Memory, 11*(3), 261–275.

Crovitz, H. F. (1979). Memory retraining in brain-damaged patients: The airplane list. *Cortex, 15*(1), 131–134.

Cullen, C. N. (1976). Errorless learning with the retarded. *Nursing Times, 72*(12), 45–47.

Cutajar, R., Ferriani, E., Scandellari, C., Sabattini, L., Trocino, C., Marchello, L. P., et al. (2000). Cognitive function and quality of life in multiple sclerosis patients. *Journal of Neurology, 6,* 186–190.

Dalgleish, T., & Cox, S. (2002). Memory and emotional disorder. In A. D. Baddeley, M. D. Kopelman, & B. A. Wilson (Eds.), *The handbook of memory disorders.* Chichester, UK: Wiley.

Davis, A., Davis, S., Moss, N., Marks, J., McGrath, J., Hovard, L., et al. (1992). First steps towards an interdisciplinary approach to rehabilitation. *Clinical Rehabilitation, 6*(3), 237–244.

Dawson, K. S., Batchelor, J., Meares, S., Chapman, J., & Marosszeky, J. E. (2007). Applicability of neural reserve theory in mild traumatic brain injury. *Brain Injury, 21*(9), 943–949.

De Renzi, E., & Vignolo, L. A. (1962). The Token Test: A sensitive test to detect receptive disturbances in aphasics. *Brain, 85,* 665–678.

DeGutis, J. M., Bentin, S., Robertson, L. C., & D'Esposito, M. (2007). Functional plasticity in ventral temporal cortex following cognitive rehabilitation of a congenital prosopagnosic. *Journal of Cognitive Neuroscience, 19*(11), 1790–1802.

Delis, D. C., Kramer, J. H., Kaplan, E., & Ober, B. A. (1987). *California Verbal Learning Test: Adult version.* San Antonio, TX: Psychological Corporation.

Della Sala, S., Gray, C., Baddeley, A. D., Allamano, N., & Wilson, L. (1999). Pattern span: A tool for unwelding visuo-spatial memory. *Neuropsychologia, 37*(10), 1189–1199.

Della Sala, S., Gray, C., Baddeley, A. D., & Wilson, L. (1997). *Visual pattern test.* Bury St. Edmunds, UK: Thames Valley Test Company.

Della Sala, S., & Logie, R. H. (2002). Neuropsychological impairments of visual and spatial working memory. In A. D. Baddeley & M. D. Kopelman (Eds.), *Handbook of memory disorders* (2nd ed.). New York: Wiley.

Derogatis, L. R., Lipman, R. S., & Covi, L. (1973). SCL-90: An outpatient psychiatric rating scale—Preliminary report. *Psychopharmacology Bulletin, 9*(1), 13–28.

Dewar, B., & Gracey, F. (2007). "Am not was": Cognitive-behavioural therapy for adjustment and identity change following herpes simplex encephalitis. *Neuropsychological Rehabilitation, 17*(4–5), 602–620.

Dewar, B., Patterson, K., Wilson, B. A., & Graham, K. S. (in press). Reacquisition of person knowledge in semantic memory disorders. *Neuropsychological Rehabilitation.*

Dewar, B., & Williams, H. (2007). *Encephalitis: Assessment and rehabilitation across the lifespan* (1st ed.). Hove, UK: Psychology Press.

Dewar, B., & Wilson, B. A. (2006). Training face identification in prosopagnosia. *Brain Impairment, 7*(2), 160.

Dhanushkodi, A., & Shetty, A. K. (2008). Is exposure to enriched environment beneficial for functional post-lesional recovery in temporal lobe epilepsy? *Neuroscience and Biobehavioral Reviews, 32*(4), 657–674.

Diehl-Schmid, J., Pohl, C., Ruprecht, C., Wagenpfeil, S., Foerstl, H., & Kurz, A. (2007). The Ekman 60 Faces Test as a diagnostic instrument in frontotemporal dementia. *Archives of Clinical Neuropsychology, 22*(4), 459–464.

Diesfeldt, H. F., & Smits, J. C. (1991). [Faces get names—cognitive training for psychogeriatric patients for remembering names and faces]. *Tijdschrift Voor Gerontologie En Geriatrie, 22*(6), 221–227.

Diller, L. (1976). A model for cognitive retraining in rehabilitation. *The Clinical Psychologist, 26,* 13–15.

Dixon, R. A., & Bäckman, L. (1999). Principles of compensation in cognitive neurorehabilitation. In D. T. Stuss, G. Winocur, & I. H. Robertson (Eds.), *Cognitive neurorehabilitation: A comprehensive approach.* New York: Cambridge University Press.

Döbrössy, M. D., & Dunnett, S. B. (2004). The influence of environment and experience on neural grafts. *Nature Reviews Neuroscience, 2*(12), 871–879.

Donaghy, S., & Williams, W. (1998). A new protocol for training severely impaired patients in the usage of memory journals. *Brain Injury, 12*(12), 1061–1076.

Downes, J. J., Kalla, T., Davies, A. D. M., Flynn, A., Ali, H., & Mayes, A. R. (1997). The pre-exposure technique: A novel method for enhancing the effects of imagery in face-name association learning. *Neuropsychological Rehabilitation, 7*(3), 195–214.

Dunn, J., & Clare, L. (2007). Learning face–name associations in early-stage dementia: Comparing the effects of errorless learning and effortful processing. *Neuropsychological Rehabilitation, 17*(6), 735–754.

Ehlhardt, L., Sohlberg, M. M., Kennedy, M., Coelho, C., Ylvisaker, M., Turkstra, L., et al. (2008). Evidence-based practice guidelines for instructing individuals with neurogenic memory impairments: What have we learned in the past 20 years? *Neuropsychological Rehabilitation, 18*(3), 300–342.

Eichenbaum, H., & Cohen, N. J. (2001). *From conditioning to conscious recollection: Memory systems of the brain.* New York: Oxford University Press.

Ekman, P., & Friesen, W. V. (1971). Constants across cultures in the face and emotion. *Journal of Personality and Social Psychology, 17*(2), 124–129.

Elkins, J. S., Longstreth, W. T., Manolio, T. A., Newman, A. B., Bhadelia, R. A., & Johnston, S. C. (2006). Education and the cognitive decline associated with MRI-defined brain infarct. *Neurology, 67*(3), 435–440.

Ellis, J. A. (1996). Prospective memory or the realization of delayed intentions: A conceptual framework for research. In M. A. Brandimonte, G. O. Einstein, & M. A. McDaniel (Eds.), *Prospective memory: Theory and applications.* Mahwah, NJ: Erlbaum.

Emslie, H., Wilson, B. A., Quirk, K., Evans, J. J., & Watson, P. (2007). Using a paging system in the rehabilitation of encephalitic patients. *Neuropsychological Rehabilitation, 17*(4–5), 567–581.

Ericcson, K. A., Chase, W. G., & Faloon, S. (1980). Acquisition of a memory skill. *Science, 208*(4448), 1181–1182.

Eriksson, P. S., Perfilieva, E., Björk-Eriksson, T., Alborn, A. M., Nordborg, C., Peterson, D. A., et al. (1998). Neurogenesis in the adult human hippocampus. *Nature Medicine, 4*, 1313–1317.

Eslinger, P. J. (2002). *Neuropsychological interventions: Clinical research and practice* (1st ed.). New York: Guilford Press.

Evans, J. J. (2005). Can executive impairments be effectively treated? In P. W. Halligan & D. Wade (Eds.), *The effectiveness of rehabilitation for cognitive deficits.* Oxford, UK: Oxford University Press.

Evans, J. J. (in press). The cognitive group, part two: Memory. In B. A. Wilson, F. Gracey, J. J. Evans, & A. Bateman (Eds.), *Neuropsychological rehabilitation: Theory, models, therapy and outcome.* Cambridge, UK: Cambridge University Press.

Evans, J. J., Emslie, H. C., & Wilson, B. A. (1998). External cueing systems in the rehabilitation of executive impairments of action. *Journal of the International Neuropsychological Society, 4*(4), 399–408.

Evans, J. J., & Williams, W. H. (in press). Caroline: PTSD after traumatic brain injury. In B. A. Wilson, F. Gracey, J. J. Evans, & A. Bateman (Eds.), *Neuropsychological rehabilitation: Theory, models, therapy and outcome.* Cambridge, UK: Cambridge University Press.

Evans, J. J., & Wilson, B. A. (1992). A memory group for individuals with brain injury. *Clinical Rehabilitation, 6*(1), 75–81.

Evans, J. J., Wilson, B. A., Calder, A. J., & Bateman, A. (2007). Frequency and nature of deficits in facial emotion perception after brain injury. *Journal of the International Neuropsychological Society, 13*(S2), 13.

Evans, J. J., Wilson, B. A., Needham, P., & Brentnall, S. (2003). Who makes good use of memory aids? Results of a survey of people with acquired brain injury. *Journal of the International Neuropsychological Society, 9*, 925–935.

Evans, J. J., Wilson, B. A., Schuri, U., Andrade, J., Baddeley, A. D., Bruna, O., et al. (2000). A comparison of errorless and trial-and-error learning methods for teaching individuals with acquired memory deficits. *Neuropsychological Rehabilitation, 10*(1), 67–101.

Farace, E., & Alves, W. M. (2000). Do women fare worse? A meta-analysis of gender differences in outcome after traumatic brain injury. *Neurosurgical Focus, 8*(1), e6.

Feeney, D. M., & Baron, J. C. (1986). Diaschisis. *Stroke, 17*(5), 817–830.

Feredoes, E., & Postle, B. R. (2007). Localization of load sensitivity of working memory storage: Quantitatively and qualitatively discrepant results yielded by single-subject and group-averaged approaches to fMRI group analysis. *NeuroImage, 35*(2), 881–903.

Ferrans, C. E. (1990). Development of a quality of life index for patients with cancer. *Oncology Nursing Forum, 17*(3, Suppl.), 15–19.

Ferrans, C. E., & Powers, M. J. (1992). Psychometric assessment of the Quality of Life Index. *Research in Nursing and Health, 15*(1), 29–38.

Fillingham, J. K., Hodgson, C., Sage, K., & Lambon-Ralph, M. A. (2003). The application of errorless learning to aphasic disorders: A review of theory and practice. *Neuropsychological Rehabilitation, 13*(3), 337–363.

Fillingham, J. K., Sage, K., & Lambon-Ralph, M. A. (2005a). Treatment of anomia using errorless versus errorful learning: Are frontal executive skills and feedback important? *International Journal of Language and Communication Disorders, 40*(4), 505–523.

Fillingham, J. K., Sage, K., & Lambon-Ralph, M. A. (2005b). Further explorations and an overview of errorless and errorful therapy for aphasic word-finding difficulties: The number of naming attempts during therapy affects outcome. *Aphasiology, 19*(7), 597–614.

Fillingham, J. K., Sage, K., & Lambon Ralph, M. A. (2006). The treatment of anomia using errorless learning. *Neuropsychological Rehabilitation, 16*(2), 129–154.

Fish, J., Evans, J. J., Nimmo, M., Martin, E., Kersel, D., Bateman, A., et al. (2007). Rehabilitation of executive dysfunction following brain injury: "Content-free" cueing improves everyday prospective memory performance. *Neuropsychologia, 45*(6), 1318–1330.

Fish, J., Manly, T., Emslie, H., Evans, J. J., & Wilson, B. A. (2008). Compensatory strategies for acquired disorders of memory and planning: Differential effects of a paging system for patients with brain injury of traumatic versus cerebrovascular aetiology. *Journal of Neurology, Neurosurgery, and Psychiatry, 79*(8), 930–935.

Fish, J., Manly, T., & Wilson, B. A. (2008a). Rehabilitation for prospective memory problems resulting from acquired brain injury. In M. Oddy & A. Worthington (Eds.), *Rehabilitation of executive disorders: A guide to theory and practice*. Oxford, UK: Oxford University Press.

Fish, J., Manly, T., & Wilson, B. A. (2008b). Long-term compensatory treatment of organizational deficits in a patient with bilateral frontal lobe damage. *Journal of the International Neuropsychological Society, 14*(1), 154–163.

Fisk, J. D., & Rockwood, K. (2005). Outcomes of incident mild cognitive impairment in relation to case definition. *Journal of Neurology, Neurosurgery, and Psychiatry, 76*(8), 1175–1177.

Fleminger, S. (2008). Long-term psychiatric disorders after traumatic brain injury. *European Journal of Anaesthesiology Supplement, 42*, 123–130.

Fleminger, S., Oliver, D. L., Williams, W. H., & Evans, J. J. (2003). The neuropsychiatry of depression after brain injury. *Neuropsychological Rehabilitation, 13*(1–2), 65–87.

Foa, E. B., Huppert, J. D., Leiberg, S., Langner, R., Kichic, R., Hajcak, G., et al. (2002). The Obsessive–Compulsive Inventory: Development and validation of a short version. *Psychological Assessment, 14*(4), 485–496.

Folsom, J. (1968). Reality orientation for the elderly mental patient. *Journal of Geriatric Psychiatry, 1,* 291–307.

Foulkes, S. H. (1965). *Group psychotherapy.* New York: Penguin.

Franzen, K. M., Roberts, M. A., Schmits, D., Verduyn, W., & Manshadi, F. (1996). Cognitive remediation in pediatric traumatic brain injury. *Child Neuropsychology, 2*(3), 176–184.

Frattali, C., & LaPointe, L. L. (2004). An errorless learning approach to treating dysnomia in frontotemporal dementia. *Journal of Medical Speech–Language Pathology, 12,* 21–24.

Freed, D. M., Corkin, S., & Cohen, N. J. (1987). Forgetting in H. M.: A second look. *Neuropsychologia, 25*(3), 461–471.

Fridriksson, J., Holland, A. L., Beeson, P., & Morrow, L. (2005). Spaced retrieval treatment of anomia. *Aphasiology, 19*(2), 99–109.

Frith, C. (2007). *Making up the mind: How the brain creates our mental world* (1st ed.). Oxford, UK: Blackwell.

Gainotti, G. (1993). Emotional and psychosocial problems after brain injury. *Neuropsychological Rehabilitation, 3*(3), 259–277.

Gainotti, G. (2003). Assessment and treatment of emotional disorders. In P. W. Halligan, U. Kischka, & J. C. Marshall (Eds.), *Handbook of clinical neuropsychology.* Oxford, UK: Oxford University Press.

Gainotti, G., Azzoni, A., Razzano, C., Lanzillotta, M., & Gasparini, F. (1997). The Post-Stroke Depression Rating Scale: A test specifically designed to investigate affective disorders of stroke patients. *Journal of Clinical and Experimental Neuropsychology, 19,* 340–356.

Galton, F. (1907). *Inquiries into human faculty and its development.* London: Dent.

Gardner, H. Y. (1977). *The shattered mind: The person after brain damage.* London: Routledge & Kegan Paul.

Garske, G. G., & Thomas, K. R. (1992). Self-reported self-esteem and depression: Indexes of psychosocial adjustment following severe traumatic brain injury. *Rehabilitation Counseling Bulletin, 36*(1), 44–52.

Gatz, M., Fiske, A., Fox, L. S., Kaskie, B., Kasl-Godley, J. E., McCallurn, T. J., et al. (1998). Empirically validated psychological treatments for older adults. *Journal of Mental Health and Aging, 4,* 9–46.

Gauggel, S., & Billino, J. (2002). The effects of goal setting on the arithmetic performance of brain-damaged patients. *Archives of Clinical Neuropsychology, 17*(3), 283–294.

Gauggel, S., & Fischer, S. (2001). The effect of goal setting on motor performance and motor learning in brain-damaged patients. *Neuropsychological Rehabilitation, 11*(1), 33–44.

Gauggel, S., Leinberger, R., & Richardt, M. (2001). Goal setting and reaction time performance in brain-damaged patients. *Journal of Clinical and Experimental Neuropsychology, 23*(3), 351–361.

Gentry, T. (2008). PDAs as cognitive aids for people with multiple sclerosis. *American Journal of Occupational Therapy, 62*(1), 18–27.

Gentry, T., Wallace, J., Kvarfordt, C., & Lynch, K. B. (2008). Personal digital assistants as cognitive aids for individuals with severe traumatic brain injury: A community-based trial. *Brain Injury, 22*(1), 19–24.

Giacino, J. T., Ashwal, S., Childs, N., Cranford, R., Jennett, B., Katz, D. I., et al. (2002). The minimally conscious state: Definition and diagnostic criteria. *Neurology, 58*, 349–353.

Gianutsos, R., & Gianutsos, J. (1987). Single case experimental approaches to the assessment of interventions in rehabilitation psychology. In B. Caplan (Ed.), *Rehabilitation psychology*. Rockville, MD: Aspen Corporation.

Gibbs, W. (2000, November). As we may live. *Scientific American, 283*, 36, 40.

Glasgow, R. E. (1977). Case studies on remediating memory deficits in brain-damaged individuals. *Journal of Clinical Psychology, 33*(4), 1049–1054.

Glisky, E. L. (1992). Acquisition and transfer of declarative and procedural knowledge by memory-impaired patients: A computer data-entry task. *Neuropsychologia, 30*(10), 899–910.

Glisky, E. L., & Delaney, S. M. (1996). Implicit memory and new semantic learning in posttraumatic amnesia. *The Journal of Head Trauma Rehabilitation, 11*(2), 31–42.

Glisky, E. L., & Schacter, D. L. (1988). Long-term retention of computer learning by patients with memory disorders. *Neuropsychologia, 26*(1), 173–178.

Glisky, E. L., & Schacter, D. L. (1989). Extending the limits of complex learning in organic amnesia: Computer training in a vocational domain. *Neuropsychologia, 27*, 107–120.

Glisky, E. L., Schacter, D. L., & Tulving, E. (1986). Computer learning by memory-impaired patients: Acquisition and retention of complex knowledge. *Neuropsychologia, 24*(3), 313–328.

Godden, D. R., & Baddeley, A. D. (1975). Context-dependent memory in two natural environments: On land and underwater. *British Journal of Psychology, 66*, 325–331.

Goldenberg, G., Schuri, U., Gromminger, O., & Arnold, U. (1999). Basal forebrain amnesia: Does the nucleus accumbens contribute to human memory? *Journal of Neurology, Neurosurgery, and Psychiatry, 67*(2), 163.

Goldstein, K., & Denny-Brown, D. (1942). *Aftereffects of brain injuries in war: Their evaluation and treatment: The application of psychologic methods in the clinic*. New York: Grune & Stratton.

Goodman, W. K., Price, L. H., Rasmussen, S. A., Mazure, C., Fleischmann, R. L., Hill, C. L., et al. (1989). The Yale–Brown Obsessive Compulsive Scale. *Archives of General Psychiatry, 46*, 1006–1016.

Gracey, F. (2002). Mood and affective problems after traumatic brain injury. *Advances in Clinical Neuroscience and Rehabilitation, 2*, 18–19.

Gracey, F., Yeates, G., Palmer, S., & Psaila, K. (in press). The psychological support group. In B. A. Wilson, F. Gracey, J. J. Evans, & A. Bateman (Eds.), *Neuropsychological rehabilitation: Theory, models, therapy and outcome.* Cambridge, UK: Cambridge University Press.

Grady, C. L., & Kapur, S. (1999). The use of imaging in neurorehabilitative research. In D. T. Stuss, G. Winocur, & I. H. Robertson (Eds.), *Cognitive neurorehabilitation: A comprehensive approach.* Cambridge, UK: Cambridge University Press.

Graf, P., & Schacter, D. L. (1985). Implicit and explicit memory for new associations in normal and amnesic subjects. *Journal of Experimental Psychology: Learning, Memory, and Cognition, 11*(3), 501–518.

Graf, P., Squire, L. R., & Mandler, G. (1984). The information that amnesic patients do not forget. *Journal of Experimental Psychology. Learning, Memory, and Cognition, 10,* 164–177.

Graham, K. S., & Hodges, J. R. (1997). Differentiating the roles of the hippocampal complex and the neocortex in long-term memory storage: Evidence from the study of semantic dementia and Alzheimer's disease. *Neuropsychology, 11*(1), 77–89.

Graham, K. S., Kropelnicki, A., Goldman, W. P., & Hodges, J. R. (2003). Two further investigations of autobiographical memory in semantic dementia. *Cortex, 39*(4–5), 729–750.

Graham, K. S., Patterson, K., Pratt, K. H., & Hodges, J. R. (2001). Can repeated exposure to "forgotten" vocabulary help alleviate word-finding difficulties in semantic dementia? An illustrative case study. *Neuropsychological Rehabilitation, 11*(3), 429–454.

Grandmaison, E., & Simard, M. (2003). A critical review of memory stimulation programs in Alzheimer's disease. *Journal of Neuropsychiatry and Clinical Neurosciences, 15*(2), 130–144.

Greenfield, E., Nannery, R., & Wilson, B. A. (2007). You learn something new every day—Or do you? *Brain Impairment, 8*(2), 182–183.

Griesbach, G. S., Hovda, D. A., Molteni, R., Wu, A., & Gomez-Pinilla, F. (2004). Voluntary exercise following traumatic brain injury: Brain-derived neurotrophic factor upregulation and recovery of function. *Neuroscience, 125*(1), 129–139.

Groot, Y. C. T., Wilson, B. A., Evans, J. J., & Watson, P. (2002). Prospective memory functioning in people with and without brain injury. *Journal of the International Neuropsychological Society, 8*(5), 645–654.

Grubb, N. R., Fox, K. A. A., Smith, K., Best, J., Blane, A., Ebmeier, K. P., et al. (2000). Memory impairment in out-of-hospital cardiac arrest survivors is associated with global reduction in brain volume, not focal hippocampal injury. *Stroke, 31,* 1509–1514.

Hagen, I. (2007). Technology in dementia care [Special issue]. *Technology and Disability, 19*(2–3).

Hall, J. F. (1971). *Verbal learning and retention.* New York: Lippincott.

Hamilton, M. (1960). A rating scale for depression. *Journal of Neurology, Neurosurgery, and Psychiatry, 23,* 56–62.

Harris, J. E. (1980). Memory aids people use: Two interview studies. *Memory and Cognition, 8*(1), 31–38.

Harris, J. E. (1984). Remembering to do things: A forgotten topic. In J. E. Harris & P. E. Morris (Eds.), *Everyday memory, actions, and absentmindedness.* London: Academic Press.

Hart, T., & Evans, J. J. (2006). Self-regulation and goal theories in brain injury rehabilitation. *Journal of Head Trauma Rehabilitation, 21*(2), 142–155.

Hart, T., Hawkey, K., & Whyte, J. (2002). Use of a portable voice organizer to remember therapy goals in traumatic brain injury rehabilitation: A within-subjects trial. *Journal of Head Trauma Rehabilitation, 17*(6), 556–570.

Hay, L. R. (1982). Teaching behavioral assessment to clinical psychology students. *Behavioral Assessment, 4,* 35–40.

Hebb, D. O. (1949). *The organization of behavior: A neuropsychological theory.* Chichester, UK: Wiley.

Helmstaedter, C., & Kockelmann, E. (2006). Cognitive outcomes in patients with chronic temporal lobe epilepsy. *Epilepsia, 47*(Suppl. 2), 96–98.

Herrmann, D. J., & Neisser, U. (1978). An inventory of everyday memory experiences. In M. M. Gruneberg, P. Morris, & R. N. Sykes (Eds.), *Practical aspects of memory.* London: Academic Press.

Hersen, M., & Barlow, D. (1982). *Single case experimental designs.* Oxford, UK: Pergamon Press.

Hibbard, M. R., Uysal, S., Kepler, K., Bogdany, J., & Silver, J. (1998). Axis I psychopathology in individuals with traumatic brain injury. *Journal of Head Trauma Rehabilitation, 13*(4), 24–39.

Hillary, F. G., Schultheis, M. T., Challis, B. H., Millis, S. R., Carnevale, G. J., Galshi, T., et al. (2003). Spacing of repetitions improves learning and memory after moderate and severe TBI. *Journal of Clinical and Experimental Neuropsychology, 25*(1), 49–58.

Hillis, A. E., & Caramazza, A. (1991). Category-specific naming and comprehension impairment: A double dissociation. *Brain, 114*(Pt. 5), 2081–2094.

Hirono, N., Mori, E., Ikejiri, Y., Imamura, T., Shimomura, T., Ikeda, M., et al. (1997). Procedural memory in patients with mild Alzheimer's disease. *Dementia and Geriatric Cognitive Disorders, 8*(4), 210–216.

Hochhalter, A. K., Overmier, J. B., Gasper, S. M., Bakke, B. L., & Holub, R. J. (2004). A comparison of spaced retrieval to other schedules of practice for people with dementia. *Experimental Aging Research, 31*(2), 101–118.

Hodder, K., & Haslam, C. (2006, July). *Errorless learning: A comparison with other memory rehabilitation techniques.* Paper presented at the International Neuropsychological Society Satellite Meeting on Neuropsychological Rehabilitation, Triesenberg, Liechtenstein.

Hodges, J. R., & McCarthy, R. A. (1993). Autobiographical nokamnesia resulting from bilateral paramedian thalamic infarction: A case study in cognitive neurobiology. *Brain, 116*(4), 921–940.

Hodges, J. R., Patterson, K., Oxbury, S., & Funnell, E. (1992). Semantic dementia. Progressive fluent aphasia with temporal lobe atrophy. *Brain, 115*(Pt. 6), 1783–1806.

Holliday, R. C., Cano, S., Freeman, J. A., & Playford, E. D. (2007). Should patients participate in clinical decision making? An optimised balance block design controlled study of goal setting in a rehabilitation unit. *Journal of Neurology, Neurosurgery, and Psychiatry, 78*(6), 576–580.

Holmes, T. H., & Rahe, R. H. (1967). The Social Readjustment Rating Scale. *Journal of Psychosomatic Research, 11*(2), 213–218.

Hong, K. S., Lee, S. K., Kim, K. K., & Nam, H. (2000). Visual working memory revealed by repetitive transcranial magnetic stimulation. *Journal of the Neurological Sciences, 181*(1–2), 50–55.

Hopper, T., Mahendra, N., Kim, E., Azuma, T., Bayles, K. A., Cleary, S. J., et al. (2005). Evidence-based practice recommendations for working with individuals with dementia: Spaced-retrieval training. *Journal of Medical Speech Language Pathology, 13*(4), 27–34.

Horner, M. D., Selassie, A. W., Lineberry, L., Ferguson, P. L., & Labbate, L. A. (2008). Predictors of psychological symptoms 1 year after traumatic brain injury: A population-based, epidemiological study. *The Journal of Head Trauma Rehabilitation, 23*(2), 74–83.

Houts, P. S., & Scott, R. A. (1975). *Goal planning with developmentally disabled persons: Procedures for developing and individual client plant.* Hershey: Department of Behavioral Science, Pennsylvania State University College of Medicine.

Howard, D., & Patterson, K. (1992). *The Pyramids and Palm Trees Test.* Bury St. Edmunds, UK: Thames Valley Test Company.

Hunkin, N. M., & Parkin, A. J. (1995). The method of vanishing cues: An evaluation of its effectiveness in teaching memory-impaired individuals. *Neuropsychologia, 33*(10), 1255–1279.

Hunkin, N. M., Parkin, A. J., Bradley, V. A., Burrows, E. H., Aldrich, F. K., Jansari, A., et al. (1995). Focal retrograde amnesia following closed head injury: A case study and theoretical account. *Neuropsychologia, 33*(4), 509–523.

Hunkin, N. M., Squires, E. J., Parkin, A. J., & Tidy, J. A. (1998). Are the benefits of errorless learning dependent on implicit memory? *Neuropsychologia, 36*(1), 25–36.

Hurn, J., Kneebone, I., & Cropley, M. (2006). Goal setting as an outcome measure: A systematic review. *Clinical Rehabilitation, 20*(9), 756–772.

Isaacs, E., Lucas, A., Chong, W., Wood, S., Johnson, C., Marshall, C., et al.

(2000). Hippocampal volume and everyday memory in children of very low birth weight. *Pediatric Research, 47*(6), 713–720.

Isaacs, E. B., Vargha-Khadem, F., Watkins, K. E., Lucas, A., Mishkin, M., & Gadian, D. G. (2003). Developmental amnesia and its relationship to degree of hippocampal atrophy. *Proceedings of the National Academy of Sciences, 100*(22), 13060–13063.

Jacoby, L. L., & Dallas, M. (1981). On the relationship between autobiographical memory and perceptual learning. *Journal of Experimental Psychology: General, 110*, 306–340.

Jang, S. H., You, S. H., & Ahn, S. H. (2007). Neurorehabilitation-induced cortical reorganization in brain injury: A 14-month longitudinal follow-up study. *Neurorehabilitation, 22*(2), 117–122.

Jennett, B., & Bond, M. (1975). Assessment of outcome after severe brain damage. *Lancet, 1*(7905), 480–484.

Jennett, B., Snoek, J., Bond, M. R., & Brooks, N. (1981). Disability after severe head injury: Observations on the use of the Glasgow Outcome Scale. *Journal of Neurology, Neurosurgery, and Psychiatry, 44*(4), 285–293.

Jennett, S. M., & Lincoln, N. B. (1991). An evaluation of the effectiveness of group therapy for memory problems. *International Disability Studies, 13*(3), 83–86.

Johnson, M. K., Kim, J. K., & Risse, G. (1985). Do alcoholic Korsakoff's syndrome patients acquire affective reactions? *Journal of Experimental Psychology: Learning, Memory, and Cognition, 11*, 22–36.

Jones, M. K. (1974). Imagery as a mnemonic aid after left temporal lobectomy: Contrast between material-specific and generalized memory disorders. *Neuropsychologia, 12*(1), 21–30.

Jones, R. S. P., & Eayrs, C. B. (1992). The use of errorless learning condition procedures in teaching people with a learning disability. *Mental Handicap Research, 5*, 304–312.

Jorge, R. E., Robinson, R. G., Arndt, S. V., Starkstein, S. E., Forrester, A. W., & Geisler, F. (1993). Depression following traumatic brain injury: A 1 year longitudinal study. *Journal of Affective Disorders, 27*(4), 233–243.

Judd, T. (1999). *Neuropsychotherapy and community integration: Brain illness, emotions, and behaviour.* New York: Kluwer Academic/Plenum.

Kanfer, F. H. (1970). Self regulation: Research issues and speculations. In C. Neuringer & M. L. Michael (Eds.), *Behavior modification in clinical psychology.* New York: Appleton-Century-Crofts.

Kanfer, F. H., & Saslow, G. (1969). Behavioral diagnosis. In C. Franks (Ed.), *Behavior therapy: Appraisal and status.* New York: Appleton-Century-Crofts.

Kapur, N. (1993). Focal retrograde amnesia in neurological disease: A critical review. *Cortex, 29*(2), 217–234.

Kapur, N. (1999). Syndromes of retrograde amnesia: A conceptual and empirical synthesis. *Psychological Bulletin, 125*, 800–825.

Kapur, N. (2008). *Cambridge memory manual: A manual for improving everyday memory skills.* Cambridge, UK: Addenbrooke's Hospital.

Kapur, N., Glisky, E. L., & Wilson, B. A. (2002). External memory aids and computers in memory rehabilitation. In A. D. Baddeley, M. D. Kopelman, & B. A. Wilson (Eds.), *Handbook of memory disorders* (2nd ed.). Chichester, UK: Wiley.

Kapur, N., Glisky, E. L., & Wilson, B. A. (2004). Technological memory aids for people with memory deficits. *Neuropsychological Rehabilitation, 14*(1/2), 41–60.

Kapur, N., & Graham, K. S. (2002). Recovery of memory function in neurological disease. In A. D. Baddeley, M. D. Kopelman, & B. A. Wilson (Eds.), *The handbook of memory disorders.* Chichester, UK: Wiley.

Kapur, N., & Pearson, D. (1983). Memory systems and memory performance of neurological patients. *British Journal of Psychology, 74,* 409–415.

Kapur, N., Thompson, S., Cook, P., Lang, D., & Brice, J. (1996). Anterograde but not retrograde memory loss following combined mammillary body and medial thalamic lesions. *Neuropsychologia, 34*(1), 1–8.

Kaschel, R. (2003). [Rehabilitation of memory disorders.] *Sprache Stimme Gehor, 27*(1), 18–23.

Kaschel, R., Della Sala, S., Cantagallo, A., Fahlböck, A., Laaksonen, R., & Kazen, M. (2002). Imagery mnemonics for the rehabilitation of memory: A randomised group controlled trial. *Neuropsychological Rehabilitation, 12*(2), 127–153.

Katzman, R., Terry, R., DeTeresa, R., Brown, T., Davies, P., Fuld, P., et al. (1988). Clinical, pathological, and neurochemical changes in dementia: A subgroup with preserved mental status and numerous neocortical plaques. *Annals of Neurology, 23*(2), 138–144.

Kauschal, P. I., Zetin, M., & Squire, L. R. (1981). A psychosocial study of chronic circumscribed amnesia. *Journal of Nervous and Mental Disease, 169,* 383–389.

Kazdin, A. E. (1982). *Single case research designs.* New York: Oxford University Press.

Keith, R. A., Granger, C. V., Hamilton, B. B., & Sherwin, F. S. (1987). The functional independence measure: A new tool for rehabilitation. *Advances in Clinical Rehabilitation, 1,* 6–18.

Kennard, M. A. (1940). Relation of age to motor impairment in man and subhuman primates. *Archives of Neurology and Psychiatry, 44,* 377–397.

Kertesz, A., & Gold, B. T. (2003). Recovery of cognition. In K. M. Heilman & E. Valenstein (Eds.), *Clinical neuropsychology* (4th ed.). New York: Oxford University Press.

Kesler, S. R., Adams, H. F., Blasey, C. M., & Bigler, E. D. (2003). Premorbid intellectual functioning, education, and brain size in traumatic brain injury: An investigation of the cognitive reserve hypothesis. *Applied Neuropsychology, 10*(3), 153–162.

Kessels, R. P. C., Boekhorst, S. T., & Postma, A. (2005). The contribution of implicit and explicit memory to the effects of errorless learning: A comparison between young and older adults. *Journal of the International Neuropsychological Society, 11*(2), 144–151.

Kessels, R. P. C., & de Haan, E. H. F. (2003). Implicit learning in memory rehabilitation: A meta-analysis on errorless learning and vanishing cues methods. *Journal of Clinical and Experimental Neuropsychology, 25*(6), 805–814.

Khan-Bourne, N., & Brown, R. G. (2003). Cognitive behaviour therapy for the treatment of depression in individuals with brain injury. *Neuropsychological Rehabilitation, 13*(1–2), 89–107.

Kime, S. K. (2006). *Compensating for memory deficits using a systematic approach.* Bethesda, MD: AOTA Press.

Kime, S. K., Lamb, D. G., & Wilson, B. A. (1996). Use of a comprehensive program of external cuing to enhance procedural memory in a patient with dense amnesia. *Brain Injury, 10,* 17–25.

King, N. S. (1997). Post-traumatic stress disorder and head injury as a dual diagnosis: "Islands" of memory as a mechanism. *Journal of Neurology, Neurosurgery, and Psychiatry, 62*(1), 82–84.

Kiresuk, T. J., & Sherman, R. E. (1968). Goal attainment scaling: A general method for evaluating comprehensive community mental health programs. *Community Mental Health Journal, 4*(6), 443–453.

Kixmiller, J. S. (2002). Evaluation of prospective memory training for individuals with mild Alzheimer's disease. *Brain and Cognition, 49*(2), 237–241.

Klonoff, P. S. (1997). Individual and group psychotherapy in milieu-oriented neurorehabilitation. *Applied Neuropsychology, 4*(2), 107–118.

Klonoff, P. S., Watt, L. M., Dawson, L. K., Henderson, S. W., Gehrels, J., & Wethe, J. V. (2006). Psychosocial outcomes 1–7 years after comprehensive milieu-oriented neurorehabilitation: The role of pre-injury status. *Brain Injury, 20*(6), 601–612.

Kolb, B. (1995). *Brain plasticity and behaviour.* Hillsdale, NJ: Erlbaum.

Kolb, B. (2003). Overview of cortical plasticity and recovery from brain injury. *Physical Medicine and Rehabilitation Clinics of North America, 14*(1), S7–S25.

Koltai, D. C., Welsh-Bohmer, K. A., & Schmechel, D. E. (2001). Influence of anosognosia on treatment outcome among dementia patients. *Neuropsychological Rehabilitation, 11*(3), 455–475.

Komatsu, S. I., Mimura, M., Kato, M., Wakamatsu, N., & Kashima, H. (2000). Errorless and effortful processes involved in the learning of face-name associations by patients with alcoholic Korsakoff's syndrome. *Neuropsychological Rehabilitation, 10*(2), 113–132.

Kopelman, M. D. (2000). Focal retrograde amnesia and the attribution of causality: An exceptionally critical view. *Cognitive Neuropsychology, 17*(7), 585–621.

Kopelman, M. D. (2004). Psychogenic amnesia. In A. D. Baddeley, M. D.

Kopelman, & B. A. Wilson (Eds.), *The essential handbook of memory disorders for clinicians.* Chichester, UK: Wiley.

Kopelman, M. D., & Crawford, S. (1996). Not all memory clinics are dementia clinics. *Neuropsychological Rehabilitation, 6,* 187–202.

Kopelman, M. D., Stanhope, N., & Kingsley, D. (1999). Retrograde amnesia in patients with diencephalic, temporal lobe or frontal lesions. *Neuropsychologia, 37*(8), 939–958.

Kopelman, M. D., Wilson, B. A., & Baddeley, A. D. (1990). *The Autobiographical Memory Interview.* Bury St. Edmunds, UK: Thames Valley Test Company.

Kotler-Cope, L. (1990). *Memory impairment in older adults: The interrelationships between objective and subjective clinical and everyday assessment.* Paper presented at the annual meeting of the Southern Society for Philosophy and Psychology, Louisville, KY.

Kreutzer, J. S., Seel, R. T., & Gourley, E. (2001). The prevalence and symptom rates of depression after traumatic brain injury: A comprehensive examination. *Brain Injury, 15*(7), 563–576.

Laatsch, L., Jobe, T., Sychra, J., Lin, Q., & Blend, M. (1997). Impact of cognitive rehabilitation therapy on neuropsychological impairments as measured by brain perfusion SPECT: A longitudinal study. *Brain Injury, 11*(12), 851–863.

Laatsch, L., Pavel, D., Jobe, T., Lin, Q., & Quintana, J. C. (1999). Incorporation of SPECT imaging in a longitudinal cognitive rehabilitation therapy programme. *Brain Injury, 13*(8), 555–570.

Laatsch, L. K., Thulborn, K. R., Krisky, C. M., Shobat, D. M., & Sweeney, J. A. (2004). Investigating the neurobiological basis of cognitive rehabilitation therapy with fMRI. *Brain Injury, 18*(10), 957–974.

Lambon-Ralph, M. A., & Patterson, K. (2008). Generalization and differentiation in semantic memory: Insights from semantic dementia. *Annals of the New York Academy of Sciences, 1124,* 61–76.

Landauer, T. K., & Bjork, R. A. (1978). Optimum rehearsal patterns and name learning. In M. M. Gruneberg, P. Morris, & R. N. Sykes (Eds.), *Practical aspects of memory.* London: Academic Press.

Latham, G. P., & Seijts, G. H. (1999). The effects of proximal and distal goals on performance on a moderately complex task. *Journal of Organizational Behavior, 20*(4), 421–429.

Laurence, S., & Stein, D. G. (1978). Recovery after brain damage and the concept of localization of function. In S. Finger (Ed.), *Recovery from brain damage.* New York: Plenum Press.

Lekeu, F., Wojtasik, V., Van der Linden, M., & Salmon, E. (2002). Training early Alzheimer patients to use a mobile phone. *Acta Neurologica Belgica, 102*(3), 114–121.

Leng, N. R., & Copello, A. G. (1990). Rehabilitation of memory after brain injury: Is there an effective technique? *Clinical Rehabilitation, 4,* 63–69.

Leong, K. C., Chen, W. S., Leong, K. W., Mastura, I., Mimi, O., Sheikh, M. A., et al. (2006). The use of text messaging to improve attendance in primary care: A randomized controlled trial. *Family Practice, 23*(6), 699–705.

LeVere, T. E. (1980). Recovery of function after brain damage: A theory of the behavioral deficit. *Physiological Psychology, 8*, 297–308.

Levin, H. S. (2006). Neuroplasticity and brain imaging research: Implications for rehabilitation. *Archives of Physical Medicine and Rehabilitation, 87*(12,S2), S1.

Levin, H. S., & Hanten, G. (2004). Posttraumatic amnesia and residual memory deficit after closed head injury. In A. D. Baddeley, M. D. Kopelman, & B. A. Wilson (Eds.), *The essential handbook of memory disorders for clinicians*. Chichester, UK: Wiley.

Lezak, M. D. (1976). *Neuropsychological assessment*. New York: Oxford University Press.

Lezak, M. D. (1979). Recovery of memory and learning functions following traumatic brain injury. *Cortex, 15*, 63–72.

Lezak, M. D., Howieson, D. B., Loring, D. W., Hannay, H. J., & Fischer, J. S. (2004). *Neuropsychological assessment* (4th ed.). New York: Oxford University Press.

Lindgren, M., Österberg, K., Ørbæk, P., & Rosén, I. (1997). Solvent-induced toxic encephalopathy: Electrophysiological data in relation to neuropsychological findings. *Journal of Clinical and Experimental Neuropsychology, 19*(5), 772–783.

Lishman, W. A. (1998). *Organic psychiatry: The psychological consequences of cerebral disorder* (3rd ed.). Oxford, UK: Blackwell.

Locke, E. A., & Latham, G. P. (2002). Building a practically useful theory of goal setting and task motivation: A 35-year odyssey. *American Psychologist, 57*, 705–717.

Long, T., Cameron, K., Harju, B., Lutz, J., & Means, L. (1999). Women and middle-aged individuals report using more prospective memory aids. *Psychological Reports, 85*, 1139–1153.

Lorge, I. (1930). *Influence of regularly interpolated time intervals upon subsequent learning*. New York: Teachers College, Columbia University.

Loukavenko, E. A., Ottley, M. C., Moran, J. P., Wolff, M., & Dalrymple-Alford, J. C. (2007). Towards therapy to relieve memory impairment after anterior thalamic lesions: Improved spatial working memory after immediate and delayed postoperative enrichment. *European Journal of Neuroscience, 26*(11), 3267–3276.

Lu, Z. L., & Sperling, G. (2003). Measuring sensory memory: Magnetoencephalography habituation and psychophysics. In Z. L. Lu & L. Kaufman (Eds.), *Magnetic source imaging of the human brain*. Mahwah, NJ: Erlbaum.

Luria, A. R. (1968). *The mind of a mnemonist*. Cambridge, MA: Harvard University Press.

Luria, A. R. (1975). *The man with a shattered world.* Cambridge, MA: Harvard University Press.

Macniven, J. A., Poz, R., Bainbridge, K., Gracey, F., & Wilson, B. A. (2003). Emotional adjustment following cognitive recovery from "persistent vegetative state": Psychological and personal perspectives. *Brain Injury, 17*(6), 525–533.

Mahoney, F. I., & Barthel, D. W. (1965). Functional evaluation: The Barthel Index. *Maryland State Medical Journal, 14,* 61–65.

Mai, N. (1992). Evaluation in constructing neuropsychological treatments. In N. Von Steinbüchel, D. Y. Cramon, & E. Pöppel (Eds.), *Neuropsychological Rehabilitation.* Berlin: Springer-Verlag.

Malec, J. F. (1999). Goal attainment scaling in rehabilitation. *Neuropsychological Rehabilitation, 9*(3), 253–275.

Malec, J. F. (2004). The Mayo–Portland Participation Index: A brief and psychometrically sound measure of brain injury outcome. *Archives of Physical Medicine and Rehabilitation, 85*(12), 1989–1996.

Malec, J. F. (2008, June). *Mayo brain injury rehabilitation: What we've learned in the in the last twenty years.* Paper presented at the Fifteenth Annual Brain Injury Conference, Rochester, MN.

Malec, J. F., Smigielski, J. S., & DePompolo, R. W. (1991). Goal attainment scaling and outcome measurement in postacute brain injury rehabilitation. *Archives of Physical Medicine and Rehabilitation, 72*(2), 138–143.

Malley, D., Bateman, A., & Gracey, F. (in press). Practically based project groups. In B. A. Wilson, F. Gracey, J. J. Evans, & A. Bateman (Eds.), *Neuropsychological rehabilitation: Theory, models, therapy and outcome.* Cambridge, UK: Cambridge University Press.

Markowitsch, H. J. (2003). Functional neuroanatomy of learning and memory. In P. W. Halligan, U. Kischka, & J. C. Marshall (Eds.), *Handbook of clinical neuropsychology.* Oxford, UK: Oxford University Press.

Markowitsch, H. J. (2005). The neuroanatomy of memory. In P. W. Halligan & D. T. Wade (Eds.), *Effectiveness of rehabilitation for cognitive deficits.* Oxford, UK: Oxford University Press.

Marshall, J. F. (1985). Neural plasticity and recovery of function after brain injury. *International Review of Neurobiology, 26,* 201–247.

Masters, R. S. W., & Maxwell, J. P. (2004). Implicit motor learning, reinvestment and movement disruption: What you don't know won't hurt you. In A. M. Williams & N. J. Hodges (Eds.), *Skill acquisition in sport: Research, theory and practice.* Abingdon, UK: Routledge.

Mateer, C. A., Sira, C. S., & O'Connell, M. E. (2005). Putting Humpty Dumpty together again: The importance of integrating cognitive and emotional interventions. *Journal of Head Trauma Rehabilitation, 20*(1), 62–75.

Mateer, C. A., Sohlberg, M. M., & Crinean, J. (1987). Focus on clinical research: Perceptions of memory function in individuals with closed-head injury. *Journal of Head Trauma Rehabilitation, 2*(3), 74–84.

May, L. A., & Warren, S. (2001). Measuring quality of life of persons with spinal cord injury: Substantive and structural validation. *Quality of Life Research, 10*(6), 503–515.

McCarthy, R. A., Kopelman, M. D., & Warrington, E. K. (2005). Remembering and forgetting of semantic knowledge in amnesia: A 16–year follow-up investigation of RFR. *Neuropsychologia, 43*(3), 356–372.

McClelland, J. L., Thomas, A. G., McCandliss, B. D., & Fiez, J. A. (1999). Understanding failures of learning: Hebbian learning, competition for representational space, and some preliminary experimental data. *Progress in Brain Research, 121*, 75–80.

McDonald, S., Flanagan, S., & Rollins, J. (2002). *The Awareness of Social Inference test (T.A.S.I.T.)*. San Antonio, TX: Psychological Corporation.

McGrath, J., & Adams, L. (1999). Patient-centred goal planning: A systemic psychological therapy? *Topics in Stroke Rehabilitation, 6*, 43–50.

McKenna, P. (1998). *Category-Specific Names Test.* Hove, UK: Psychology Press.

McKenna, P., & Gerhand, S. (2002). Preserved semantic learning in an amnesic patient. *Cortex, 38*(1), 37–58.

McKitrick, L. A., & Camp, C. J. (1993). Relearning the names of things: The spaced-retrieval intervention implemented by a caregiver. *Clinical Gerontologist, 14*(2), 60–62.

McKitrick, L. A., Camp, C. J., & Black, W. (1992). Prospective memory intervention in Alzheimers' disease. *Journal of Gerontology: Psychological Sciences, 47*, 337–343.

McLellan, D. L. (1991). Functional recovery and the principles of disability medicine. In M. Swash & J. Oxbury (Eds.), *Clinical neurology.* Edinburgh, Scotland: Churchill Livingstone.

McMillan, T. M. (1996). Post-traumatic stress disorder following minor and severe closed head injury: 10 single cases. *Brain Injury, 10*(10), 749–758.

McMillan, T. M., Robertson, I. H., & Wilson, B. A. (1999). Neurogenesis after brain injury: Implications for neurorehabilitation. *Neuropsychological Rehabilitation, 9*(2), 129–133.

McMillan, T. M., & Sparkes, C. (1999). Goal planning and neurorehabilitation: The Wolfson Neurorehabilitation Centre approach. *Neuropsychological Rehabilitation, 9*(3), 241–251.

McMillan, T. M., Williams, W. H., & Bryant, R. (2003). Post-traumatic stress disorder and traumatic brain injury: A review of causal mechanisms, assessment, and treatment. *Neuropsychological Rehabilitation, 13*(1–2), 149–164.

McNair, D. M., Lorr, M., & Droppleman, L. F. (1992). *Profile of Mood States.* San Diego, CA: Educational and Industrial Testing Service.

Meeberg, G. A. (1993). Quality of life: A concept analysis. *Journal of Advanced Nursing, 18*(1), 32–38.

Ment, L. R., & Constable, R. T. (2007). Injury and recovery in the developing brain: Eidence from functional MRI studies of prematurely born children. *Nature Clinical Practice. Neurology, 3*(10), 558–571.

Merians, A. S., Poizner, H., Boian, R., Burdea, G., & Adamovich, S. (2006). Sensorimotor training in a virtual reality environment: Des it improve functional recovery poststroke? *Neurorehabilitation and Neural Repair, 20*(2), 252–267.

Metzler-Baddeley, C., & Snowden, J. S. (2005). Brief report: Erorless versus errorful learning as a memory rehabilitation approach in Alzheimer's dsease. *Journal of Clinical and Experimental Neuropsychology, 27*(8), 1070–1079.

Middleton, J. A. (2004). Assessment and management of memory problems in children. In A. D. Baddeley, M. D. Kopelman, & B. A. Wilson (Eds.), *The essential handbook of memory disorders for clinicians*. Chichester, UK: Wiley.

Milders, M. V., Berg, I. J., & Deelman, B. G. (1995). Four-year follow-up of a controlled memory training study in closed head injured patients. *Neuropsychological Rehabilitation, 5*(3), 223–238.

Miller, G. A. (1956). The magical number seven plus or minus two: Some limits on our capacity for processing information. *Psychological Review, 63*, 81–97.

Milner, B. (1965). Visually-guided maze learning in man: Effects of bilateral hippocampal, bilateral frontal, and unilateral cerebral lesions. *Neuropsychologia, 3*(3), 317–338.

Milner, B. (1968). Visual recognition and recall after right temporal lobe excision in man. *Neuropsychologia, 6*, 191–209.

Milner, B. (1971). Interhemispheric differences in the localisation of psychological processes in man. *British Medical Bulletin, 27*(3), 272–277.

Mischel, W. (1968). *Personality and assessment*. New York: Wiley.

Mitchell, D. B., & Schmitt, F. A. (2006). Short- and long-term implicit memory in aging and Alzheimer's disease. *Neuropsychology, Development, and Cognition, Section B: Aging, Neuropsychology and Cognition, 13*(3–4), 611–635.

Mitrushina, M. N., Boone, K. B., Razani, L. J., & D'Elia, L. F. (2005). *Handbook of normative data for neuropsychological assessment* (2nd ed.). New York: Oxford University Press.

Moffat, N. (1984). Strategies of memory therapy. In B. A. Wilson & N. Moffat (Eds.), *Clinical management of memory problems*. Beckenham, UK: Croom Helm.

Moffat, N. (1989). Home-based cognitive rehabilitation with the elderly. In L. W. Poon, D. C. Rubin, & B. A. Wilson (Eds.), *Everyday cognition in adulthood and later life*. Cambridge, UK: Cambridge University Press.

Mohr, D. C., Boudewyn, A. C., Goodkin, D. E., Bostrom, A., & Epstein, L. (2001). Comparative outcomes for individual cognitive-behavior therapy, supportive-expressive group psychotherapy, and sertraline for the treatment of depression in multiple sclerosis. *Journal of Consulting and Clinical Psychology, 69,* 942–949.

Monakov, C. von (1914). *Die Lokalisation im Grosshirn und der Abbau der Funktion durch kortikale Herde* [Localization in the large brain and the removal of cortical function]. Wiesbaden, Germany: Bergmann.

Moore, A., Stambrook, M., & Peters, L. (1993). Centripetal and centrifugal family life cycle factors in long-term outcome following traumatic brain injury. *Brain Injury, 7*(3), 247–255.

Moradi, A. R., Neshat-Doost, H. T. N., Taghavi, M. R., Yule, W., & Dalgleish, T. (1999). Everyday memory deficits in children and adolescents with PTSD: Performance on the Rivermead Behavioural Memory Test. *Journal of Child Psychology and Psychiatry, 40*(3), 357–361.

Murphy, G., & Goodall, E. (1980). Measurement error in direct observations: A comparison of common recording methods. *Behaviour Research and Therapy, 18*(2), 147–150.

Naccache, L., & Dehaene, S. (2001). The priming method: Imaging unconscious repetition priming reveals an abstract representation of number in the parietal lobes. *Cerebral Cortex, 11*(10), 966–974.

Nadel, L., & Moscovitch, M. (1997). Memory consolidation, retrograde amnesia and the hippocampal complex. *Current Opinion in Neurobiology, 7*(2), 217–227.

Nair, K. P., & Wade, D. T. (2003). Life goals of people with disabilities due to neurological disorders. *Clinical Rehabilitation, 17*(5), 521–527.

Nannery, R., Greenfield, E., Wilson, B. A., Sopena, S., & Rous, R. (2007). Memory without memory: Assessing the integrity of implicit memory using the Implicit Memory Test. *Brain Impairment, 8*(2), 216.

National Institutes of Health. (1998). Rehabilitation of persons with traumatic brain injury. *NIH Consensus Statement, 16*(1), 1–41.

Nelson, H. E., & Willison, J. R. (1991). *National Adult Reading Test (NART).* Windsor, UK: NFER-Nelson.

Nelson, R. O., & Hayes, S. C. (1979). The nature of behavioral assesssment: A commentary. *Journal of Applied Behavior Analysis, 12,* 491–500.

Nichols, K., & Jenkinson, J. (1990). *Leading a support group.* Cheltenham, UK: Nelson Thornes Ltd.

Nicolson, R. I., & Fawcett, A. J. (2007). Procedural learning difficulties: Reuniting the developmental disorders? *Trends in Neurosciences, 30*(4), 135–141.

Norman, D. A. (1988). *The psychology of everyday things.* New York: Basic Books.

Noulhiane, M., Piolino, P., Hasboun, D., Clemenceau, S., Baulac, M., & Samson, S. (2007). Autobiographical memory after temporal lobe resection: Neuropsychological and MRI volumetric findings. *Brain, 130*(Pt. 12), 3184–3199.

O'Carroll, R. E., Russell, H. H., Lawrie, S. M., & Johnstone, E. C. (1999).

Errorless learning and the cognitive rehabilitation of memory-impaired schizophrenic patients. *Psychological Medicine, 29*(1), 105–112.

O'Connell, R. G., Bellgrove, M. A., Dockree, P. M., Lau, A., Fitzgerald, M., & Robertson, I. H. (2008). Self-alert training: Volitional modulation of autonomic arousal improves sustained attention. *Neuropsychologia, 46*(5), 1379–1390.

O'Connor, M. G., Cermak, L. S., & Seidman, L. J. (1995). Social and emotional characteristics of a profoundly amnesic post encephalitic patient. In R. Campbell & M. R. Conway (Eds.), *Broken memories: Case studies in memory impairment.* Oxford, UK: Blackwell.

Ogden, J. A. (1996). *Fractured minds.* Oxford, UK: Oxford University Press.

Ogden, J. A. (2000). Neurorehabilitation in the third millenium: New roles for our environment, behaviors, and mind in brain damage and recovery? *Brain and Cognition, 42*(1), 110–112.

Olsson, E., Wik, K., Ostling, A., Johansson, M., & Andersson, G. (2006). Everyday memory self-assessed by adult patients with acquired brain damage and their significant others. *Neuropsychological Rehabilitation, 16*(3), 257–271.

Osman, M., Wilkinson, L., Beigi, M., Castaneda, C. S., & Jahanshahi, M. (2008). Patients with Parkinson's disease learn to control complex systems via procedural as well as non-procedural learning. *Neuropsychologia, 46*(9), 2355–2363.

Ottenbacher, K. J., & Cusick, A. (1990). Goal attainment scaling as a method of clinical service evaluation. *American Journal of Occupational Therapy, 44*(6), 519–525.

Padesky, C. A., & Greenberger, D. (1995). *Clinician's guide to mind over mood.* New York: Guilford Press.

Page, M., Wilson, B. A., Shiel, A., Carter, G., & Norris, D. (2006). What is the locus of the errorless-learning advantage? *Neuropsychologia, 44*(1), 90–100.

Palmer, S., Psaila, K., & Yeates, G. (in press). Simon: Brain injury and the family—The inclusion of children, family members and wider systems in the rehabilitation process. In B. A. Wilson, F. Gracey, J. J. Evans, & A. Bateman (Eds.), *Neuropsychological rehabilitation: Theory, models, therapy and outcome.* Cambridge, UK: Cambridge University Press.

Park, D., Smith, A., & Cavanaugh, J. (1990). Metamemories of memory researchers. *Memory and Cognition, 18*(3), 321–327.

Parkin, A. J., Hunkin, N. M., & Squires, E. J. (1998). Unlearning John Major: The use of errorless learning in the reacquisition of proper names following herpes simplex encephalitis. *Cognitive Neuropsychology, 15*(4), 361–375.

Peck, K. K., Moore, A. B., Crosson, B. A., Gaiefsky, M., Gopinath, K. S., White, K., et al. (2004). Functional magnetic resonance imaging before and after aphasia therapy: Shifts in hemodynamic time to peak during an overt language task. *Stroke, 35*(2), 554–559.

Pérez, M., & Godoy, J. (1998). Comparison between a "traditional" memory test and a "behavioral" memory battery in Spanish patients. *Journal of Clinical and Experimental Neuropsychology, 20*(4), 496–502.

Perlesz, A., Kinsella, G., & Crowe, S. (1999). Impact of traumatic brain injury on the family: A critical review. *Rehabilitation Psychology, 44*, 6–35.

Petchprapai, N., & Winkelman, C. (2007). Mild traumatic brain injury: Determinants and subsequent quality of life. A review of the literature. *Journal of Neuroscience Nursing, 39*(5), 260–272.

Pewter, S. M., Williams, W. H., Haslam, C., & Kay, J. M. (2007). Neuropsychological and psychiatric profiles in acute encephalitis in adults. *Neuropsychological Rehabilitation, 17*(4–5), 478–505.

Phillips, W. A. (1983). Short-term visual memory. *Philosophical Transactions of the Royal Society of London, Series B: Biological Sciences, 302*, 295–309.

Philpot, V. D., & Madonna, S. (1993). Fluctuations in mood state and learning and retrieval. *Psychological Reports, 73*(1), 203–208.

Pizzamiglio, L., Perani, D., Cappa, S. F., Vallar, G., Paolucci, S., Grassi, F., et al. (1998). Recovery of neglect after right hemispheric damage: H2(15)O positron emission tomographic activation study. *Archives of Neurology, 55*(4), 561–568.

Ponds, R., & Hendriks, M. (2006). Cognitive rehabilitation of memory problems in patients with epilepsy. *Seizure: European Journal of Epilepsy, 15*(4), 267–273.

Ponsford, J. L., Myles, P. S., Cooper, D. J., McDermott, F. T., Murray, L. J., Laidlaw, J., et al. (2008). Gender differences in outcome in patients with hypotension and severe traumatic brain injury. *Injury, 39*(1), 67–76.

Powell, G. E. (1981). *Brain function therapy.* Aldershot, UK: Gower Press.

Powell, J. H., Beckers, K., & Greenwood, R. J. (1998). Measuring progress and outcome in community rehabilitation after brain injury with a new assessment instrument—The BICRO-39 scales. *Archives of Physical Medicine and Rehabilitation, 79*(10), 1213–1225.

Powell, J. H., Heslin, J., & Greenwood, R. (2002). Community based rehabilitation after severe traumatic brain injury: A randomised controlled trial. *Journal of Neurology, Neurosurgery, and Psychiatry, 72*(2), 193–202.

Prigatano, G. P. (1986). Personality and psychosocial consequences of brain injury. In G. P. Prigatano, D. J. Fordyce, H. K. Zeiner, J. R. Roueche, M. Pepping, & B. C. Wood (Eds.), *Neuropsychological rehabilitation after brain injury.* Baltimore, MD: The Johns Hopkins University Press.

Prigatano, G. P. (1994). Individuality, lesion location and psychotherapy after brain injury. In A. L. Christensen & B. P. Uzzell (Eds.), *Brain injury and neuropsychological rehabilitation.* Hillsdale, NJ: Erlbaum.

Prigatano, G. P. (1995). Personality and social aspects of memory rehabilitation. In A. D. Baddeley, B. A. Wilson, & F. N. Watts (Eds.), *Handbook of memory disorders.* Chichester, UK: Wiley.

Prigatano, G. P. (1999). *Principles of neuropsychological rehabilitation*. New York: Oxford University Press.

Prigatano, G. P., Klonoff, P. S., O'Brien, K. P., Altman, I. M., Amin, K., Chiapello, D., et al. (1994). Productivity after neuropsychologically oriented milieu rehabilitation. *Journal of Head Trauma Rehabilitation, 9*(1), 91–102.

Prince, L., Keohane, C., Gracey, F., Cope, J., Connell, S., & Threadgold, C. (in press). Lorna: Applying models of language, calculation, and learning within holistic rehabilitation—From dysphasia and dyscalculia to independent cooking and travel. In B. A. Wilson, F. Gracey, J. J. Evans, & A. Bateman (Eds.), *Neuropsychological rehabilitation: Theory, models, therapy and outcome.* Cambridge, UK: Cambridge University Press.

Psaila, K., & Gracey, F. (in press). The mood management group. In B. A. Wilson, F. Gracey, J. J. Evans, & A. Bateman (Eds.), *Neuropsychological rehabilitation: Theory, models, therapy and outcome.* Cambridge, UK: Cambridge University Press.

Rader, S. K., Holmes, J. L., & Golob, E. J. (2008). Auditory event-related potentials during a spatial working memory task. *Clinical Neurophysiology, 119*(5), 1176–1189.

Radice-Neumann, D., Zupan, B., Babbage, D. R., & Willer, B. (2007). Overview of impaired facial affect recognition in persons with traumatic brain injury. *Brain Injury, 21*(8), 807–816.

Randall, K. E., & McEwen, I. R. (2000). Writing patient-centered functional goals. *Physical Therapy, 80*(12), 1197–1203.

Ratcliff, J. J., Greenspan, A. I., Goldstein, F. C., Stringer, A. Y., Bushnik, T., Hammond, F. M., et al. (2007). Gender and traumatic brain injury: Do the sexes fare differently? *Brain Injury, 21*(10), 1023–1030.

Reed, J. M., & Squire, L. R. (1998). Retrograde amnesia for facts and events: Findings from four new cases. *Journal of Neuroscience, 18*(10), 3943–3954.

Rey, A. (1941). L'examen psychologique dans les cás d'encephalopathie traumatique. *Archives de Psychologie, 28*, 286–340.

Ribot, T. (1881). *Les maladies de la memoire* [Diseases of memory]. New York: Appleton-Century-Crofts.

Richards, M., & Deary, I. J. (2005). A life course approach to cognitive reserve: Amodel for cognitive aging and development? *Annals of Neurology, 58*(4), 617–622.

Riley, G. A., & Heaton, S. (2000). Guidelines for the selection of a method of fading cues. *Neuropsychological Rehabilitation, 10*, 133–149.

Riley, G. A., Sotiriou, D., & Jaspal, S. (2004). Which is more effective in promoting implicit and explicit memory: The method of vanishing cues or errorless learning without fading? *Neuropsychological Rehabilitation, 14*(3), 257–283.

Robertson, I. H. (1999). Theory-driven neuropsychological rehabilitation:

The role of attention and competition in recovery of function after brain damage. In D. Gopher & A. Koriat (Eds.), *Attention and performance XVI*. Cambridge, MA: MIT Press.

Robertson, I. H. (2002). Cognitive neuroscience and brain rehabilitation: A promise kept. *Journal of Neurology, Neurosurgery, and Psychiatry, 73*, 357–357.

Robertson, I. H., & Murre, J. M. J. (1999). Rehabilitation of brain damage: Brain plasticity and principles of guided recovery. *Psychological Bulletin, 125*, 544–575.

Robinson, F. B. (1970). *Effective study*. New York: Harper & Row.

Robinson, M. D. (1997). Neuropsychiatric consequences of stroke. *Annual Reviews in Medicine, 48*(1), 217–229.

Rockwood, K., Joyce, B., & Stolee, P. (1997). Use of goal attainment scaling in measuring clinically important change in cognitive rehabilitation patients. *Journal of Clinical Epidemiology, 50*(5), 581–588.

Rojas Vega, S., Abel, T., Lindschulten, R., Hollmann, W., Bloch, W., & Strüder, H. K. (2008). Impact of exercise on neuroplasticity-related proteins in spinal cord injured humans. *Neuroscience, 153*(4), 1064–1070.

Roof, R. L., & Hall, E. D. (2000). Gender differences in acute CNS trauma and stroke: Neuroprotective effects of estrogen and progesterone. *Journal of Neurotrauma, 17*(5), 367–388.

Rose, F. D., Brooks, B. M., Attree, E. A., Parslow, D. M., Leadbetter, A. G., McNeil, J. E., et al. (1999). A preliminary investigation into the use of virtual environments in memory retraining after vascular brain injury: Indications for future strategy? *Disability and Rehabilitation, 21*(12), 548–554.

Rose, F. D., Brooks, B. M., & Rizzo, A. A. (2005). Virtual reality in brain damage rehabilitation: Review. *CyberPsychology and Behavior, 8*(3), 241–262.

Rowntree, D. (1982). *Learn how to study*. New York: Harper & Row.

Royle, J., & Lincoln, N. B. (2008). The Everyday Memory Questionnaire-Revised: Development of a 13-item scale. *Disability and Rehabilitation, 30*(2), 114–121.

Ruis, C., & Kessels, R. P. C. (2005). Effects of errorless and errorful face-name associative learning in moderate to severe dementia. *Aging Clinical and Experimental Research, 17*(6), 514–517.

Ryan, T. V., & Ruff, R. M. (1988). The efficacy of structured memory retraining in a group comparison of head trauma patients. *Archives of Clinical Neuropsychology, 3*(2), 165–179.

Sacchett, C., & Humphreys, G. W. (1992). Calling a squirrel a squirrel but a canoe a wigwam: A category-specific deficit for artefactual objects and body parts. *Cognitive Neuropsychology, 9*(1), 73–86.

Sanavio, E. (1988). Obsessions and compulsions: The Padua Inventory. *Behaviour Research and Therapy, 26*(2), 169–177.

Sander, A. (2002). *Picking up the pieces after TBI: A guide for family members.* Houston, TX: Baylor College of Medicine.

Sander, A. (2008, June). *Intervening with caregivers to improve the outcomes of persons with traumatic brain injury.* Paper presented at the Fifteenth Annual Brain Injury Conference, Rochester, MN.

Sbordone, R. J., & Liter, J. C. (1995). Mild traumatic brain injury does not produce post-traumatic stress disorder. *Brain Injury, 9*(4), 405–412.

Sbordone, R. J., & Long, C. J. (1996). *Ecological validity of neuropsychological testing.* Delray Beach, FL: GR Press/St. Lucie Press.

Schacter, D. L., & Crovitz, H. F. (1977). Memory function after closed head injury: A review of the quantitative research. *Cortex, 13*(2), 150–176.

Schacter, D. L., Rich, S. A., & Stampp, M. S. (1985). Remediation of memory disorders: Experimental evaluation of the spaced-retrieval technique. *Journal of Clinical and Experimental Neuropsychology, 7*(1), 79–96.

Scherer, M. (2005). Assessing the benefits of using assistive technologies and other supports for thinking, remembering and learning. *Disability and Rehabilitation, 27*(13), 731–739.

Scheutzow, M. H., & Wiercisiewski, D. R. (1999). Panic disorder in a patient with traumatic brain injury: A case report and discussion. *Brain Injury, 13*(9), 705–714.

Schultheis, M. T., & Rizzo, A. A. (2001). The application of virtual reality technology in rehabilitation. *Rehabilitation Psychology, 46*(3), 296–311.

Schwartz, A. F., & McMillan, T. M. (1989). Assessment of everyday memory problems after severe head injury. *Cortex, 25,* 665–671.

Scott, J., & Clare, L. (2003). Do people with dementia benefit from psychological interventions offered on a group basis? *Clinical Psychology and Psychotherapy, 10*(3), 186–196.

Scoville, W. B. (1968). Amnesia after bilateral mesial temporal-lobe excision: Introduction to case HM. *Neuropsychologia, 6*(21), 1–213.

Scoville, W. B., & Milner, B. (1957). Loss of recent memory after hippocampal lesions. *Journal of Neurology, Neurosurgery, and Psychiatry, 20,* 11–21.

Scoville, W. B., & Milner, B. (1957). Loss of recent memory after bilateral hippocampal lesions. *Journal of Neuropsychiatry and Clinical Neurosciences, 12,* 103–113.

Selzer, M., Clarke, S., Cohen, L., Duncan, P., & Gage, F. (2006). *Textbook of neural repair and rehabilitation: Medical neurorehabilitation* (1st ed., Vols. 1–2). Cambridge, UK: Cambridge University Press.

Shallice, T., & Burgess, P. W. (1991). Higher-order cognitive impairments and frontal lobe lesions in man. In H. S. Levin, H. M. Eisenberg, & A. L. Benton (Eds.), *Frontal lobe function and dysfunction.* New York: Oxford University Press.

Shallice, T., & Warrington, E. K. (1970). Independent functioning of verbal memory stores: A neuropsychological study. *Quarterly Journal of Experimental Psychology, 22*(2), 261–273.

Sidman, M., & Stoddard, L. T. (1967). The effectiveness of fading in programming a simultaneous form discrimination for retarded children. *Journal of the Experimental Analysis of Behavior, 10*(1), 3–15.

Siegert, R. J., Weatherall, M., & Bell, E. M. (2008). Is implicit sequence learning impaired in schizophrenia? A meta-analysis. *Brain and Cognition, 67*(3), 351–359.

Sim, A., Terryberry-Spohr, L., & Wilson. (2008). Prolonged recovery of memory functioning after mild traumatic brain injury in adolescent athletes. *Journal of Neurosurgery, 108*(3), 511–516.

Small, G. W., Rabins, P. V., Barry, P. P., Buckholtz, N. S., DeKosky, S. T., & Ferris, S. H. (1997). Diagnosis and treatment of Alzheimer disease and related disorders: Consensus statement of the American Association for Geriatric Psychiatry, the Alzheimer's Association and the American Geriatric Society. *Journal of the American Medical Association, 278*, 1363–1371.

Snaith, R. P., Ahmed, S. N., Mehta, S., & Hamilton, M. (1971). Assessment of the severity of primary depressive illness. Wakefield Self-Assessment Depression Inventory. *Psychological Medicine, 1*(2), 143–149.

Snowden, J. S. (2002). Disorders of semantic memory. In A. D. Baddeley, M. D. Kopelman, & B. A. Wilson (Eds.), *The handbook of memory disorders.* Chichester, UK: Wiley.

Snowden, J. S., Griffiths, H., & Neary, D. (1994). Semantic dementia: Autobiographical contribution to preservation of meaning. *Cognitive Neuropsychology, 11*(3), 265–288.

Snowden, J. S., Griffiths, H. L., & Neary, D. (1996). Semantic-episodic memory interactions in semantic dementia: Implications for retrograde memory function. *Cognitive Neuropsychology, 13*(8), 1101–1139.

Snowden, J. S., & Neary, D. (2002). Relearning of verbal labels in semantic dementia. *Neuropsychologia, 40*(10), 1715–1728.

Snowden, J. S., Neary, D., Mann, D. M., Goulding, P. J., & Testa, H. J. (1992). Progressive language disorder due to lobar atrophy. *Annals of Neurology, 31*(2), 174–183.

Sohlberg, M. M. (2005). External aids for management of memory impairment. In W. High, A. Sander, K. M. Struchen, & K. A. Hart (Eds.), *Rehabilitation for traumatic brain injury.* New York: Oxford University Press.

Sohlberg, M. M., & Kennedy, M., Avery, J., Coelho, C., Turkstra, L., Ylvisaker, M., & Yorkston, K. (2007). Evidence-based practice for the use of external aids as a memory compensation technique. *Journal of Medical Speech–Language Pathology, 15*(1) xv–li.

Sohlberg, M. M., & Mateer, C. A. (1989a). *Prospective Memory Screening Test (ProMS).* Gaylord, MI: National Rehabilitation Services.

Sohlberg, M. M., & Mateer, C. A. (1989b). *Introduction to cognitive rehabilitation: Theory and practice.* New York: Guilford Press.

Sohlberg, M. M., & Mateer, C. A. (1989c). Training use of compensatory memory books: A three stage behavioral approach. *Journal of Clinical and Experimental Neuropsychology, 11*, 871–891.

Spector, A., Orrell, M., Davies, S., & Woods, R. T. (2007). Reality orientation for dementia. *Cochrane Database of Systematic Reviews* (Issue No. 3), CD001119.

Sprengelmeyer, R., Rausch, M., Eysel, U. T., & Przuntek, H. (1998). Neural structures associated with recognition of facial expressions of basic emotions. *Proceedings of the Royal Society, Section B: Biological Sciences, 265*(1409), 1927–1931.

Squire, L. R., & Alvarez, P. (1995). Retrograde amnesia and memory consolidation: A neurobiological perspective. *Current Opinion in Neurobiology, 5*(2), 169–177.

Squires, E. J., Aldrich, F. K., Parkin, A. J., & Hunkin, N. M. (1998). Errorless learning condition and the acquisition of word processing skills. *Neuropsychological Rehabilitation, 8,* 433–449.

Squires, E. J., Hunkin, N. M., & Parkin, A. J. (1996). Memory notebook training in a case of severe amnesia: Generalising from paired associate learning to real life. *Neuropsychological Rehabilitation, 6*(1), 55–66.

Squires, E. J., Hunkin, N. M., & Parkin, A. J. (1997). Errorless learning of novel associations in amnesia. *Neuropsychologia, 35*(8), 1103–1111.

Stapleton, S., Adams, M., & Atterton, L. (2007). A mobile phone as a memory aid for individuals with traumatic brain injury: A preliminary investigation. *Brain Injury, 21*(4), 401–411.

Stark, C., Stark, S., & Gordon, B. (2005). New semantic learning and generalization in a patient with amnesia. *Neuropsychology, 19*(2), 139–151.

Starkstein, S. E., & Robinson, R. G. (1988). Aphasia and depression. *Aphasiology, 2,* 1–20.

Starr, J. M., & Lonie, J. (2008). Estimated pre-morbid IQ effects on cognitive and functional outcomes in Alzheimer disease: A longitudinal study in a treated cohort. *BMC Psychiatry, 8,* 27.

Steadman-Pare, D., Colantonio, A., Ratcliff, G., Chase, S., & Vernich, L. (2001). Factors associated with perceived quality of life many years after traumatic brain injury. *Journal of Head Trauma Rehabilitation, 16*(4), 330–342.

Steinvorth, S., Levine, B., & Corkin, S. (2005). Medial temporal lobe structures are needed to re-experience remote autobiographical memories: Evidence from H. M. and W. R. *Neuropsychologia, 43*(4), 479–496.

Steketee, G., & Nziroglu, F. (2003). Assessment of obsessive–compulsive disorder and spectrum disorders. *Brief Treatment and Crisis Intervention, 3*(2), 169–186.

Stenset, V., Grambaite, R., Reinvang, I., Hessen, E., Cappelen, T., Bjornerud, A., et al. (2007). Diaschisis after thalamic stroke: A comparison of metabolic and structural changes in a patient with amnesic syndrome. *Acta Neurologica Scandinavica, 115*(s187), 68–71.

Stern, Y. (2006). Cognitive reserve and Alzheimer disease. *Alzheimer Disease and Associated Disorders, 20*(3, Suppl. 2), S69–S74.

Stern, Y. (2007). *Cognitive reserve: Theory and applications*. London: Taylor & Francis.

Stewart, A. L., & King, A. C. (1994). Conceptualizing and measuring quality of life in older populations. In R. P. Abeles, H. C. Gift, & M. G. Ory (Eds.), *Aging and quality of life*. New York: Springer.

Stilwell, P., Stilwell, J., Hawley, C., & Davies, C. (1999). The national traumatic brain injury study: Assessing outcomes across settings. *Neuropsychological Rehabilitation, 9*(3), 277–293.

Strangman, G. E., O'Neil-Pirozzi, T. M., Goldstein, R., Kelkar, K., Katz, D. I., Burke, D., et al. (2008). Prediction of memory rehabilitation outcomes in traumatic brain injury by using functional magnetic resonance imaging. *Archives of Physical Medicine and Rehabilitation, 89*(5), 974–981.

Strauss, E., Sherman, E. M. S., & Spreen, O. (2006). *A compendium of neuropsychological tests: Administration, norms, and commentary* (3rd ed.). New York: Oxford University Press.

Sundberg, N. D., & Tyler, L. E. (1962). *Clinical psychology*. New York: Appleton-Century-Crofts.

Sunderland, A., Harris, J. E., & Baddeley, A. D. (1983). Do laboratory tests predict everyday memory? A neuropsychological study. *Journal of Verbal Learning and Verbal Behavior, 22*, 341–357.

Sunderland, A., Harris, J. E., & Gleave, J. (1984). Memory failures in everyday life following severe head injury. *Journal of Clinical and Experimental Neuropsychology, 6*(2), 127–142.

Swinnen, S. P., Puttemans, V., & Lamote, S. (2005). Procedural memory in Korsakoff's disease under different movement feedback conditions. *Behavioural Brain Research, 159*(1), 127–133.

Symonds, C. P. (1937). Mental disorder following head injury. *Proceedings of the Royal Society of Medicine, 30*(9), 1081–1094.

Szakács, R., Kálmán, J., Barzó, P., Sas, K., & Janka, Z. (2007). [Amnesic syndrome following lesion of the fornix or does reversible Korsakow's syndrome exist?] *Neuropsychopharmacologia Hungarica, 9*(1), 39–43.

Tailby, R., & Haslam, C. (2003). An investigation of errorless learning in memory-impaired patients: Improving the technique and clarifying theory. *Neuropsychologia, 41*(9), 1230–1240.

Tate, R. L. (1997). Beyond one-bun, two-shoe: Recent advances in the psychological rehabilitation of memory disorders after acquired brain injury. *Brain Injury, 11*(12), 907–918.

Tate, R. L. (2003). Impact of pre-injury factors on outcome after severe traumatic brain injury: Does post-traumatic personality change represent an exacerbation of premorbid traits? *Neuropsychological Rehabilitation, 13*(1–2), 43–64.

Tate, R. L. (2004). Emotional and social consequences of memory. In A. D. Baddeley, M. D. Kopelman, & B. A. Wilson (Eds.), *The essential handbook of memory disorders for clinicians*. Chichester, UK: Wiley.

Teasdale, G., & Jennett, B. (1974). Assessment of coma and impaired consciousness. A practical scale. *Lancet, 2*(7872), 81–84.

Teasdale, G., & Jennett, B. (1976). Assessment and prognosis of coma after head injury. *Acta Neurochirurgica, 34*(1–4), 45–55.

Teasdale, T. W., Christensen, A. L., Willmes, K., Deloche, G., Braga, L., Stachowiak, F., et al. (1997). Subjective experience in brain injured patients and their close relatives: A European Brain Injury Questionnaire study. *Brain Injury, 11*(8), 543–564.

Teasdale, T. W., & Engberg, A. W. (2001a). Suicide after a stroke: A population study. *Journal of Neurology, Neurosurgery, and Psychiatry, 55*, 863–866.

Teasdale, T. W., & Engberg, A. W. (2001b). Suicide after traumatic brain injury: A population study. *Journal of Neurology, Neurosurgery, and Psychiatry, 71*(4), 436–440.

Tennant A. (2007). Goal attainment scaling: Current methodological issues. *Disability Rehabilitation, 29*, 20–21.

Terrace, H. S. (1963). Errorless transfer of a discrimination across two continua. *Journal of the Experimental Analysis of Behavior, 6*(2), 223–232.

Terrace, H. S. (1966). Stimulus control. In W. K. Honig (Ed.), *Operant behavior: Areas of research and application.* New York: Appleton-Century-Crofts.

Testa, J. A., Malec, J. F., Moessner, A. M., & Brown, A. W. (2005). Outcome after traumatic brain injury: Effects of aging on recovery. *Archives of Physical Medicine and Rehabilitation, 86*(9), 1815–1823.

Thase, M. E., & Denko, T. (2008). Pharmacotherapy of mood disorders . In S. Nolen-Hoeksema, T. D. Cannon, & T. Widiger (Eds.), *Annual reviews in clinical psychology.* Palo Alto, CA: Annual Reviews.

Thickpenny-Davis, K. L., & Barker-Collo, S. L. (2007). Evaluation of a structured group format memory rehabilitation program for adults following brain injury. *Journal of Head Trauma Rehabilitation, 22*(5), 303–313.

Thoene, A. I., & Glisky, E. L. (1995). Learning of name-face associations in memory impaired patients: A comparison of different training procedures. *Journal of the International Neuropsychological Society, 1*(1), 29–38.

Thomsen, I. V. (1984). Late outcome of very severe blunt head trauma: A 10–15 year second follow-up. *Journal of Neurology, Neurosurgery, and Psychiatry, 47*(3), 260–268.

Troyer, A. K., Murphy, K. J., Anderson, N. D., Moscovitch, M., & Craik, F. I. M. (2008). Changing everyday memory behaviour in amnestic mild cognitive impairment: A randomised controlled trial. *Neuropsychological Rehabilitation, 18*(1), 65–88.

Tulving, E. (1972). Episodic and semantic memory. In E. Tulving & W. Donaldson (Eds.), *Organization of memory.* New York: Academic Press.

Tulving, E. (1983). *Elements of episodic memory.* Oxford, UK: Oxford University Press.

Tulving, E., & Schacter, D. L. (1990). Priming and human memory systems. *Science, 247*(4940), 301–306.

Turkstra, L. S., & Bourgeois, M. (2005). Intervention for a modern day HM: Errorless learning of practical goals. *Journal of Medical Speech Language Pathology, 13*(3), 205–212.

Turner, S., & Lee, D. (1998). *Measures in post traumatic stress disorder: A practitioner's guide.* Windsor, UK: NFER-Nelson.

Turner-Stokes, L., Disler, P. B., Nair, A., & Wade, D. T. (2005). Multidisciplinary rehabilitation for acquired brain injury in adults of working age. *Cochrane Database of Systematic Reviews, 3.*

Turner-Stokes, L., & Hassan, N. (2002). Depression after stroke: A review of the evidence base to inform the development of an integrated care pathway: Part 2. Treatment alternatives. *Clinical Rehabilitation, 16*(3), 248–260.

Tyerman, A., & Humphrey, M. (1984). Changes in self-concept following severe head injury. *International Journal of Rehabilitation Research, 7*(1), 11–23.

Tyerman, A., & King, N. (2004). Interventions for psychological problems after brain injury. In L. H. Goldstein & J. E. McNeil (Eds.), *Clinical neuropsychology: A practical guide to assessment and management for clinicians.* Chichester, UK: Wiley.

Vakil, E., & Herishanu-Naaman, S. (1998). Declarative and procedural learning in Parkinson's disease patients having tremor or bradykinesia as the predominant symptom. *Cortex, 34*(4), 611–620.

Vallar, G., & Papagno, C. (2002). Neuropsychological impairments of verbal short-term memory. In A. D. Baddeley, M. D. Kopelman, & B. A. Wilson (Eds.), *Handbook of memory disorders* (2nd ed.). Chichester, UK: Wiley.

Van der Linden, M., Meulemans, T., & Lorrain, D. (1994). Acquisition of new concepts by two amnesic patients. *Cortex, 30*(2), 305–317.

Van Hulle, A., & Hux, K. (2006). Improvement patterns among survivors of brain injury: Three case examples documenting the effectiveness of memory compensation strategies. *Brain Injury, 20*(1), 101–109.

Vanhalle, C., Van der Linden, M., Belleville, S., & Gilbert, B. (1997). Putting names on faces: Use of a spaced retrieval strategy in a patient with dementia of the Alzheimer's type. *Perspectives on Neurophysiology and Neurogenic Speech and Language Disorders, 2,* 17–21.

Vargha-Khadem, F., Carr, L. J., Isaacs, E., Brett, E., Adams, C., & Mishkin, M. (1997). Onset of speech after left hemispherectomy in a nine-year-old boy. *Brain, 120*(1), 159–182.

Vargha-Khadem, F., Gadian, D. G., & Mishkin, M. (2001). Dissociations in cognitive memory: The syndrome of developmental amnesia. *Philosophical Transactions of the Royal Society of London, Series B: Biological Sciences, 356*(1413), 1435–1440.

Vargha-Khadem, F., Gadian, D. G., Watkins, K. E., Connelly, A., Van Paesschen, W., & Mishkin, M. (1997). Differential effects of early hippocampal pathology on episodic and semantic memory. *Science, 277*(5324), 376–380.

Varney, N. R., Martzke, J. S., & Roberts, R. J. (1987). Major depression in patients with closed head injury. *Neuropsychology, 1*, 7–9.

Verfaellie, M., Rajaram, S., Fossum, K., & Williams, L. (2008). Not all repetition is alike: Different benefits of repetition in amnesia and normal memory. *Journal of the International Neuropsychological Society, 14*(3), 365–372.

Vicari, S., Finzi, A., Menghini, D., Marotta, L., Baldi, S., & Petrosini, L. (2005). Do children with developmental dyslexia have an implicit learning deficit? *Journal of Neurology, Neurosurgery, and Psychiatry, 76*(10), 1392–1397.

Victor, M., Adams, R. D., & Collins, G. H. (1989). *The Wernicke-Korsakoff syndrome and related neurologic disorders due to alcoholism and malnutrition* (2nd ed.). Worcester, MA: Davis Publications.

Von Cramon, D. Y., Mathes Von Cramon, G. M., & Mai, N. (1991). Problem-solving deficits in brain-injured patients: A therapeutic approach. *Neuropsychological Rehabilitation, 1*(1), 45–64.

Wade, D. T. (1999). Goal planning in stroke rehabilitation: What? *Topics in Stroke Rehabilitation, 6*(2), 8–15.

Walsh, B. F., & Lamberts, F. (1979). Errorless discrimination and fading as techniques for teaching sight words to TMR students. *American journal of Mental Deficiency, 83*, 473–479.

Walsh, K. (1978). *Neuropsychology: A clinical approach* New York: Churchill Livingstone.

Warner, M. (2000). *Alzheimer's proofing your home.* West Lafeyette, IN: Purdue University Press.

Warrington, E. K. (1975). The selective impairment of semantic memory. *Quarterly Journal of Experimental Psychology, 27*(4), 635–657.

Warrington, E. K. (1984). *Recognition Memory Test.* Windsor, UK: NFER-Nelson.

Warrington, E. K. (1996). *The Camden Memory Tests.* Hove, UK: Psychology Press.

Warrington, E. K., & Shallice, T. (1984). Category specific semantic impairments. *Brain, 107*(3), 829–853.

Warrington, E. K., & Weiskrantz, L. (1968). A study of learning and retention in amnesic patients. *Neuropsychologia, 6*(3), 283–291.

Warrington, E. K., & Weiskrantz, L. (1982). Amnesia: A disconnection syndrome? *Neuropsychologia, 20*(3), 233–248.

Wearing, D. (1992). Self-help groups. In B. A. Wilson & N. Moffat (Eds.), *Clinical management of memory problems* (2nd ed.). London: Chapman & Hall.

Wearing, D. (2005). *Forever today: A memoir of love and amnesia.* London: Doubleday.

Wechsler, D. (1945). A standardised memory scale for clinical use. *Journal of Psychology, 19,* 87–85.

Wechsler, D. (1987). *Wechsler Memory Scale—Revised.* New York: Psychological Corporation.

Wechsler, D. (1997). *Wechsler Memory Scale–III.* San Antonio, TX: Psychological Corporation.

Weiskopf, N., Scharnowski, F., Veit, R., Goebel, R., Birbaumer, N., & Mathiak, K. (2004). Self-regulation of local brain activity using real-time functional magnetic resonance imaging (fMRI). *Journal of Physiology–Paris, 98*(4–6), 357–373.

Weiskrantz, L., & Warrington, E. K. (1979). Conditioning in amnesic patients. *Neuropsychologia, 17*(2), 187–194.

West, R. L. (1995). Compensatory strategies for age-associated memory impairment. In A. D. Baddeley, F. N. Watts, & B. A. Wilson (Eds.), *Handbook of memory disorders.* Chichester, UK: Wiley.

Westmacott, R., Leach, L., Freedman, M., & Moscovitch, M. (2001). Different patterns of autobiographical memory loss in semantic dementia and medial temporal lobe amnesia: A challenge to consolidation theory. *Neurocase, 7*(1), 37–55.

Westmacott, R., & Moscovitch, M. (2002). Temporally-graded retrograde memory loss for famous names and vocabulary terms in amnesia and semantic dementia: Further evidence for opposite gradients using implicit memory tasks. *Cognitive Neuropsychology, 19,* 135–163.

Whalley, L. J., Deary, I. J., Appleton, C. L., & Starr, J. M. (2004). Cognitive reserve and the neurobiology of cognitive aging. *Ageing Research Reviews, 3,* 369–382.

Williams, A. (1990). EuroQol—A new facility for the measurement of health-related quality of life. *Health Policy, 16,* 199–208.

Williams, W. H. (2003). Neurorehabilitation and cognitive behaviour therapy for emotional disorders in acquired brain injury. In B. A. Wilson (Ed.), *Neuropsychological rehabilitation: Theory and practice.* Lisse, The Netherlands: Swets & Zeitlinger.

Williams, W. H., Evans, J. J., & Wilson, B. A. (2003). Neurorehabilitation for two cases of post-traumatic stress disorder following traumatic brain injury. *Cognitive Neuropsychiatry, 8*(1), 1–18.

Williams, W. H., Evans, J. J., Wilson, B. A., & Needham, P. (2002). Brief report: Prevalence of post-traumatic stress disorder symptoms after severe traumatic brain injury in a representative community sample. *Brain Injury, 16*(8), 673–679.

Wilson, B. A. (1984). *Cognitive rehabilitation after brain damage.* Unpublished doctoral dissertation, University of London.

Wilson, B. A. (1987). *Rehabilitation of memory.* New York: Guilford Press.

Wilson, B. A. (1989). Improving recall of health service information. *Clinical Rehabilitation, 3,* 275–279.

Wilson, B. A. (1991). Long-term prognosis of patients with severe memory disorders. *Neuropsychological Rehabilitation, 1*(2), 117–134.

Wilson, B. A. (1992). Memory therapy in practice. In B. A. Wilson & N. Moffat (Eds.), *Clinical management of memory problems* (2nd ed.). London: Chapman & Hall.

Wilson, B. A. (1997). Semantic memory impairments following nonprogressive brain injury: A study of four cases. *Brain Injury, 11*(4), 259–270.

Wilson, B. A. (1998). Recovery of cognitive functions following nonprogressive brain injury. *Current Opinion in Neurobiology, 8*(2), 281–287.

Wilson, B. A. (1999). *Case studies in neuropsychological rehabilitation.* New York: Oxford University Press.

Wilson, B. A. (2000). Compensating for cognitive deficits following brain injury. *Neuropsychology Review, 10*(4), 233–243.

Wilson, B. A. (2002a). Towards a comprehensive model of cognitive rehabilitation. *Neuropsychological Rehabilitation, 12*(2), 97–110.

Wilson, B. A. (2003a). The natural recovery and treatment of learning and memory disorders. In J. Gurd & U. Kischka (Eds.), *Handbook of clinical neuropsychology.* Oxford, UK: Oxford University Press.

Wilson, B. A. (2003b). Rehabilitation of memory deficits. In B. A. Wilson (Ed.), *Neuropsychological rehabilitation: Theory and practice.* Lisse, The Netherlands: Swets & Zeitlinger.

Wilson, B. A. (2004). Assessment of memory disorders. In A. D. Baddeley, M. D. Kopelman, & B. A. Wilson (Eds.), *The essential handbook of memory disorders for clinicians.* Chichester, UK: Wiley.

Wilson, B. A. (2008). Neuropsychological rehabilitation. In S. Nolen-Hoeksema, T. D. Cannon, & T. Widiger (Eds.), *Annual reviews in clinical psychology.* Palo Alto, CA: Annual Reviews.

Wilson, B. A. (in press). The natural recovery and treatment of learning and memory disorders. In J. Gurd & U. Kischka (Eds.), *Handbook of clinical neuropsychology.* Oxford, UK: Oxford University Press.

Wilson, B. A., & Baddeley, A. D. (1988). Semantic, episodic, and autobiographical memory in a postmeningitic amnesic patient. *Brain and Cognition, 8*(1), 31–46.

Wilson, B. A., & Baddeley, A. D. (1993). Spontaneous recovery of impaired memory span: Does comprehension recover? *Cortex, 29*(1), 153–159.

Wilson, B. A., Baddeley, A. D., Evans, J. J., & Shiel, A. (1994). Errorless learning in the rehabilitation of memory impaired people. *Neuropsychological Rehabilitation, 4,* 307–326.

Wilson, B. A., Baddeley, A. D., & Kapur, N. (1995). Dense amnesia in a professional musician following herpes simplex virus encephalitis. *Journal of Clinical and Experimental Neuropsychology, 17*(5), 668–681.

Wilson, B. A., Baddeley, A. D., & Young, A. W. (1999). LE, a person who lost her "mind's eye." *Neurocase, 5*(2), 119–127.

Wilson, B. A., Clare, L., Cockburn, J., Baddeley, A. D., Tate, R., & Watson, P. (1999). *The Rivermead Behavioural Memory Test—Extended Version.* Bury St. Edmunds, UK: Thames Valley Test Company.

Wilson, B. A., Cockburn, J., & Baddeley, A. D. (1985). *The Rivermead Behavioural Memory Test.* Bury St. Edmunds, UK: Thames Valley Test Company.

Wilson, B. A., Cockburn, J., Baddeley, A. D., & Hiorns, R. (1989). The development and validation of a test battery for detecting and monitoring everyday memory problems. *Journal of Clinical and Experimental Neuropsychology, 11,* 855–870.

Wilson, B. A., Emslie, H., Foley, J., Shiel, A., Watson, P., Hawkins, K., et al. (2005). *The Cambridge Prospective Memory Test.* London: Harcourt Assessment.

Wilson, B. A., Emslie, H. C., Quirk, K., & Evans, J. J. (2001). Reducing everyday memory and planning problems by means of a paging system: A randomised control crossover study. *Journal of Neurology, Neurosurgery, and Psychiatry, 70*(4), 477–482.

Wilson, B. A., & Evans, J. J. (1996). Error free learning in the rehabilitation of individuals with memory impairments. *Journal of Head Trauma Rehabilitation, 11*(2), 54–64.

Wilson, B. A., & Evans, J. J. (2000). Practical management of memory problems. In G. E. Berrios & J. R. Hodges (Eds.), *Memory disorders in psychiatric practice.* Cambridge, UK: Cambridge University Press.

Wilson, B. A., Evans, J. J., Emslie, H., Balleny, H., Watson, P. C., & Baddeley, A. D. (1999). Measuring recovery from post traumatic amnesia. *Brain Injury, 13*(7), 505–520.

Wilson, B. A., Evans, J. J., Emslie, H., & Malinek, V. (1997). Evaluation of NeuroPage: A new memory aid. *Journal of Neurology, Neurosurgery, and Psychiatry, 63,* 113–115.

Wilson, B. A., Evans, J. J., & Keohane, C. (2002). Cognitive rehabilitation: A goal-planning approach. *Journal of Head Trauma Rehabilitation, 17*(6), 542–555.

Wilson, B. A., Forester, S., Bryant, T., & Cockburn, T. (1990). Performance of 11–14 year olds on the Rivermead Behavioural Memory Test. *Clinical Psychology Forum, 30,* 8–10.

Wilson, B. A., Gracey, F., Evans, J. J., & Bateman, A. (2009). *Neuropsychological rehabilitation: Theory, models, therapy and outcome.* Cambridge, UK: Cambridge University Press.

Wilson, B. A., Green, R., Teasdale, T., Beckers, K., Della Sala, S., Kaschel, R., et al. (1996). Implicit learning in amnesic subjects: A comparison with a large group of normal control subjects. *The Clinical Neuropsychologist, 10*(3), 279–292.

Wilson, B. A., Greenfield, E., Clare, L., Baddeley, A. D., Cockburn, J., Watson, P., et al. (2008). *The Rivermead Behavioural Memory Test–3.* London: Pearson Assessment.

Wilson, B. A., Herbert, C. M., & Shiel, A. (2003). *Behavioural approaches in neuropsychological rehabilitation: Optimising rehabilitation procedures.* Hove, UK: Psychology Press.

Wilson, B. A., JC, & Hughes, E. (1997). Coping with amnesia: The natural history of a compensatory memory system. *Neuropsychological Rehabilitation, 7,* 43–56.

Wilson, B. A., & Ivani-Chalian, R. (1995). Performance of adults with Down's syndrome on the children's version of the Rivermead Behavioural Memory Test: A brief report. *British Journal of Clinical Psychology, 34,* 85–88.

Wilson, B. A., Ivani-Chalian, R., & Aldrich, F. (1991). *The Rivermead Behavioural Memory Test for children aged 5 to 10 years.* Bury St. Edmunds, UK: Thames Valley Test Company.

Wilson, B. A., & Kapur, N. (2008). Memory rehabilitation for people with brain injury. In D. T. Stuss, G. Winocur, & I. H. Robertson (Eds.), *Cognitive neurorehabilitation* (2nd ed.). Cambridge, UK: Cambridge University Press.

Wilson, B. A., Kopelman, M. D., & Kapur, N. (2008). Prominent and persistent loss of self-awareness in amnesia: Delusion, impaired consciousness or coping strategy? *Neuropsychological Rehabilitation, 18,* 527–540.

Wilson, B. A., & Moffat, N. (1984). Rehabilitation of memory for everyday life. In J. E. Harris & P. Morris (Eds.), *Everyday memory: Actions and absentmindedness.* London: Academic Press.

Wilson, B. A., & Moffat, N. (1992). *Clinical management of memory problems* (2nd ed.). London: Chapman & Hall.

Wilson, B. A., Rous, R., & Sopena, S. (2008). The current practice of neuropsychological rehabilitation in the United Kingdom. *Applied Neuropsychology, 15,* 229–240.

Wilson, B. A., & Watson, P. C. (1996). A practical framework for understanding compensatory behaviour in people with organic memory impairment. *Memory, 4*(5), 465–486.

Wilson, B. A., Watson, P., Baddeley, A. D., Emslie, H., & Evans, J. J. (2000). Improvement or simply practice? The effects of twenty repeated assessments on people with and without brain injury. *Journal of the International Neuropsychological Society, 6*(4), 469–479.

Wilson, F. C., & Manly, T. (2003). Sustained attention training and errorless learning facilitates self-care functioning in chronic ipsilesional neglect following severe traumatic brain injury. *Neuropsychological Rehabilitation, 13*(5), 537–548.

Wright, D. W., Kellermann, A. L., Hertzberg, V. S., Clark, P. L., Frankel, M., Goldstein, F. C., et al. (2007). ProTECT: A randomized clinical trial of progesterone for acute traumatic brain injury. *Annals of Emergency Medicine, 49*(4), 391–402.

Wright, P., Bartram, C., Rogers, N., Emslie, H., Evans, J. J., Wilson, B. A., et al. (2000). Text entry on handheld computers by older users. *Ergonomics, 43*(6), 702–716.

Yalom, I. D. (1975). *Theory and practice of group psychotherapy.* New York: Basic Books.

Yates, F. (1966). *The art of memory.* London: Routledge & Kegan Paul.

Yeates, G. (2007). Awareness of disability after acquired brain injury and the family context. *Neuropsychological Rehabilitation, 17*(2), 151–173.

Ylvisaker, M., & Feeney, T. (2000). Reconstruction of identity after brain injury. *Brain Impairment, 1*(1), 12–28.

Yoo, S. S., O'Leary, H. M., Fairneny, T., Chen, N. K., Panych, L. P., Park, H. W., et al. (2006). Increasing cortical activity in auditory areas through neurofeedback functional magnetic resonance imaging. *NeuroReport, 17*(12), 1273–1278.

Young, A. W., Perrett, D. I., Calder, A. J., Sprengelmeyer, R., & Ekman, P. (2002). *Facial expressions of emotion: Stimuli and tests (FEEST).* Bury St. Edmunds, UK: Thames Valley Test Company.

Young, C. A., Manmathan, G. P., & Ward, J. C. R. (2008). Perceptions of goal setting in a neurological rehabilitation unit: A qualitative study of patients, carers and staff. *Journal of Rehabilitation Medicine, 40*(3), 190–194.

Yule, W., & Carr, J. (1987). *Behaviour modification for people with mental handicaps* (3rd ed.). Cheltenham, UK: Nelson Thornes Ltd.

Zangwill, O. L. (1947). Psychological aspects of rehabilitation in cases of brain injury. *British Journal of Psychology, 37*, 60–69.

Zarit, S. H., Zarit, J., & Reever, K. E. (1982). Memory training for severe memory loss: Effects on senile dementia patients and their families. *Gerontologist, 22*(4), 373–377.

Zeisel, J. (2006). *Inquiry by design* (rev. ed.). New York: Norton.

Zencius, A., Wesolowski, M. D., Krankowski, T., & Burke, W. H. (1991). Memory notebook training with traumatically brain-injured clients. *Brain Injury, 5*(3), 321–325.

Zhang, L., Abreu, B. C., Seale, G. S., Masel, B., Christiansen, C. H., & Ottenbacher, K. J. (2003). A virtual reality environment for evaluation of a daily living skill in brain injury rehabilitation: Reliability and validity. *Archives of Physical Medicine and Rehabilitation, 84*(8), 1118–1124.

Zietlow, R., Lane, E. L., Dunnett, S. B., & Rosser, A. E. (2008). Human stem cells for CNS repair. *Cell and Tissue Research, 331*(1), 301–322.

Zigmond, A. S., & Snaith, R. P. (1983). The Hospital Anxiety and Depression Scale. *Acta Psychiatrica Scandinavica, 67*(6), 361–370.

Zung, W. (1965). A self rating depression scale. *Archives of General Psychiatry, 12*, 63–70.

Zweber, B., & Malec, J. F. (1990). Goal attainment scaling in post acute out patient brain injury rehabilitation. *Occupational Therapy in Health Care, 7*, 45–53.

# Index

Note. *t*, table; *f*, figure

ABC assessment (functional analysis), 49–50
Activities, as motivators, 170
AD. *See* Alzheimer's disease
Adult Memory and Information Processing Battery (AMIPB), 40
Age
  at insult, recovery and, 23, 24
  as predictor of memory aid use, 59
Alarms
  checklist for using, 174, 175*f*
  as reminders, 31*t*, 161
  training for, 69–70
Alzheimer's disease (AD)
  cognitive reserve and, 28
  early, identification of, 45
  errorless learning for, 93
  goal setting, 161
  loss of emotional control and, 129–130
  procedural learning deficits, 7–8
  recovery, 25
  semantic memory deficits, 6
  spaced retrieval with errorless learning for, 98–99
Alzheimer's Society, 112, 114
AMIPB (Adult Memory and Information Processing Battery), 40
Amnesia
  anterograde, 14–15, 15*f*, 193
  classic syndrome, 1, 5, 6*t*, 9, 16

episodic buffer and, 4
episodic memory impairment, 7
errorless learning for, 92
from herpes simplex encephalitis, 17
H. M. clinical case, 7, 26
implicit memory, 44
improvement over time, 43
memory aids for, 68, 79–80
pattern of learning, 44
priming and, 12
recovery from, 23–24
rhyming associations, use of, 76
vanishing cues for, 90, 101–102
Animal studies, 33
Anomia (word-finding difficulties), 32, 94
Anterograde amnesia, 14–15, 15*f*, 193
Anxiety disorders
  assessment tools, 131, 133*t*
  cognitive-behavioral therapy, 140, 141
  coping strategies, 146*t*
  memory groups and, 111
  prevalence, after brain damage, 127, 129–130, 203
Apathy, in memory-impaired patients, 129–130
Aphasia, vanishing cues and, 102
Assessment, 34–51
  Behavioral. *See* Behavioral assessment
  in children, lines of inquiry for, 37–38
  definition of, 34–35, 195

275

Assessment *(cont.)*
  effort of testee, 48–49
  of emotional/mood disorders, 130–135
  of facial expression recognition, 132
  factors in, 38–46
  functional, 35, 37, 196
  of immediate memory, 38–39, 39*t*
  implicit memory, 42–43
  of memory aid benefit, 59–60
  memory function range of, 38–39, 39*t*
  new episodic verbal learning, 41
  nonverbal learning, 42
  questions in, 35–38
  for rehabilitation, 38
  results, 50
  standardized tests for. *See* Standardized
    tests
  subjective, of quality of life, 186–187
Assessment tools. *See also specific assessment
    tools*
  for anxiety and depression, 131, 133*t*
  for emotions, 132, 133*t*–134*t*, 134–135
  for obsessive–compulsive disorder, 132
  for posttraumatic stress disorder,
    131–132, 133*t*
  prose passages in, 40
Auditory cortex, 16
Auditory priming tasks, 44
The Awareness of Social Inference Test,
    134–135

Backward chaining, 101, 201
Backward digit span, 38
Barthel Index (BI), 154
Basal forebrain disease, 47
Basal ganglia, 17
Beck Anxiety Inventory, 133*t*
Beck Depression Inventory, 131, 133*t*
Beck Hopelessness Scale, 133*t*
Behavioral assessment
  for identifying memory problems, 49–51
  interviews, 167–168
  observations, 169–170
  relationship with treatment, 50
  techniques, 170
  in treatment process, 51
  types of measurement, 165–167
  *vs.* behavioral treatment, 49
Behavioral therapy. *See* Cognitive-
    behavioral therapy
Behavior problem, defining, for treatment
    purposes, 181
Benton Visual Retention Test (BVRT), 40

BI (Barthel Index), 154
Brain damage
  cause, recovery and, 24
  edema/swelling, resolution of, 24
  emotional disorders after. *See* Mood
    disorders
  hypoxic, 24
  number of insults, recovery and, 23
  recovery of memory functions. *See*
    Recovery
  traumatic. *See* Traumatic brain injury
Brain imaging, 29–30, 30, 72
Brain Injury Community Rehabilitation
    Outcomes, 155
BVRT (Benton Visual Retention Test), 40

California Verbal Learning Test (CVLT),
    41
Cambridge Memory Aids Resource
    Centre, 61, 61*f*
Cambridge Prospective Memory Test, 45
Cameras, as memory aids, 72, 173
CAPS (Clinician-Administered PTSD
    Scale), 131–132
Cardiac failure, 47
Caregivers, working with, 123–124, 186
CBT. *See* Cognitive-behavioral therapy
Central executive, 3
Central executive disorders (dysexecutive
    syndrome), 3
Central nervous system regeneration, 22
Cerebral artery aneurysm, 14
Cerebrovascular accident, 24
Cerebrovascular infarcts, cognitive
    reserve and, 28
Checklists, as treatment strategies, 169,
    174, 175*f*, 176
Children, RBMT for, 47
CISS (Coping Inventory for Stressful
    Situations), 133*t*
Clinical interview, in assessing emotional
    difficulties, 131
Clinician-Administered PTSD Scale
    (CAPS), 131–132
Cognition, compensation. *See*
    Compensation
Cognitive-behavioral therapy (CBT),
    138–144
  applications, 140
  behavioral experiments in, 141–142
  for comorbidity, 140–141
  components of, 139, 143
  *vs.* cognitive rehabilitation, 140

Cognitive deficits, 125
Cognitive maps, 36, 36t
Cognitive recovery. See Recovery
Cognitive rehabilitation. See
    Rehabilitation
Cognitive reserve, 28–29
Coma, 19
*Compensating for Memory Deficits Using a
    Systematic Approach* (Kime), 172
Compensation
    definition of, 53
    memory aids for. See Memory aids
    strategies, 52, 185–186
    vs. recovery, 31, 31f
Concept memory aids, 62
Consolidation theory, 15–16
Continuous recording, observational, 165
Conventional methods, 105
Coping Inventory for Stressful Situations
    (CISS), 133t
Coping strategies, for stress, anxiety and
    panic, 146t
Corsi blocks, 38
Cortical sensory memory systems, 16
CVLT (California Verbal Learning Test),
    41

Daily Living Scales, 151
Datebooks (personal organizers), 66,
    68–69, 173–174
Day patients
    memory groups for, 119–121, 119t
    Oliver Zangwill Centre day
        rehabilitative program, 158–159
Definition of memory, 1
Delayed memory
    definition of, 4–5
    episodic, assessment of, 39, 39t
Dementia
    Alzheimer's. See Alzheimer's disease
    with anomia, errorless learning for, 94
    diagnosis, 47
    executive deficits, 9
    memory groups for, 121–122
    progressive semantic, 6
    spaced retrieval for, 100
    vanishing cues and, 102
Denial, 115
Depression
    assessment tools, 131, 133t
    cognitive-behavioral therapy, 140
    memory groups and, 111
    prevalence of, 126–127

Diagnostic criteria, 131
Diaries, as memory aids, 66
Diaschisis, 20
Dictaphones, 66, 196
Dimension, quality of life, 186
Disability Rating Scale, 151
Distributed practice, 9, 98, 200
Domain, quality of life, 186
Doors and People Test, 39–41
Dorset outpatient memory group, 116–117
Dowell, Elaine, 112
Down syndrome, 47
Duration recording, observational, 166
Dysexecutive Questionnaire, 158
Dysexecutive syndrome, 3
Dysphagia patients, goals for, 159–160,
    159t
Dyspraxia, 40

Easton, Ava, 113
EBIQ (European Brain Injury
    Questionnaire), 155, 158
Echoic sensory memory, 3
Education, cognitive reserve and, 28
Ekman Faces, 132, 134
Elaboration, 10, 75–76
Elderly without dementia, memory groups
    for, 122–123
Electronic memory aids, 55, 56t, 57
EL learning. See Errorless learning
Emotions. See also Mood disorders; *specific
    emotional problems*
    assessment tools, 132, 133t–134t,
        134–135
    facial expressions, recognition of, 132,
        134
    loss of expression, 130
    perception after brain injury,
        treatment of, 143–144
Encephalitis, 14, 24, 47, 130, 140, 193
Encephalitis Society (Encephalitis
    Support Group), 112, 113f,
        114–115
Encoding, 9–10, 193
Environmental management strategies,
    54t, 185–186
Epileptic seizures, 14
Episodic buffer, 4
Episodic memory
    deficits, 6–7
    definition of, 6–7, 192
    delayed, assessment of, 39, 39t
    semantic memory and, 7

Errorless learning (EL), 89–106
    advantage of, 95
    for anomia, 94
    benefits of, 93–94
    for day patients, 160
    definition of, 89, 199
    explicit and implicit memory and,
        94–96, 95t
    principles of, 9
    selection of, 172–173
    with spaced retrieval, 97–99, 100
    studies with memory-impaired persons,
        92–94
    for teaching new information, 105–106
    theoretical background, 89–92, 91f
    vanishing cues and, 103–104
    vs. errorful or trial and error learning,
        9, 90–96, 199–200
European Brain Injury Questionnaire
        (EBIQ), 155, 158
European Quality of Life Scale
        (EuroQol), 187
Evaluation of memory rehabilitation,
        147–162, 187–189
Event recording, observational, 165–166
Everyday Memory Symptoms
        Questionnaire, 168–169
Executive deficits, 9, 137
Executive function, 13
Expanded rehearsal. See Spaced retrieval
Explicit memory
    definition of, 11, 193
    errorless learning and, 94–96, 95t, 200

Face–name learning, imagery and, 80
Faces
    emotional expressions, recognition of,
        132, 134
    familiar, inability to recall, 32
Facial Expressions of Emotions: Stimuli
        and Tests, 134, 135f
FAM (Functional Assessment Measure),
        154
Family/families
    denial, 115
    goal setting and, 153
    memory groups for, 123–124
    working with, 186
Famous faces/events tests, 44–45
Filofaxes, 31t, 66
FIM (Functional Independence
        Measure), 154

First-letter mnemonics, 81
Formulation, 155–156, 171, 185
Fractionation of memory, 1
Fragmented pictures, 43
Functional assessment, 35, 37, 196
Functional Assessment Measure (FAM),
        154
Functional Independence Measure
        (FIM), 154

GAS (goal attainment scaling), 149–151
Gender differences, in recovery, 27–28
Generalizations
    enhancement of, 180
    evidence of, 32–33
    planning for, 179, 183
    in training program, 199
    types of, 179–180
    vanishing cues and, 104–105
Generalized anxiety disorder, in brain-
        injured patients, 127
Generalized Anxiety Disorder Scale, 133t
Glasgow Outcome Scale (GOS), 18, 154
Glasgow Outcome Scale—Extended
        (GOSE), 154
Goal attainment scaling (GAS), 149–151
Goals for rehabilitation, 147–162, 181
    attainment as outcome measure,
        154–155
    definition of, 147–148
    functionally relevant, 184–185
    identifying, 152–154, 156–157
    for inpatients, 160–161
    long-term, 148, 152, 159–160, 171, 204
    meaningful, 184–185
    provisional, 171
    reviewing, 153, 157
    setting, 152–154
        advantages of, 149, 203
        in clinical practice, 155–162, 156f,
            158t
        disadvantages of, 149
        for Memory Rehabilitation Program,
            170–172
        negotiation in, 153–154, 171, 204
        SMARTER principles for, 157
        SMART principles for, 156–157, 204
        stages in, 153–154, 156f
        theories of, 151–152
        use of, 148–151
    short-term, 157, 159, 204
    specificity of, 151

strategy selection, 172–176
typical, 153
ultimate, 52
GOS (Glasgow Outcome Scale), 18, 154
GOSE (Glasgow Outcome Scale—
    Extended), 154
Groingen group, 117–119
Group therapy
    advantages of, 107–108, 201–202
    description of, 136–137
    facilitator for, 137
    procedures in, 136
    self-help organizations and, 112

HADS (Hospital Anxiety and Depression
    Scale), 131, 133t
Hamilton Depression Rating Scale, 131
Headway, 112–113
Hebbian learning, 92
Hebbian plasticity, 91–92
Hemianopia, 22
Herpes simplex encephalitis, amnesia
    from, 17
Hippocampus, 15, 16, 22, 24, 29
Hospital Anxiety and Depression Scale
    (HADS), 131, 133t
Huntington's disease, 7, 25, 132

Iconic memory (visual sensory), 3
Imagery, 77–78, 80
Immediate memory, 3, 38–39, 39t
Immediate visuospatial span, 38
Implicit learning, 90
Implicit memory
    assessment, 39t, 42–44
    definition of, 11, 193
    errorless learning and, 94–96, 95t, 200
    procedural memory, 11–12
    subtypes, 43
    vanishing cues and, 103
Implicit memory tests, 44
Infants, premature, 24
Information
    length of storage time for, 2, 192
    new, teaching strategies for, 105–106,
        172, 199, 201
    retention, rehearsal strategies for, 10
    retrieval. See Retrieval
    type to be remembered, 5–8
Information display items, as memory
    aids, 31t, 64–65
Inhibition, 20–21

Inpatients
    goals for, 160–161
    memory groups, 115–116
Instruction, systematic and conventional,
    105–106
Interval recording, 166
"Islands of memory," 128

Kapur's Dead and Alive Test, 45
Kennard principle, 23
Korean melodies, 44
Korsakoff's syndrome
    cognitive-behavioral therapy, 142
    imagery and, 80
    PQRST strategy for, 85
    procedural learning deficits, 7
    recovery, 25
    retrograde amnesia and, 14, 193
    rhyming associations, 76
    vanishing cues method for, 102

Language difficulties, errorless learning
    for, 94
Learning
    face–name, imagery and, 80
    new, enhancement of, 185
    transfer of. See Generalizations
Learning (EL)
    Errorless. See Errorless learning
Levels of processing, 9–10
Life Events Scale, 132
Limbic encephalitis, 30, 47
Limbic system, 17. See also Hippocampus
"Little and often rule" (distributed
    practice), 9, 98, 200
Location, remembering, 78–79
Location detection memory aids, 62, 72
Long-term store (long-term memory),
    4–5

Malec, Jim, "Mayo Brain Injury
    Rehabilitation: What We've
    Learned in the Past 20 years,"
    204–205
Malingering, 48–49
The Man with a Shattered World (Luria), 27
Massed practice, 98, 200
"Mayo Brain Injury Rehabilitation: What
    We've Learned in the Past 20
    years" (Malec), 204–205
Mayo–Portland Adaptability Inventory,
    154–155

Measurement. *See also* Assessment tools
  baseline, 181–182
  outcome, 148–151, 154–155
Medial temporal lobe, 16, 17
Memory. *See also specific types of memory*
  classification of, 192–193
  definition of, 8, 192
  functional changes, following
    intervention or rehabilitation,
    30–33
  tips, 163, 164*t*
Memory aids, 52–73. *See also specific memory
    aids*
  assessing use during rehabilitation, 70
  cataloging of, 63–64
  compliance, 64, 71
  context for, 53
  efficacy of, 57–58, 70
  efficient use of, 53, 58–59, 196
  electronic, 65–66, 196–197
  environmental, 197–198
  external, 185, 196–197
  frequently used, 55, 56*f*, 57
  in future, 71–73
  generalization and, 64, 71
  nonelectronic, 196–197
  preinjury/illness use of, 57
  selection of, 173
  successful use, predictors of, 59–60
  teaching use of, 67–70
  typology of, 31*t*, 54–55
Memory aids clinics
  advertising, 64
  audit, 63
  cataloging of aids, 63–64
  compliance, 64
  finding/purchasing memory aids, 63
  funding for, 61–62
  generalization, 64
  range of aids/support materials, 62–63
  research and development, 64
  setting up, 60–64, 61*f*
  staffing, 62
Memory books, 68
Memory groups, 107–124
  advantages of, 107–108
  in clinical practice, 115–124
  efficacy of, 110–112
  evaluation studies, 110–112
  open *vs.* closed, 108
  participants, 108–109
  sessions, number/duration of, 109

  structure of, 108–110
  therapist involvement, 109–110
  types of, 202
Memory impairments, 1–17. *See also specific
    impairments*
  assessment of. *See* Assessment
  baseline measurement, 181–182
  compensating for. *See* Memory aids
  self-perceptions of, 165
Memory Rehabilitation Program, 163–183
  behavioral assessment, 165
  behavioral interviews, 167–168
  behavioral observations, 169
  case example of Jay, 176–179
  checklists, 169
  goal setting, 170–172
  lead person, 157
  neuropsychological assessment, 165
  planning, 163–164, 204
  planning framework for, 180–183, 204
  pre-planning, 163
  questionnaires, 168
  rating scales, 168–169
  self-monitoring techniques, 169
  transfer of learning, 179–180
Memory strategy training, 111
Memory system
  neuroanatomical structures in, 193
  stages of, 8–11, 192–193. *See also*
    Encoding; Retrieval; Storage
Memory training, *vs.* problem-solving
    training, 189
Method of loci, 78–79
Mild cognitive impairment, memory
    groups for, 122–123
Mirror tracing, 44
Mnemonics, 74–81
  definition of, 74, 198
  efficacy, enhancement of, 199
  examples of, 75*t*
  success, in memory rehabilitation,
    80–81
  using, advice for, 81
  verbal, 74–77, 198
  visual, 77–79, 198
Mobile phones, as memory aids, 31*t*, 72
Modality-specific memory, 8
Mood, influence on ability to remember, 11
Mood disorders, 125–146. *See also specific
    mood disorders*
  assessment of, 130–135
  assessment tools, 203

group treatments, 135–138
individual psychological therapy,
    137–144
prevalence after brain injury, 126–139
treatment in clinical practice, 144–146,
    145*f*, 146*t*
Mood disorders (emotional problems),
    strategies for, 173
Mood management group, 136, 137
Motivators, for rehabilitation, 13, 182
Motor movements, as memory aids, 79–80
Multiple sclerosis, 47
Multiple trace theory, 15

Names, remembering, 77–78, 172
National Adult Reading Test, 38
National Brain Injuries Association. *See*
    Headway
National Head Injuries Group. *See*
    Headway
Negotiation, in setting goals, 153–154,
    171, 204
Nervous system changes, recovery and, 20
Neural shock, secondary, 20
Neuroanatomy, of memory, 16–17
Neurogenesis, 22, 29
NeuroPage paging system, 58, 70
Neuropsychological assessment. *See*
    Assessment
New episodic memory, assessment, 39*t*, 41
Nonelectronic memory aids, efficacy of,
    58
Nonverbal learning, assessment, 42
Novel Task subtest, 41, 42*f*

Object names, relearning, 32
Observations, in behavioral assessment,
    131, 169–170
Obsessive–compulsive disorder (OCD)
    assessment, 145
    assessment tools, 132
    cognitive-behavioral therapy, 140
    posttraumatic, 127–128
    treatment formulation, 145–146
Obsessive–Compulsive Inventory, 132
Oliver Zangwill Centre day rehabilitative
    program, 158–159
Oliver Zangwill Memory Group, 119–121,
    119*t*
Operational definitions, 181
Organic memory deficits, 12
Organic memory impairment, 38, 50

Orientation, assessment of, 39*t*, 46
Outcome measures, 148–151, 154–155
Outpatient memory groups, 116–117
Outpatients, goal setting, 161

Padua Inventory, 132
Panic disorders, 127, 128, 146*t*
Parietal areas, 16
Parkinson's disease, 7, 47
Pattern recognition tasks, 39
PDS (Posttraumatic Stress Diagnostic
    Scale), 133*t*
Perceptual priming (fragmented
    pictures), 44
Personality change, 130
Personal organizers (datebooks), 66,
    68–69, 173–174
Pharmacotherapy, for mood disorders,
    135–136
Phobias, after brain injury, 127, 128
Phonological loop, 3
Phonological loop disorders, 3–4
Photophones, 66, 67*f*
Pillboxes, 66–67
Place remembering, 78–79
Planning, rehabilitative, 147–162
Planning problems, 40
Plasticity, 21, 52, 91–92
Post-it Notes, 31*t*, 66
Post Stroke Depression Rating Scale,
    131
Posttraumatic amnesia (PTA), 24, 26,
    160–161
Posttraumatic Cognition Inventory
    (PTCI), 133*t*
Posttraumatic Stress Diagnostic Scale
    (PDS), 133*t*
Posttraumatic stress disorder (PTSD)
    assessment tools, 131–132, 133*t*
    characteristics of, 47, 141
    cognitive-behavioral therapy, 140–143
    with memory impairment, goals for,
        161–162
    RBMT and, 47
PQRST method
    in clinical practice, 87–88, 117
    encoding specificity and, 87
    evaluation studies, 83–86, 85*f*
    levels of processing and, 87
    modifications, 83
    procedure, 82–83, 199
    retrieval cues and, 86–87

Pragmatic memory training, *vs.* visual imagery, 80–81
Prefrontal cortex, 17
Premorbid functioning, assessment tool for, 38
Premorbid strategy use, as predictor of memory aid use, 59
Primary memory, 3
Priming, 12
Problem-solving training (PST), 189
Procedural memory
    deficits, 7–8
    definition of, 7, 11–12, 192
    neuroanatomy, 17
Profile of Mood States, 132
Prosopaganosia, 32, 141
Prospective memory
    assessment, 39*t*, 45
    components of, 13
    deficits, 193
    definition of, 12–13, 193
    neuroanatomy, 17
Prospective Memory Screening Tool, 45
Psychological interventions, 185
    group, 136–138
    individual, 137–144, 203
*The Psychology of Everyday Things* (Norman), 197
Psychoses, after brain injury, 128–129
Psychosocial difficulties, 125–126, 202–203
PTA (posttraumatic amnesia), 24, 26, 160–161
PTCI (Posttraumatic Cognition Inventory), 133*t*
Purdue Pegboard Test, 151
Pyramids and Palm Trees Test (PPT), 46

Quality of life (QOL), 186–187
Questionnaires, 168

RA battery, 44
Randomized controlled trials, 189
Rating scales, 168–169
RBMT. *See* Rivermead Behavioural Memory Test
Reality orientation therapy (RO), 110, 121
Recall, of familiar faces, 32
Recency effect, in free recall, 39
Recent memory, definition of, 4–5
Recognition Memory Test (RMT), 40
Recording, 170

Recovery, 18–33
    definition of, 18–19, 18*t*, 194
    evidence of, 25
    extent of, 25–29
    gender differences in, 27–28
    influencing factors, 23–24, 194
    mechanisms of, 20–24, 194
    for multiple circuit deficits, 22
    natural, improving on, 29–30
    types, after brain injury, 22
    *vs.* compensation, 31, 31*f*
Rehabilitation
    assessment for. *See* Assessment
    changing treatment, 183
    evaluation of, 187–189
    formulation, factors in, 144–145, 145*f*
    goals. *See* Goals for rehabilitation
    goals of, 181
    improvements, 30
    main area of concern, 8
    memory function changes, 30–33
    motivators, 182
    outcome measures, 148–149
    planning, stages, 182–183
    principles of, 184–186
    quality of life and, 186–187
    reinforcers, 182
    teamwork and, 205
    theoretical models of, 190, 191*f*, 192
    through memory groups. *See* Memory groups
    treatment planning framework, 180–183, 204
    *vs.* cognitive-behavioral therapy, 140
Rehearsal strategies
    definition of, 82–83, 199
    for information retention, 10
    PQRST. *See* PQRST method
    rote or simple repeating, 82–83, 199
    SQR3, 82
Reinforcers, for rehabilitation, 182
Remote memory, 4–5, 39*t*, 44
Repeated practice, 82–83
Representational memory aids, 55
Response Styles Questionnaire (RSQ), 134*t*
Retraining, 186
Retrieval, 9–11, 193
Retrograde amnesia, 14–15, 15*f*, 193
Retrospective memory, 12, 193
Rey Auditory Verbal Learning Test, 41
Rey–Osterrieth Complex Figure, 40

Rhymes, 76
Rivermead Behavioural Memory Test
  (RBMT)
  for children, 24, 47
  extended version, 40, 45, 48
  limitations of, 46, 48
  original design of, 47
  sensitivity of, 48
  subtests, 48
  validation study, 47
  version 3, 40–42, 42*f*, 45, 48
Rivermead Life Goals Questionnaire,
  157–158, 158*t*
Rivermead Memory Group for inpatients,
  115–116
RO (reality orientation therapy), 110, 121
Robson Self-Concept Questionnaire, 134*t*
Role play, 170
Rote rehearsal, 82–83, 85–86, 85*f*
Royal Society for Mentally Handicapped
  Children and Adults, 112
RSQ (Response Styles Questionnaire),
  134*t*

Schizophrenia, after brain injury, 129
Secondary memory. *See* Long-term store
  (long-term memory)
Self-help and support groups
  advantages of, 114–115
  aims/goals of, 115, 202
  for family/caregivers, 123–124
  historical perspective, 112–115, 113*f*
Self-monitoring techniques, 169
Semantic dementia, 14, 32
Semantic memory
  assessment, 39*t*
  deficits, 5–6, 45–46
  definition of, 5, 192
  episodic memory and, 7
  temporal lobe and, 16, 17
Semantic memory battery, 45–46
Sensory memory, 2–3, 16
Severity of impairment, as predictor of
  memory aid use, 59
Shaping procedures, 97. *See also* Spaced
  retrieval
Shared understanding, 185
Short-term memory (STM), 1, 3, 25
Simulated observations, 170
Single-case experimental designs, 188
Skills retraining, 186
SMARTER principles, 157

Smart homes, 71
SMART principles, 156–157, 171–172, 180
Social cognitive theory, 151
Spaced retrieval (expanded rehearsal)
  for Alzheimer's disease patients, 93
  in clinical practice, 100
  definition of, 96–97, 200
  distributed practice and, 9, 98
  with errorless learning, 97–99
  rationale for, 97–98
  selection of, 172
  for teaching new information, 105–
    106
  used alone, 99–100
Span plus two task, 42
Specificity of deficit, as predictor of
  memory aid use, 59
Specific Names Test, 46
Speed and Capacity of Language
  Processing Test, 38
Spot-the-Word test, 38
SQR3, 82
Standardized tests. *See also specific
    standardized tests*
  limitations of, 37, 49, 195–196
  as outcome measures, 148–149
  questions answered by, 195
  questions for, 36–37
  relationship with treatment, 50–51
  *vs.* functional analysis, 50
State-dependent learning, 11
State of mind, influence on ability to
  remember, 11
State–Trait Anger Expression
  Inventory—2 (STAXI-2), 134*t*
Stationery items, as memory aids, 66
STAXI-2 (State–Trait Anger Expression
  Inventory—2), 134*t*
Stem cells, 29
Stem completion, 103
STM (short-term memory), 1, 3, 25
Storage, 9, 193
Story method of elaboration, 75–76
Stress, coping strategies for, 146*t*
Stroke, 129–130
The Stroke Association, 112
Sturge–Weber syndrome, 22–23
Support groups. *See* Self-help and support
  groups
Symptom Checklist-90—Revised (SCL-
  90-R), 134*t*
Systematic methods, 105

TBI. *See* Traumatic brain injury
Teaching of new information, to memory-
    impaired people, 105–106, 172,
    199, 201
Temporal gradient, 15
Temporal lobe atrophy, 17
Temporal lobectomy, unilateral, 8
Temporal lobe epilepsy, cognitive reserve
    and, 28
Theoretical models, of cognitive
    rehabilitation, 190, 191*f*, 192
Therapeutic milieu, 184
Therapist, in memory group, 109–110
Time-dependent memory, 2–5
Time sampling, 166–167
"Tip-of-the-tongue" phenomenon, 10
Toilet use, 161, 174, 176
Token Test, 39
Toxic encephalopathy, 30
Transfer of learning. *See* Generalizations
Traumatic brain injury (TBI)
    apathy/loss of emotion and, 129–130
    cognitive reserve and, 28
    coma patients, 128
    conscious state, 19
    emotional problems after. *See* Mood
        disorders; *specific emotional problems*
    executive deficits, 9
    quality of life after, 187
    recovery, 25–28
    secondary neural shock, 20
    semantic memory deficits, 5–6
    vegetative or minimally conscious state,
        19
    verbal implicit memory, 44
Treatment, rehabilitative. *See*
    Rehabilitation
Triage of spontaneous recovery, 22
Trial-and-error learning (errorful
    learning), 9, 90–96, 199–200
Triggers, behavioral, 167–168

Unilateral neglect, 22, 30, 40

Vanishing cues (VC)
    in clinical practice, 104–105
    definition of, 101

description of, 90, 200–201
    errorless learning and, 103–104
    evaluation studies, 90, 101–102
    generalization and, 104–105
    implicit memory and, 103
    limitations of, 104, 201
    meta-analysis of, 102–104
    selection of, 172
    for teaching new information, 105–106
    use after 6-week delay, 103
Verbal memory, 192
Verbal memory deficits, 8
Verbal mnemonics, 74–77
Verbal recall, 39
Verbal recognition, 39
Virtual reality procedures, cognitive-
    rehabilitative, 73
Visual imagery, 77–78, 80–81
Visual memory, 192
Visual memory deficits, 8
Visual mnemonics, 77–79, 102
Visual object agnosia, 6
Visual Patterns Test, 38–39
Visual peg method, 78
Visual recall, 39
Visual recall tests, 40
Visual recognition, 39
Visual sensory memory (iconic), 3
Visuospatial sketchpad, 3
Visuospatial sketchpad disorders, 4, 38

Wakefield Self Assessment Depression
    Scale, 131
Way-finding devices, 65–66
Wechsler Memory Scales (WMS), 38, 40,
    41, 46
Well-Being Questionnaire, 134*t*
Wimbleton Self Report Scale, 131
WMS (Wechsler Memory Scales), 38, 40,
    41, 46
Word-finding difficulties (anomia), 32, 94
Working memory, 2*f*, 3–4

Yale–Brown Obsessive Compulsive Scale,
    132

Zung Self Rating Depression Scale, 131